Management of Spastic Conditions of the Upper Extremity

Editor

JOSHUA M. ADKINSON

HAND CLINICS

www.hand.theclinics.com

Consulting Editor
KEVIN C. CHUNG

November 2018 • Volume 34 • Number 4

ELSEVIER

1600 John F. Kennedy Boulevard • Suite 1800 • Philadelphia, Pennsylvania, 19103-2899

http://www.theclinics.com

HAND CLINICS Volume 34, Number 4
November 2018 ISSN 0749-0712, ISBN-13: 978-0-323-64151-7

Editor: Lauren Boyle
Developmental Editor: Kristen Helm

Hand Clinics (ISSN 0749-0712) is published quarterly by Elsevier Inc., 360 Park Avenue South, New York, NY 10010-1710. Months of publication are February, May, August, and November. Business and Editorial Offices: 1600 John F. Kennedy Blvd., Ste. 1800, Philadelphia, PA 19103-2899. Customer Service Office: 3251 Riverport Lane, Maryland Heights, MO 63043. Periodicals postage paid at New York, NY and at additional mailing offices. Subscription price is $422.00 per year (domestic individuals), $772.00 per year (domestic institutions), $100.00 per year (domestic students/residents), $481.00 per year (Canadian individuals), $898.00 per year (Canadian institutions), $541.00 per year (international individuals), $898.00 per year (international institutions), and $256.00 per year (international and Canadian students/residents). Foreign air speed delivery is included in all *Clinics* subscription prices. All prices are subject to change without notice. **POSTMASTER:** Send address changes to *Hand Clinics*, Elsevier Health Sciences Division, Subscription Customer Service, 3251 Riverport Lane, Maryland Heights, MO 63043. Customer Service (orders, claims, online, change of address): Elsevier Health Sciences Division, Subscription **Customer Service, 3251 Riverport Lane, Maryland Heights, MO 63043. Tel: 1-800-654-2452 (U.S. and Canada); 314-447-8871 (outside U.S. and Canada). Fax: 314-447-8029. E-mail: journalscustomerservice-usa@elsevier.com (for print support);** **journalsonlinesupport-usa@elsevier.com (for online support).**

Reprints. For copies of 100 or more of articles in this publication, please contact the Commercial Reprints Department, Elsevier Inc., 360 Park Avenue South, New York, New York 10010-1710. Tel.: 212-633-3874; Fax: 212-633-3820; E-mail: reprints@elsevier.com.

Hand Clinics is covered in *MEDLINE/PubMed (Index Medicus), Current Contents/Clinical Medicine, EMBASE/Excerpta Medica,* and *ISI/BIOMED.*

Contributors

CONSULTING EDITOR

KEVIN C. CHUNG, MD, MS
Chief of Hand Surgery, University of Michigan
Health System, Charles B.G. de Nancrede
Professor of Plastic Surgery and Orthopaedic
Surgery, Department of Surgery, Assistant
Dean for Faculty Affairs, Associate Director of
Global REACH, University of Michigan Medical
School, Ann Arbor, Michigan, USA

EDITOR

JOSHUA M. ADKINSON, MD
Assistant Professor, Division of Plastic Surgery,
Department of Surgery, Indiana University
School of Medicine, Indianapolis, Indiana, USA

AUTHORS

JOSHUA M. ADKINSON, MD
Assistant Professor, Division of Plastic
Surgery, Department of Surgery, Indiana
University School of Medicine, Indianapolis,
Indiana, USA

FRANCISCO J. ANGULO-PARKER, MD
Assistant Professor, Physical Medicine and
Rehabilitation, Department of Pediatrics,
Indiana University School of Medicine,
Indianapolis, Indiana, USA

KARL BALSARA, MD
Clinical Instructor, Section of Pediatric
Neurosurgery, Department of Neurosurgery,
Goodman Campbell Brain and Spine, Riley
Hospital for Children, Indiana University School
of Medicine, Indianapolis, Indiana, USA

AARON BERGER, MD, PhD
Voluntary Assistant Professor, Department of
Orthopaedic Surgery, University of Miami Miller
School of Medicine, Clinical Assistant Professor
(Voluntary), Division of Plastic Surgery, Florida
International University, Herbert Wertheim
College of Medicine, Miami, Florida, USA

LAURA BLACK, MD, MPH
Shirley Ryan AbilityLab, Department of
Physical Medicine and Rehabilitation,
Northwestern University Feinberg School of
Medicine, Chicago, Illinois, USA

KEVIN C. CHUNG, MD, MS
Chief of Hand Surgery, University of Michigan
Health System, Charles B.G. de Nancrede
Professor of Plastic Surgery and Orthopaedic
Surgery, Department of Surgery, Assistant
Dean for Faculty Affairs, Associate Director of
Global REACH, University of Michigan Medical
School, Ann Arbor, Michigan, USA

AARON DALUISKI, MD
Associate Attending Orthopedic Surgeon,
Departments of Pediatric Orthopaedic Surgery
and Hand and Upper Extremity, Hospital for
Special Surgery, New York, New York, USA

STEPHEN P. DUQUETTE, MD
Resident, Division of Plastic Surgery,
Department of Surgery, Indiana University
School of Medicine, Indianapolis, Indiana,
USA

JAN FRIDÉN, MD, PhD
Department of Hand Surgery, Swiss Paraplegic
Centre, Nottwil, Switzerland; Institute of
Clinical Sciences, Center for Advanced
Reconstruction of Extremities, University of
Gothenburg, Gothenburg, Sweden

DEBORAH GAEBLER-SPIRA, MD
Shirley Ryan AbilityLab, Department of
Physical Medicine and Rehabilitation,
Northwestern University Feinberg School of
Medicine, Chicago, Illinois, USA

MICHAEL S. GART, MD
Plastic and Reconstructive Surgery, Hand and
Upper Extremity Surgery, OrthoCarolina Hand
Center, Charlotte, North Carolina, USA

ANDREAS GOHRITZ, MD
Department of Hand Surgery, Swiss Paraplegic
Centre, Nottwil, Switzerland; Department of
Plastic, Reconstructive and Aesthetic Surgery,
Hand Surgery, Universitätsspital, Basel,
Switzerland

ANDREW JEA, MD
Professor, Division Chief, Section of Pediatric
Neurosurgery, Department of Neurosurgery,
Goodman Campbell Brain and Spine, Riley
Hospital for Children, Indiana University School
of Medicine, Indianapolis, Indiana, USA

TASOS KARAKOSTAS, MS, MPT, PhD BEng
Associate Director, Research Scientist,
Adjunct Professor, Computerized Motion
Analysis Laboratory, Orthopaedic Surgery,
Shirley Ryan AbilityLab, Ann & Robert H. Lurie
Children's Hospital of Chicago, Northwestern
University, Chicago, Illinois, USA

KAITLIN KIERAS, MS, OTR/L
Occupational Therapist II, Ann & Robert H.
Lurie Children's Hospital of Chicago, Chicago,
Illinois, USA

ERIK C. KING, MS, MD
Pediatric Orthopaedic Surgeon, Associate
Professor, Orthopaedic Surgery, Ann & Robert
H. Lurie Children's Hospital of Chicago,
Northwestern University, Chicago, Illinois, USA

CAROLINE LECLERCQ, MD
Institut de la Main, Clinique Bizet, Paris,
France

KEVIN J. LITTLE, MD
Director, Pediatric Hand and Upper Extremity
Center, Cincinnati Children's Hospital Medical
Center, Associate Professor of Orthopaedic
Surgery, University of Cincinnati School of
Medicine, Cincinnati, Ohio, USA

MONICA PAYARES-LIZANO, MD
Attending Surgeon, Department of
Orthopaedic Surgery, Nicklaus Children's
Hospital, Miami, Florida, USA

JANESE PETUCHOWSKI, MS, OTR/L, CHT
Occupational Therapist, Certified Hand
Therapist, Solace Health Care, Denver,
Colorado, USA

JEFFREY S. RASKIN, MS, MD
Assistant Professor, Section of Pediatric
Neurosurgery, Department of Neurosurgery,
Goodman Campbell Brain and Spine, Riley
Hospital for Children, Indiana University School
of Medicine, Indianapolis, Indiana, USA

SAOUSSEN SALHI, MD, FRCSC
Attending Surgeon, Division of Plastic
Surgery, Nicklaus Children's Hospital, Miami,
Florida, USA

MITCHEL SERUYA, MD
Clinical Assistant Professor, Division of Plastic
and Maxillofacial Surgery, Keck School of
Medicine of USC, Children's Hospital Los
Angeles, Los Angeles, California, USA

KRISTINA STEIN, MS, OTR/L
Clinical Coordinator, Occupational Therapy,
Ann & Robert H. Lurie Children's Hospital of
Chicago, Chicago, Illinois, USA

GENEVA V. TRANCHIDA, MD
Orthopedic Surgery Resident, Department of
Orthopaedic Surgery, University of Minnesota,
Minneapolis, Minnesota, USA

SAMIR K. TREHAN, MD
Fellow, Pediatric Hand and Upper Extremity
Center, Cincinnati Children's Hospital Medical
Center, Cincinnati, Ohio, USA

ANN E. VAN HEEST, MD
Professor, Department of Orthopaedic
Surgery, University of Minnesota, Minneapolis,
Minnesota, USA

JENNIFER F. WALJEE, MD, MPH
Associate Professor, Department of
Surgery, Section of Plastic Surgery,
Michigan Medicine, Ann Arbor, Michigan,
USA

KELSEY WATTERS, BS, OTR/L
Occupational Therapist, Think and Speak Lab,
Shirley Ryan AbilityLab, Chicago, Illinois,
USA

KRISTI S. WOOD, MD, MSc, FRCSC
Clinical Fellow, Department of Pediatric
Orthopaedic Surgery, Hospital for Special
Surgery, New York, New York, USA

DAN A. ZLOTOLOW, MD
Adjunct Clinical Associate Professor, The
Hospital for Special Surgery, New York City,
New York, USA; Attending Surgeon, Shriners
Hospital for Children–Philadelphia,
Philadelphia, Pennsylvania, USA

JENNIFER F. WALJEE, MD, MPH
Associate Professor, Department of Surgery, Section of Plastic Surgery, Michigan Medicine, Ann Arbor, Michigan, USA

KELSEY WATTERS, BS, OTR/L
Occupational Therapist, Think and Speak Lab, Shirley Ryan AbilityLab, Chicago, Illinois, USA

KRISTI S. WOOD, MD, MSc, FRCSC
Clinical Fellow, Department of Pediatric Orthopaedic Surgery, Hospital for Special Surgery, New York, New York, USA

DAN A. ZLOTOLOW, MD
Adjunct Clinical Associate Professor, The Hospital for Special Surgery, New York, New York, USA; Attending Surgeon, Shriners Hospital for Children-Philadelphia, Philadelphia, Pennsylvania, USA

Contents

Preface: Upper Extremity Spasticity   xiii

Joshua M. Adkinson

Common Etiologies of Upper Extremity Spasticity   437

Francisco J. Angulo-Parker and Joshua M. Adkinson

Spasticity is a motor disorder that manifests as a component of the upper motor neuron syndrome. It is associated with paralysis and can cause significant disability. The most common causes leading to spasticity include stroke, traumatic brain injury, multiple sclerosis, spinal cord injury, and cerebral palsy. This article discusses the pathophysiology and clinical findings associated with each of the most common etiologies of upper extremity spasticity.

Assessment of the Spastic Upper Limb with Computational Motion Analysis   445

Tasos Karakostas, Kelsey Watters, and Erik C. King

This article presents the current status of integrating 3-dimensional motion analysis and electromyography to assess upper extremity function clinically. The authors used their approach to establish a normative database for 5 Shriners Hospital Upper Extremity Evaluation tasks, which provides ranges of motion at the point of task achievement. Also, the interjoint correlations are provided to understand the movement coordination required for each task. Distal upper extremity motion is strongly related to proximal function, supporting the idea that treatment of the proximal upper extremity deficits may be best preceded by treatment of the more distal upper extremity segments.

Nonsurgical Treatment Options for Upper Limb Spasticity   455

Laura Black and Deborah Gaebler-Spira

There are many nonsurgical treatment options for patients with upper limb spasticity. This article presents an algorithmic approach to management, encompassing evidence-based rehabilitation therapies, medications, and promising new orthotic and robotic innovations.

Considerations in the Management of Upper Extremity Spasticity   465

Michael S. Gart and Joshua M. Adkinson

Spasticity is a movement disorder characterized by a velocity-dependent increase in muscle tone and a hyperexcitable stretch reflex. Common causes of spasticity include cerebral palsy, spinal cord injury, and stroke. Surgical treatment plans for spasticity must be highly individualized and based on the characteristics of patients and the spasticity to maximize functional gains. Candidates for surgery must be carefully selected. In this article, the authors review the pathophysiology of spasticity and discuss general considerations for surgical management with an emphasis on patient factors and spasticity characteristics. Specific considerations for the common causes of spasticity are presented.

Surgical Management of Spasticity of the Thumb and Fingers   473

Jennifer F. Waljee and Kevin C. Chung

Spasticity of the hand profoundly limits an individual's independent ability to accomplish self-care and activities of daily living. Surgical procedures should be tailored to patients' needs and functional ability, and even patients with severe cognitive injuries and poor upper extremity function may benefit from surgery to improve appearance and hygiene. Careful preoperative examination and planning are needed, and consideration is given to the potential unintended detrimental effect of a surgical procedure on hand function.

Surgical Management of Spasticity of the Forearm and Wrist   487

Stephen P. Duquette and Joshua M. Adkinson

Upper extremity spasticity may result from a variety of types of brain injury, including cerebral palsy, stroke, or traumatic brain injury. These conditions lead to a predictable pattern of forearm and wrist deformities caused by opposing spasticity and flaccid paralysis. Upper extremity spasticity affects all ages and sociodemographics and is a complex clinical problem with a variety of treatment options depending on the patient, the underlying disease process, and postoperative expectations. This article discusses the cause, diagnosis, operative planning, operative techniques, postoperative outcomes, and rehabilitation protocols for the spastic wrist and forearm.

Surgical Management of Spasticity of the Elbow   503

Aaron Berger, Saoussen Salhi, and Monica Payares-Lizano

A spastic limb refers to one with increased tone, which commonly results from an upper motor neuron injury, which, in turn, leads to disinhibition of reflex arcs. At the level of the elbow, affected individuals typically exhibit a flexion posture secondary to spastic contracture of the biceps, brachialis, and brachioradialis muscles. Surgical treatment aims to improve access for hygiene, function, and cosmetic appearance of the affected limb. The specific surgical intervention performed depends on the degree of elbow flexion contracture and whether there is an associated joint contracture or soft tissue deficit.

Surgical Management of Spasticity of the Shoulder   511

Dan A. Zlotolow

Although spastic conditions often involve the shoulder, it is rare for surgical intervention to be required. In cases in which chemodenervation and therapy are insufficient to optimize the patient's function or minimize their care requirements, surgical options, such as tendon and joint releases, can be considered. Tendon transfers are rarely indicated. Nerve transfers, particularly contralateral C7, may play a larger role in the future as further understanding is gained into the risks, indications, and contraindications of this exciting technique.

Management of Joint Contractures in the Spastic Upper Extremity   517

Kristi S. Wood and Aaron Daluiski

Upper extremity contractures in the spastic patient may result from muscle spasticity, secondary muscle contracture, or joint contracture. Knowledge of the underlying cause is critical in planning successful treatment. Initial management consists of physical therapy and splinting. Botulinum toxin can be helpful as a therapeutic treatment in relieving spasticity and as a diagnostic tool in determining the underlying cause of the contracture. Surgical management options include release or lengthening of the causative muscle/tendon unit and joint capsular release, as required. Postoperative splinting is important to maintain the improved range of motion and protect any associated tendon lengthening or transfer.

Technical Pearls of Tendon Transfers for Upper Extremity Spasticity 529

Samir K. Trehan and Kevin J. Little

Tendon transfers are an important surgical option when treating patients with muscular imbalance due to upper extremity spasticity. A successful surgical outcome requires a thorough preoperative clinical evaluation, an understanding of tendon transfer biomechanics, appropriate donor and recipient muscle selection, technical execution, and postoperative rehabilitation. This article reviews the principles, biomechanics, and techniques for commonly performed tendon transfers in patients with upper extremity spasticity.

Selective Neurectomy for the Spastic Upper Extremity 537

Caroline Leclercq

Surgery is one element of the rehabilitative care of the spastic upper limb. Different surgical techniques have been advocated to address each of the common deformities and underlying causes, including muscle spasticity, joint contracture, and paralysis. Partial neurectomy of motor nerves has been shown to reduce spasticity in the target muscles. It is effective only for the spastic component of the deformity, which underscores the importance of a preliminary thorough clinical examination. Hyperselective neurectomy, which involves performing a partial division of each motor ramus at its entry point into the target muscle, results in improved selectivity, reliable partial muscle denervation, and durable results.

Neurosurgical Management of Spastic Conditions of the Upper Extremity 547

Karl Balsara, Andrew Jea, and Jeffrey S. Raskin

Spasticity is a hypertonic segmental reflex pathway caused by a central nervous system injury. Spasticity of the upper extremity causes loss of function, joint contracture, pain, and poor cosmesis. Treatment aims to reduce or change the pathophysiology underlying the hyperactive reflex from dorsal sensory rootlets through the intrinsic machinery of the spinal cord to the neuromuscular junction. There are many treatments for upper extremity spasticity, including oral medication, physiotherapy, intrathecal baclofen, and lesional or neuromodulatory surgical approaches. Goals of treatment must always be clearly defined, but neurosurgical management is most effective when paired with multidisciplinary therapies and caregiver participation.

Management of Spinal Cord Injury–Induced Upper Extremity Spasticity 555

Andreas Gohritz and Jan Fridén

Spasticity affects more than 80% of patients with spinal cord injury. Neural mechanisms and musculotendinous alterations lead to typical upper extremity features including shoulder adduction/internal rotation, forearm pronation, and elbow, wrist, and finger flexion. Long-standing spasticity may lead to soft tissue and joint contractures and further impairment of upper extremity function. Surgical management involves tendon lengthening, release, and transfer, as well as selective neurotomy, in an effort to reduce spastic muscle hypertonicity, restore balance, prevent further contracture, and improve posture and function. This article summarizes surgical strategies to improve function of the upper extremity in patients with tetraplegia.

Rehabilitation Strategies Following Surgical Treatment of Upper Extremity Spasticity   567

Janese Petuchowski, Kaitlin Kieras, and Kristina Stein

Upper motor neuron injuries that occur in cases such as cerebral palsy, cerebrovascular accidents, and traumatic brain injury often result in upper extremity deformity and dysfunction. Multiple surgical options are available to improve upper extremity positioning, and, in some cases, motor control. Postoperative therapeutic management is imperative to assist the patient and caregiver in maximizing potential functional gains. This article provides an overview of postoperative guidelines for commonly performed surgeries to manage upper extremity dysfunction caused by spasticity and discusses acute management as well as therapeutic techniques for functional training and improved motor control.

Outcomes After Surgical Treatment of Spastic Upper Extremity Conditions   583

Geneva V. Tranchida and Ann E. Van Heest

Surgical interventions for the spastic upper extremity aim to correct the common deformities of elbow flexion, forearm pronation, wrist flexion and ulnar deviation, and thumb-in-palm deformity. One goal is achieving optimal function and improved limb positioning. Aesthetics of the limb have a profound impact on self-esteem and satisfaction. Surgical deformity correction has not reliably been shown to improve sensory function such as stereognosis. Validated outcome measures are used to present outcomes after surgical treatment of the spastic upper extremity as it relates to motor function and limb positioning, sensory function, and self-esteem.

The Future of Upper Extremity Spasticity Management   593

Mitchel Seruya

Surgical management of upper limb spasticity has traditionally tackled the downstream effects at the muscle, tendon, and joint levels. Because this approach does not address the underlying pathologic condition within the nerve, surgical outcomes have been marked by unsatisfactory relapse over time. Future management may focus on reestablishing a normal neuronal impulse pathway to the dysfunctional musculotendinous unit. By severing the faulty γ-neuronal circuit at the C7 level, spasticity may be reduced. Transfer of the contralateral C7 nerve root to the injured C7 nerve root may open the potential for simultaneously restoring extension and improving reach and grasp functions.

HAND CLINICS

FORTHCOMING ISSUES

February 2019
Global Advances in Wide Awake Hand Surgery
Donald H. Lalonde and Jin Bo Tang, *Editors*

May 2019
Revascularization and Replantation in the Hand
Kyle R. Eberlin and Neal C. Chen, *Editors*

August 2019
Current Concepts and Controversies in Scaphoid Fracture Management
Steven L. Moran, *Editor*

RECENT ISSUES

August 2018
Dupuytren Disease
Steven C. Haase and Kevin C. Chung, *Editors*

May 2018
Current Concepts in the Management of Proximal Interphalangeal Joint Disorders
Kevin C. Chung, *Editor*

February 2018
Complex Trauma Management of the Upper Extremity
Asif M. Ilyas, *Editor*

SERIES OF RELATED INTEREST

Clinics in Plastic Surgery
Orthopedic Clinics
Physical Medicine and Rehabilitation Clinics

THE CLINICS ARE AVAILABLE ONLINE!
Access your subscription at:
www.theclinics.com

Preface
Upper Extremity Spasticity

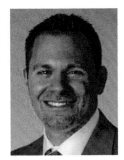

Joshua M. Adkinson, MD
Editor

Patients with upper extremity spasticity present at all ages with a variety of manifestations, ranging from isolated swan-neck deformities to contracted limbs devoid of voluntary function. These patients may be frustrated by seemingly simple activities, and their caregivers are often exhausted. Given the potentially complex clinical and social milieu in which these patients live, it is necessary to involve a multidisciplinary team with experience in caring for patients with spasticity. Many patients are effectively managed with nonoperative modalities, such as orthoses, therapy, antispastic agents, and neuromodulators, yet surgery offers the unique opportunity for a durable improvement of posture and function.

The decision making regarding surgery is no simple task. Patients with upper extremity spasticity often require serial examinations and extensive discussions with caregivers regarding the potential complexity of reconstruction and realistic postoperative outcomes. Clinicians that endeavor to treat these patients commit significant time and energy to their management. Despite the challenges, postoperative results are often satisfying and yield substantial improvements in quality of life for patients and their caregivers.

It is my distinct honor to present this issue of *Hand Clinics* as the combined effort of worldwide experts in the field of upper extremity spasticity. I would like to thank my mentor, Dr Kevin Chung, for always pushing for perfection and allowing me the opportunity to create this issue. I am confident the readers will enjoy articles written by providers in the fields of pediatric and adult upper extremity surgery, physical medicine and rehabilitation, neurosurgery, and occupational therapy. I am grateful for their time, expertise, and commitment to creating an outstanding work that represents the state-of-the-art medical and surgical care for patients with upper extremity spasticity.

Joshua M. Adkinson, MD
Division of Plastic Surgery
Department of Surgery
Indiana University School of Medicine
545 Barnhill Drive
Emerson Hall 232
Indianapolis, IN 46202, USA

E-mail address:
jadkinso@iu.edu

0749-0712/18/© 2018 Published by Elsevier Inc.

hand.theclinics.com

Common Etiologies of Upper Extremity Spasticity

Francisco J. Angulo-Parker, MD[a], Joshua M. Adkinson, MD[b],*

KEYWORDS

- Spasticity • Spastic hypertonia • Upper extremity • Motor neuron syndrome • Cerebral palsy
- Spinal cord injury • Stroke • Cerebrovascular accident

KEY POINTS

- Spasticity is a motor disorder characterized by increased muscle tone and a hyperexcitable stretch reflex.
- The most common causes of upper extremity spasticity include stroke, traumatic brain injury, multiple sclerosis, spinal cord injury, and cerebral palsy.
- The underlying pathophysiology of spasticity may vary, but the clinical manifestations are somewhat predictable and include elbow flexion, forearm pronation, wrist flexion, and thumb/digital flexion.
- The management team should understand the cause of upper extremity spasticity in order to formulate an optimal treatment plan.

INTRODUCTION

Spasticity is a motor disorder characterized by a velocity-dependent increase in tonic stretch reflexes (ie, muscle tone) with exaggerated tendon jerks resulting from hyperexcitability of the stretch reflex as one component of the upper motor neuron syndrome (UMNS).[1–4] Upper motor neurons originate in the motor region of the cerebral cortex or brain stem and carry information to the lower motor neurons, which innervate skeletal muscle. Damage to the upper motor neuron results in several clinical findings that encompass the UMNS. Some of the positive features include spasticity and dystonic hypertonia, hyperreflexia, spasms, and clonus, whereas negative features include paralysis, weakness, loss of dexterity, and muscle fatigue.[4]

Data regarding the incidence and prevalence of spasticity are scant, but the clinical impact is undeniable. Many patients with spasticity require life-long medical management and substantial assistance with activities of daily living. Upper extremity surgeons may be involved in the management of patients with spasticity in order to address joint deformities and functional deficits. In this article, the authors discuss the epidemiology and pathophysiology of the most common causes for upper extremity spasticity.

PATHOPHYSIOLOGY OF SPASTICITY

The upper motor neuron pathways originate in the brain stem or cerebral cortex. These pathways include the corticospinal (pyramidal) tract; these tracts, along with descending pathways originating in the brain stem, can directly or indirectly influence the excitability of the anterior horn cell.[4] All of these structures may play a role in the pathophysiology of positive symptoms of UMNS.

Disclosure Statement: The authors have no commercial or financial conflicts of interest regarding the content of this article.
[a] Physical Medicine and Rehabilitation, Department of Pediatrics, Indiana University School of Medicine, 705 Riley Hospital Drive, Indianapolis, IN 46202, USA; [b] Division of Plastic Surgery, Department of Surgery, Indiana University School of Medicine, 545 Barnhill Drive, Emerson Hall 232, Indianapolis, IN 46202, USA
* Corresponding author.
E-mail address: jadkinso@iu.edu

Hand Clin 34 (2018) 437–443
https://doi.org/10.1016/j.hcl.2018.06.001

The fundamental disruption leading to spasticity is in the muscle stretch reflex,[5] as evidenced byan increase in resistance during passive stretchor movement of a joint. Initial paralysis followedby aberrant motor behaviors, such as spasticity, is a result of the adaptive changes of the brain andspinal cord after damage to centralmotor pathways.The correlation between spasticity and paralysis is clinically relevant, as each manifestation results in some form of functional impairment anddisability. Recognition of the simultaneous findingsof spasticity and paralysis is also important, as they require different treatment strategies.

There is no single pathophysiologic mechanism that accounts for all aspects of spasticity. Paresis, soft tissue contracture, and muscle hypertonia are the 3 major mechanisms of motor impairment. Further, several conditions are part of spastic hypertonia, including dystonia, rigidity, myoclonus, muscle spasms, clonus, posturing, and spasticity.[6] Clinically, isolated stretch-related spasticity will be velocity-dependent and able to be tested with passive stretches. It is often assessed with examiner-dependent tools, such as the Modified Ashworth Scale, that reliably rates resistance to passive movement on a 5-point scale.[6] If left untreated, spasticity may evolve into muscle and joint contractures with limited motion and loss of function. The most common clinical manifestations are elbow flexion, forearm pronation, wrist flexion, and thumb/digital flexion (**Fig. 1**).[7,8] Optimal management of these deformities requires an understanding of the underlying cause of upper extremity spasticity and is highly individualized.

EPIDEMIOLOGY OF SPASTICITY

Upper extremity spasticity may result from several different conditions. Whereas there has been a significant amount of research into the treatment of clinically significant spasticity, the studies on the incidence and prevalence of spasticity have been limited. Most of these studies rely on patient surveys. In addition, there are differences in clinical assessment measures and diagnostic definitions,[9] which make it difficult to estimate the prevalence of spasticity.[10] Despite these limitations, existing research indicates that 17% to 38% of patients with a cerebrovascular accident (ie, stroke), 34% of patients with traumatic brain injury (TBI), 67% of patients with multiple sclerosis (MS), 68% to 78% of patients with spinal cord injury (SCI), and 85% of patients with cerebral palsy (CP) have spasticity.[10–20]

CAUSES OF UPPER EXTREMITY SPASTICITY
Cerebrovascular Accident (ie, Stroke)

A stroke is the sudden onset of neurologic deficits secondary to an acute decrease in blood flow and resultant brain hypoxia. It is a major cause of morbidity and mortality worldwide and ranks as the second-leading cause of death behind ischemic heart disease. Nearly 800,000 new cases are reported annually in the United States, where approximately 2.6 million men and 3.9 million women live with stroke.[21] Spasticity affects up to 38% of patients following a stroke.[10,11,14,18,20] Further, it is the number one cause of paralysis in the United States.[22,23]

The acute decrease in brain perfusion can be caused by 2 different mechanisms: occlusion of blood vessels (ie, ischemic stroke) and blood vessel rupture (ie, hemorrhagic stroke).[24] Hemorrhagic strokes are much less common and may be caused by hypertension, aneurysm rupture, arteriovenous malformation, anticoagulants, or tumor bleeding. The neurologic deficits present in patients who have had a stroke will depend on the area of the brain affected.[25] For example

- Unilateral ischemic injuries secondary to occlusion of the *middle cerebral artery* will result in contralateral hemiplegia. Upper extremities will be more affected than lower extremities. This lesion results in the classic clinical picture of upper extremity hemiplegia, facial palsy, and speech difficulties.
- Unilateral ischemic injuries secondary to occlusion of the *anterior cerebral artery* will result in contralateral motor deficits to the lower extremity, with little to no effect on the contralateral upper extremity.
- A central lesion to the *posterior cerebral artery* can cause contralateral hemiplegia.
- Occlusions of the *basal ganglia* result in contralateral hemiparesis.

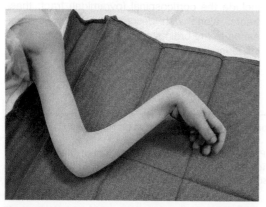

Fig. 1. Typical clinical manifestations in patients with cerebral palsy.

Although an acute stroke initially presents with flaccid paralysis, synergistic movement patterns subsequently develop. These patterns are initially generalized; as motor control recovery continues, isolated patterns of movement return to the affected extremity. As motor control returns, spastic hypertonia diminishes, but spasticity can remain problematic if motor recovery is incomplete.

Because the sensory cortex is also commonly affected, patients may have additional deficits in sensation and awareness of the affected limb in space (ie, proprioception). Furthermore, visual disturbances can occur following stroke, which may further compromise already limited upper extremity function, as an awareness of the limb in space is affected. Surgical treatment in patients after stroke tends to require more aggressive releases in order to adequately address joint deformities and contractures.

Traumatic Brain Injury

TBI is a major cause of death and disability in the United States. In 2013 alone, 2.8 million TBI-related emergency department visits, hospitalizations, and deaths occurred in the United States.[26] Approximately 80% of TBIs are considered mild, which present with a less complicated clinical picture and limited need for medical treatment. Mild injuries can have significant long-term complications, however, but do not present with significant motor findings. The remaining 20% of TBIs are divided into moderate and severe[27]; these subtypes are more commonly associated with paralysis and spasticity. Although there are limited data regarding prevalence, available research suggests that problematic spasticity affects between 34% and 84% of patients with moderate to severe TBIs.[19,27]

As with other causes of upper extremity spasticity, motor involvement depends on the location of injury. Localized, unilateral injuries due to blunt trauma present with focal patterns of spasticity (eg, monoplegia/hemiplegia), whereas diffuse axonal injuries and hypoxic/anoxic brain injuries usually present with more generalized patterns of spasticity (eg, quadriplegia). The initial care of patients with severe TBIs may be rather complex and includes intubation, coma management, and care of associated orthopedic and other injuries. The higher priority management of associated injuries may allow spasticity and upper extremity contractures to go untreated for some time. In fact, it is the authors' experience that the upper extremity manifestations of TBIs are underemphasized and few patients are referred for surgical evaluation. Facilitating range of motion should be considered a priority in early management of patients with TBIs.

Multiple Sclerosis

MS is a disease of the central nervous system (CNS) that often leads to significant impairment and disability. In fact, it is the most common cause of nontraumatic disability in the United States. With a prevalence of 0.9 per 1000, MS affects women 2 to 3 times more commonly than men; most patients are diagnosed between the third and sixth decades of life.[28]

Currently available evidence suggests that MS is an inflammatory disease, although no consensus cause has been established. It is thought to be a combination of genetic predisposition and environmental factors. MS is characterized by demyelination throughout the CNS. The demyelination in MS is not diffuse but presents in plaques that tend to have a preference for the optic nerves, periventricular white matter, brain stem, cerebellum, and cervical spinal cord.[29]

The symptoms of MS are numerous and varied and include weakness/spasticity, dysesthesias, visual changes and blindness, and cognitive deficits. There are multiple subtypes of MS, including the following:

- Relapsing-remitting MS: It is the most common type (85% of MS). This subtype is characterized by episodes of disease exacerbation with subsequent neurologic improvement. Some episodes allow for a recovery of neurologic function to baseline, whereas others lead to lasting neurologic deficits.
- Secondary progressive MS: It includes an initial period of relapsing-remitting MS with later progression of disability without an associated remission.
- Primary progressive MS: About 10% of patients with MS present with this subtype, characterized by an insidious progression without remission.
- Progressive-relapsing MS: About 5% of patients with MS present with this subtype. This type is the most aggressive form of MS and one that results in rapid progression to significant disability.

Approximately 67% of patients with MS experience spasticity, 38% of which are affected by clinically significant "problematic spasticity."[30] Further, in a study of 100 patients with MS in the United Kingdom,[31] it was found that 50% had detectable arm spasticity as measured by the commonly used Modified Ashworth Scale. Because a small percentage of patients will have a progressive variant of MS, it is essential that all patients are followed with serial examinations of range of motion, tone, and neurologic status.

Spinal Cord Injury

The National Spinal Cord Injury Statistical Center estimates the incidence of SCI to be 54 per 1,000,000, or approximately 17,000 new cases per year. Approximately 285,000 patients are living with SCI in the United States, and this condition mostly affects young males.[32–34] The most common presentation is one of incomplete tetraplegia (45.8%), followed by incomplete paraplegia (20.9%), complete paraplegia (19.7%), and complete tetraplegia (13.2%).[35] The most common cause of SCI is trauma; but spinal tumors, radiation treatment, infections, inflammatory disease (eg, transverse myelitis), and vascular diseases can also cause SCI.

Spasticity is rather common after SCI. McGuire and colleagues[30] report that the presence of spasticity after traumatic SCIs was 67% and 78% at discharge and follow-up, respectively. Of these, approximately 25% to 50% had spasticity that was problematic enough to warrant treatment. Similarly, Maynard and colleagues[15] report the presence of spasticity at discharge to be 65%, with problematic spasticity in 35% of the study population.

After initial injury, there is a period of spinal shock that causes hypotonia and a loss of muscle stretch reflexes. This process can last days to weeks and is followed by a transitional state with a progressive increase in tone. The spastic state follows and stabilizes in the months following injury. Neurologic recovery after SCI is more pronounced during the first 6 to 12 months after injury.[35]

The muscles innervated above the level of injury have normal strength. Muscles innervated below the level of injury may be either flaccid or spastic. The presence of spasticity is directly related to the level of injury; higher-level injuries (eg, cervical and high thoracic SCI) are more likely to result in upper extremity spasticity as compared with lower level injuries (eg, low thoracic and lumbar level SCI).[15,30] Further, paralysis and poor motor control of the upper extremities are characteristics of upper thoracic and cervical SCI.

Traumatic SCIs are classified according to the international standards proposed by the American Spinal Injury Association (ASIA), as follows[6]:

- ASIA A (complete injury): No sensory or motor function is preserved in the sacral segments S4 to S5.
- ASIA B (incomplete injury): Sensory but not motor function is preserved below the neurologic level and includes the sacral segments S4 to S5.
- ASIA C (incomplete injury): Motor function is preserved below the neurologic level, and

more than half of the key muscles below the neurologic level have a muscle grade less than 3.
- ASIA D (incomplete injury): Motor function is preserved below the neurologic level, and at least half of the key muscles below the neurologic level have a muscle grade greater than or equal to 3.

Patients with incomplete SCI (ASIA grades B and C) have more difficulties and limitation of function secondary to spasticity than patients with ASIA grades A and D. Although this classification system is useful in order to communicate clinical examination and prognosis among medical providers, the British Medical Research Council[36] classification of muscle strength is much more useful in planning surgical intervention in patients with SCIs (**Table 1**).

Importantly, upper extremity spasticity in SCIs does not always cause difficulties with function. Some patients leverage their spasticity to facilitate posturing and movement, in return allowing them to cooperate or perform mobility tasks, transfers, and/or activities of daily living. In patients with SCIs with problematic spasticity, function may be markedly impaired. Joint and muscle contractures can develop if left untreated. Ongoing stretching and focal therapy for specific spastic muscles are essential to preserve/improve function and to assist in the perioperative phase of care for patients that are surgical candidates. An acute change in spasticity in patients with SCIs may indicate a change in or a new medical condition, including acute infection, bowel or bladder dysfunction, urinary tract infection, pressure injury, syrinx, and deep vein thrombosis, among others.[37]

Table 1	
British Medical Research Council's muscle grading system	
Grade	Clinical Finding
0	No contraction
1	Flicker or trace of contraction
2	Active movement with gravity eliminated
3	Active movement against gravity
4	Active movement against gravity and resistance
5	Normal power

From James MA. Use of the medical research council muscle strength grading system in the upper extremity. J Hand Surg 2007;32(2):155; with permission.

Cerebral Palsy

CP is a functionally limiting group of nonprogressive, permanent disorders of movement and posture that are attributed to a disturbance of the developing fetal or infant brain.[38,39] Approximately 1.5 to 4.0 per 1000 live births are affected; it is the most common motor disability of childhood.[40] Multiple risk factors are associated with the development of CP, including low birth weight, prematurity, perinatal asphyxia, teratogens, CNS malformation, neonatal infection, and metabolic disorders.[41] In most cases, the CNS insult occurs in utero (~75%).[42]

It is estimated that spasticity is the main neuromotor impairment in nearly 80% of children with CP. Further, bilateral CP comprises nearly 70% of all patients with spasticity.[43] CP is classified clinically according to either the type of neuromotor disorder or the anatomic distribution of motor impairment[44]:

- Type of neuromotor disorder
  ○ Spastic (most common)
  ○ Dyskinetic
  ○ Hypotonic
  ○ Ataxic
  ○ Mixed forms

Hypotonic and ataxic forms of CP are rare.

- Anatomic distribution of motor impairment
  ○ Hemiparetic (hemiplegic) CP: Involvement is on one side of the body (39% of patients). Hemiplegic CP commonly presents with worse motor control and spasticity in the upper extremity as compared with the lower extremity.
  ○ Diparetic (diplegic) CP: Motor impairment is present in bilateral lower extremities (38% of patients).
  ○ Quadriparetic (quadriplegic) CP: This subtype affects the whole body (23% of patients). In other words, the upper and lower extremities as well as the central (core) muscles are impaired.
  ○ Triparetic (triplegic) CP: This subtype affects 3 extremities and is rare.

Although the CNS injury in patients with CP is nonprogressive, changes in medical and nutritional status, growth, and compliance with therapies and equipment can alter the clinical presentation. The most noticeable changes include the amount and pattern of spasticity, motor control, gait, balance, and difficulties with activities of daily living. Therefore, ongoing medical surveillance is required in order to maximize function and prevent complications. CP can also occur simultaneously with other conditions, including chronic pain, seizure disorders, intellectual disability, communication impairment, hip dislocation/subluxation, and scoliosis. These overlapping challenges require a multidisciplinary team of specialists in order to optimize medical care and outcomes.

RARE CAUSES OF UPPER EXTREMITY SPASTICITY

Spasticity may also present as part of several other less common neuromuscular diseases and can lead to marked disability.

Amyotrophic Lateral Sclerosis

Amyotrophic lateral sclerosis (ALS) is a rare disease with a prevalence of 4 to 6 per 100,000.[45] It is a disease of both upper and lower motor neurons and affects the motor cortex, brainstem, and spinal cord. The clinical course of ALS is severely debilitating and progresses rapidly with an almost inevitable death from respiratory failure. Clinically, it is common to see significant muscle wasting accompanied by hypertonia, hyperreflexia, or clonus. Spasticity in the setting of ALS can lead to substantial functional impairment. Systemic medications should be coupled with therapy in order to address the discomfort resulting from spastic hypertonia. Because of the rapid progression of the disease and limited life span after diagnosis, surgery is rarely, if ever, indicated.

Primary Lateral Sclerosis

Primary lateral sclerosis is a rare condition and usually presents in the fifth to sixth decade of life. It is a disorder of the upper motor neuron that can present with spasticity involving the upper or lower extremities. There is usually progression to involvement of the cranial nerves (ie, bulbar palsy).

SUMMARY

Upper extremity spasticity may result from several different conditions affecting the upper motor neurons. The most common causes include stroke, TBI, MS, SCI, and CP. A thorough understanding of these conditions is mandatory in order to provide an accurate prognosis and to optimize outcomes of treatment.

REFERENCES

1. Balakrishnan S, Ward A. The diagnosis and management of adults with spasticity. Handb Clin Neurol 2013;110:145–60.
2. Gormley M, O'Brien C, Yablon S. A clinical overview of treatment decisions in the management of spasticity. Muscle Nerve Suppl 1997;6:S14–20.

3. Gracies JM. Pathophysiology of spastic paresis. I: paresis and soft tissue changes. Muscle Nerve 2005;31(5):535–51.

4. Sheean G. The pathophysiology of spasticity. Eur J Neurol 2002;9(Suppl 1):3–9.

5. Dromerick AW. Clinical features of spasticity and principles of treatment. In: Gelber DA, Jeffery DR, editors. Clinical evaluation and management of spasticity. Current clinical neurology. Totowa (NJ): Humana; 2002. p. 13–26.

6. Bryce T, Ragnarsson K, Stein A. Spinal cord injury. In: Braddom R, editor. Physical medicine and rehabilitation. 4th edition. Philadelphia: Elsevier Saunders; 2011. p. 1293–346.

7. Leclercq C. General assessment of the upper limb. Hand Clin 2003;19(4):557–64.

8. Keenan M, Haider T, Stone L. Dynamic electromyography to assess elbow spasticity. J Hand Surg Am 1990;15(4):607–14.

9. Gracies J. Pathophysiology of spastic paresis. II: emergence of muscle overactivity. Muscle Nerve 2005;31(5):552–71.

10. Malhotra S, Cousins E, Pandyan A, et al. An investigation into the agreement between clinical, biomechanical and neurophysiological measures of spasticity. Clin Rehabil 2008;22(12):1105–15.

11. Sommerfeld D, Eek EU, Svensson AK, et al. Spasticity after stroke: its occurrence and association with motor impairments and activity limitations. Stroke 2004;35(1):134–9.

12. Anson C, Shepherd C. Incidence of secondary complications in spinal cord injury. Int J Rehabil Res 1996;19(1):55–66.

13. Johnson R, Gerhart KA, McCray J, et al. Secondary conditions following spinal cord injury in a population-based sample. Spinal Cord 1998;36(1): 45–50.

14. Lundstrom E, Terent A, Borg J. Prevalence of disabling spasticity 1 year after first-ever stroke. Eur J Neurol 2008;15(6):533–9.

15. Maynard F, Karunas R, Waring W. Epidemiology of spasticity following traumatic spinal cord injury. Arch Phys Med Rehabil 1990;71(8):566–9.

16. Noreau L, Proulx P, Gagnon L, et al. Secondary impairments after spinal cord injury: a population-based study. Am J Phys Med Rehabil 2000;79(6): 526–35.

17. Skold C, Levi R, Seiger A. Spasticity after traumatic spinal cord injury: nature, severity, and location. Arch Phys Med Rehabil 1999;80(12):1548–57.

18. Watkins C, Leathley MJ, Gregson JM, et al. Prevalence of spasticity post stroke. Clin Rehabil 2002; 16(5):515–22.

19. Wedekind C, Lippert-Gruner M. Long-term outcome in severe traumatic brain injury is significantly influenced by brainstem involvement. Brain Inj 2005; 19(9):681–4.

20. Welmer A, von Arbin M, Widén Holmqvist L, et al. Spasticity and its association with functioning and health-related quality of life 18 months after stroke. Cerebrovasc Dis 2006;21(4):247–53.

21. CDC. Facts about stroke. Available at: https://www.cdc.gov/stroke/facts.htm. Accessed December 1, 2017.

22. Armour B, Courtney-Long E, Fox M, et al. Prevalence and causes of paralysis–United States, 2013. Am J Public Health 2016;106(10):1855–7.

23. Leading causes of death. In: National Center for Health Statistics. Available at: https://www.cdc.gov/nchs/fastats/leading-causes-of-death.htm. Accessed December 1, 2017.

24. Harvey R, Roth E, Yu D, et al. Stroke syndromes. In: Braddom R, editor. Physical medicine and rehabilitation. 4th edition. Philadelphia: Elsevier; 2011. p. 1177–222.

25. Zorowitz R, Baerga E, Cuccurullo S. Stroke. In: Cuccurullo S, editor. Physical medicine and rehabilitation board review. 2nd edition. New York: demosMEDICAL; 2010. p. 40–87.

26. Traumatic Brain Injury and Concussion. TBI Data and Statistics. In: Centers for Disease Control and Prevention. Available at: https://www.cdc.gov/traumaticbraininjury/data/index.html. Accessed December 7, 2017.

27. Wagner A, Arenth P, Kwasnica C, et al. Traumatic brain injury. In: Braddom R, editor. Physical medicine and rehabilitation. 4th edition. Philadelphia: Elsevier; 2011. p. 1133–75.

28. Hirtz D, Thurman D, Gwinn-Hardy K, et al. How common are the 'common' neurologic disorders? Neurology 2007;68(5):326–37.

29. Kraft G, Brown T, Johnson S. Multiple sclerosis. In: Braddom R, editor. Physical medicine and rehabilitation. 4th edition. Philadelphia: Elsevier; 2011. p. 1233–52.

30. McGuire J. Epidemiology of spasticity in the adult and child. In: Brashear A, Elovic E, editors. Spasticity, diagnosis and treatment. 1st edition. New York: DemosMEDICAL; 2011. p. 5–15.

31. Barnes M, Kent R, Semlyen J, et al. Spasticity in multiple sclerosis. Neurorehabil Neural Repair 2003;17:66.

32. National Spinal Cord Injury Statistical Center. Spinal cord injury facts and figures at a glance. J Spinal Cord Med 2013;36(1):1–2.

33. Bernhard M, Gries A, Kremer P, et al. Spinal cord injury (SCI)–prehospital management. Resuscitation 2005;66(2):127–39.

34. Sekhon L, Fehlings M. Epidemiology, demographics, and pathophysiology of acute spinal cord injury. Spine (Phila Pa 1976) 2001;26(24 Suppl):S2–12.

35. Walker H, Kirshblum S. Spasticity due to disease of the spinal cord: pathophysiology, epidemiology, and

treatment. In: Brashear A, Elovic E, editors. Spasticity, diagnosis and treatment. 1st edition. New York: DemosMEDICAL; 2011. p. 313–39.

36. James M. Use of the medical research council muscle strength grading system in the upper extremity. J Hand Surg 2007;32(2):154–6.

37. Powell A, Davidson L. Pediatric spinal cord injury: a review by organ system. Phys Med Rehabil Clin N Am 2015;26:109–32.

38. Rosenbaum P, Paneth N, Leviton A, et al. A report: the definition and classification of cerebral palsy April 2006. Dev Med Child Neurol Suppl 2007;109:8–14.

39. Bax M, Goldstein M, Rosenbaum P, et al. Proposed definition and classification of cerebral palsy, April 2005. Dev Med Child Neurol 2005;47(8):571–6.

40. Winter S, Autry A, Boyle C, et al. Trends in the prevalence of cerebral palsy in a population-based study. Pediatrics 2002;110(6):1220–5.

41. McMahon M, Pruitt D, Vargus-Adams J. Cerebral palsy. In: Alexander M, Matthews D, editors. Pediatric rehabilitation. Principles and practice. 5th edition. New York: DemosMEDICAL; 2015. p. 336–72.

42. Evans K, Rigby AS, Hamilton P, et al. The relationships between neonatal encephalopathy and cerebral palsy: a cohort study. J Obstet Gynaecol 2001;21(2):114–20.

43. Durkin M, Benedict R, Yeargin-Allsopp M, et al. Prevalence of cerebral palsy among 8-year-old children in 2010 and preliminary evidence of trends in its relationship to low birthweight. Paediatr Perinat Epidemiol 2016;30(5):496–510.

44. Data and Statistics for Cerebral Palsy. In: CDC. Centers for Disease Control and Prevention. Available at: https://www.cdc.gov/ncbddd/cp/data.html. Accessed December 07, 2017.

45. Dolhun R, Donofrio P. Spasticity affecting those with neuromuscular diseases: pathology, epidemiology and treatment. In: Brashear A, Elovic E, editors. Spasticity, diagnosis and treatment. 1st edition. New York: DemosMEDICAL; 2011. p. 297–312.

Assessment of the Spastic Upper Limb with Computational Motion Analysis

Tasos Karakostas, MS, MPT, PhD BEng[a],*,
Kelsey Watters, BS, OTR/L[b], Erik C. King, MS, MD[c]

KEYWORDS

- SHUEE • Three-dimensional motion analysis • Coordination • Normative database
- Upper extremity

KEY POINTS

- Three-dimensional computerized motion analysis along with electromyography can quantify and augment clinical scales.
- Hand, wrist, forearm, and elbow function and motion are related to shoulder function and motion.
- The most optimum approach, currently, to assess upper extremity function is by combining a clinical examination, a diagnosis-specific clinical scale, and 3-dimensional data.
- It may be feasible to use the Shriners Hospital Upper Extremity Evaluation to evaluate upper extremity function for diagnoses other than hemiplegic cerebral palsy, such as obstetric brachial plexus palsy.

INTRODUCTION

There is consensus that quantifying hand and upper extremity (UE) function using 3-dimensional motion analysis (3DMA) is important.[1–5] It can facilitate clinical decision-making regarding the need and type of surgery, administration of pharmacological agents, and the focus of a therapy protocol. Furthermore, 3DMA preintervention and postintervention can quantify outcomes and assess treatment efficacy. These goals are accomplished by comparing pathological and normal movements, identifying primary and compensatory motor strategies during goal-oriented tasks, and by assessing movement quality relative to coordination. Nevertheless, there are challenges in establishing 3DMA as a means of quantifying UE function.

Although the use of 3DMA for the lower extremity (LE) during walking is an established procedure for the quantification of LE functional limitations, identifying a single, most relevant, repeatable, and cyclic activity of daily living (ADL) for the UE is difficult.[3,4] This diagnostic challenge is also compounded by the variable and complex nature of UE motion.[6]

In this article, the authors aim to provide an overview of the use of 3DMA in the evaluation of UE function to facilitate the clinical decision-making process regarding UE spasticity management. The authors also describe the approach used in their Computerized Motion Analysis (CMA) laboratory as a means of providing a more comprehensive UE clinical evaluation.

Disclosure Statement: The authors have nothing to disclose.
[a] Computerized Motion Analysis Laboratory, Orthopaedic Surgery, Shirley Ryan AbilityLab, Northwestern University, 355 East Erie Street, Chicago, IL 60611, USA; [b] Think and Speak Lab, Shirley Ryan AbilityLab, 355 East Erie Street, Chicago, IL 60611, USA; [c] Orthopaedic Surgery, Ann and Robert H. Lurie Children's Hospital of Chicago, Northwestern University, 225 East Chicago Avenue, Box 69, Chicago, IL 60611, USA
* Corresponding author.
E-mail address: tkarakosta@sralab.org

Hand Clin 34 (2018) 445–454
https://doi.org/10.1016/j.hcl.2018.06.002

CHALLENGES OF CLINICAL THREE-DIMENSIONAL MOTION ANALYSIS

Protocol

An established protocol for quantifying UE motion does not exist. There is variability in the functional tasks and ADLs selected for assessment and analysis.[1,3–9] The selected tasks must offer the ability to discern pathological from normal movement. Furthermore, they need to have validity, reproducibility, and sensitivity to clinically significant changes and they need to be predictive (ie, they need to be able to relate the 3D-based task results to the clinical findings and the outcomes of clinical assessment scales).[2]

Task variability is partly inherent in the marker-based 3DMA systems, which are considered the gold standard for computerized motion assessment.[2] For example, assessment of the fine movements of the finger joints and thumb simultaneous with other joints of the UE is difficult because of the required resolution. It is important, therefore, that all reports adequately describe the instrumentation used and the associated measurement errors. The authors' laboratory includes a 10-camera optical capture system (VICON, Los Angeles, CA, USA) with angular error of less than 1°. UE motion and analog data are captured at 120 Hz and 1080 Hz, respectively.

Biomechanical Approach

The biomechanical approach used varies between investigators. To evaluate the kinematics at a joint, one needs to start with a marker or sensor-based model. Markers are placed on specific anatomical positions to define body segments. Motion at the joint is then defined by a mathematical model determining the movement of the adjacent segments making up the joint. Some investigators select to focus on isolated UE joints,[9–11] which allows the flexibility of using mathematical models that are not applicable to all joints. Consequently, the specific mechanical approaches implemented in these investigations necessitate that the results of these studies, in conjunction with the tasks studied, may need further validation.

However, there is evidence that distal UE deficits need to be evaluated along with the other, more proximal, joints of the UE and trunk[12–14] (ie, all joints need to be assessed concurrently). In fact, Fitoussi and collaborators[12] suggested that, because of the significant effects of treatment of the distal UE on the proximal UE joints and trunk, treatment of proximal UE deficits should wait until the effects of distal UE treatment are considered. However, even among the investigators who have evaluated all joints of the UE concurrently, consensus is lacking

in terms of the manner that motion is defined mathematically. This variability is, in part, due to the complexity of the joint structures. For example, some investigators have described motion at the wrist and elbow by modeling these joints as hinged or 2 degrees of freedom joints.[6,15] Others have approached them as 3D structures. However, when considering motion in 3 dimensions, the order of rotation about each axis of motion ultimately determines the position in space. In order to address this challenge, the International Society of Biomechanics (ISB)[16] offered guidelines to standardize biomechanical modeling and reporting[1,4] of UE joint motion; these are not followed by all investigators. Most of the controversy regarding modeling revolves around the shoulder joint. Some researchers describe movement at the shoulder as motion of the humerus relative to the trunk,[6,15] which neglects the contribution of the scapulo-thoracic joint (STJ) to the motion of the shoulder complex. Although motion of the scapula is difficult to track, some investigators have tried to account for it.[1,4,9] However, all current approaches seem to neglect the contributions of the acromioclavicular joint (ACJ) and sternoclavicular joint (SCJ) to the shoulder complex motion[17,18] by considering them part of trunk movement.

The authors' CMA laboratory uses 23 passive retroreflective markers, positioned at specific, easily identifiable and reproducible, anatomical landmarks according to the Vicon PluginGait marker model (**Fig. 1**). From the markers and anthropometric measurements, the authors define the segments that comprise the UE, trunk, pelvis, and head. Each UE segment is allocated to a bone and is defined by a proximal and distal endpoint located at the center of the joint along with a third non-collinear point to describe rotational orientation. The wrist joint center is located at the midpoint of the distance between the ulnar and radial styloid processes. The elbow joint center is located at the midpoint of the distance between the medial and lateral epicondyles. The glenohumeral joint center is defined through a dynamic joint centering procedure involving humeral abduction/adduction and anterior flexion to calculate the pivot point of the instantaneous helical axes from these movements. The trunk segment is defined by the markers on the 7th cervical and 10th thoracic spinous processes, the manubrium, and the sternal notch at the xyphoid process (see **Fig. 1**). This approach allows the contributions of the STJ, ACJ, and SCJ to humeral elevation to be reflected in the shoulder complex rather than in the kinematics of the trunk.

For the purposes of the authors' analysis (focused on the hand, wrist, forearm, and elbow

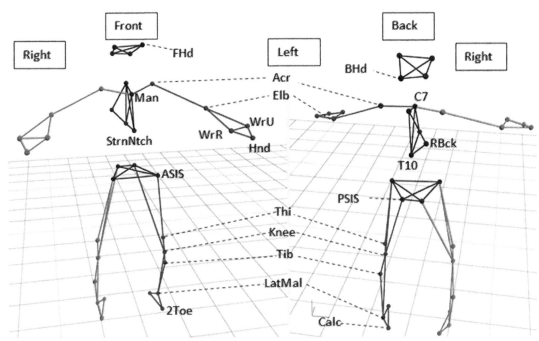

Fig. 1. Marker placement for upper extremity kinematic analysis (markers placed bilaterally): FHd, forehead; BHd, back head; Man, manubrium at the level of the interclavicular ligament; StrnNtch, sternal notch at the level of the xyphoid process; C7, seventh cervical spinous process; T10, tenth thoracic spinous process; RBck, right back at the center of the right scapula; Acr, acromion; Elb, elbow at the lateral epicondyle; WrR, WrU, wrist at the radial and ulnar styloid process; Hnd, hand proximal to the third carpometacarpal joint; ASIS, anterior superior iliac spine; PSIS, posterior superior iliac spine. Additional markers used bilaterally for lower extremity kinematic analysis include: Thi, thigh; Knee, on the lateral femoral epicondyle; Tib, tibia; LatMal, lateral malleolus; Calc, calcaneus; and 2Toe, 2nd metatarsal head.

segments), shoulder motion is defined by the position of the shoulder complex as reflected by the humeral position relative to the trunk. This approach is considered acceptable because the tasks the authors study do not focus on the shoulder joint, and they do not require frontal or sagittal shoulder elevations greater than 90°. Therefore, the STJ, ACJ, and SCJ contributions can be assumed to be negligible.[19] Subsequently, the movements that the authors report for each task are as follows:

1. For the hand, flexion/extension and radial/ulnar deviation at the wrist joint;
2. For the forearm, flexion/extension and pronation/supination at the elbow joint;
3. For the humerus, horizontal abduction/adduction (elevation plane), flexion/extension (elevation), and internal/external rotation at the shoulder joint;
4. Trunk, flexion/extension, right/left side-bending and axial rotation relative to the pelvis and relative to the fixed global/laboratory coordinate system;
5. Pelvis, anterior/posterior tilt, upward/downward obliquity, and protraction/retraction relative to the fixed global/laboratory coordinate system.

The authors' approach is inclusive of the pelvis because pelvic position can affect trunk orientation, which, in turn, can affect the entire UE kinematic chain. With the authors' biomechanical modeling approach, motion at a joint is determined from the orientation of a distal segment relative to its adjacent proximal segment. Joint motion definitions are adopted from the ISB recommendations for UE motion[16] using Euler angles.[20]

CLINICAL ASSESSMENT INSTRUMENTS

Multiple standardized, validated, and easy-to-administer clinical assessment tools are available to assess patients with UE spasticity. The clinical scales may be related to either strength,[21] function (eg, Jebsen-Taylor Hand Function scale),[22] or ADLs (eg, Functional Independence Measure for adults [FIM] and children [WeeFIM]).[23–25] However, to optimally assess the motor strategies implemented by a patient during an ADL and account for observer subjectivity, the authors believe that more objective measures are necessary.[2] Objective data derived from 3DMA have been compared with outcomes of a variety of UE assessment instruments.[7,9] Klotz and coworkers,[7] for example, found that the 3DMA UE output for the ADLs performed by their patients had a statistically significant positive correlation with the Manual Ability Classification Scale and the Disability of Arm Shoulder and Hand instrument. Rundquist and colleagues[9] reported that shoulder kinematics of their patients significantly predicted their respective shoulder and elbow subscale scores of the Fugl-Meyer Motor Assessment scale.

The Shriners Hospital Upper Extremity Evaluation (SHUEE)[26] instrument is of particular interest to the author's group because of its focus on pediatric patients with neuromuscular disorders; it has been validated for children with hemiplegic cerebral palsy (CP). The authors use the SHUEE in their CMA laboratory combined with 3DMA to accurately quantify UE functional deficits and to better formulate a plan of care. The SHUEE is a video-based assessment of the fingers, wrist, forearm, and elbow segments while a patient performs several functional tasks. The entire evaluation is divided into the 4 following sections:

a. Impairments identification, by measuring joint range of motion (ROM), spasticity and joint stability, including the shoulder joint;
b. Evaluation of spontaneous functional use (SFA) of the involved extremity to perform 9 functional tasks;
c. Assessment of dynamic positioning (DPA), or alignment, of the UE segments during 16 functional tasks; and
d. Assessment of the ability to grasp and release (GRA) a small object at 3 wrist positions (flexion, neutral, and extension).

When generating a treatment plan, the general assumption is that greater SFU and better dynamic alignment of the relevant segments predict a greater potential for improved function.[26] Performance for each task is scored and combined to calculate a total score relative to a normal maximum.

Although clinically useful, the SHUEE may be limited by its nature as a video-based assessment. The videotaping, by focusing on the task-specific UE segment of interest at any given time, may miss compensatory movements recruited by the patient to accomplish a task. Even if an observer or the videotaping captures compensatory patterns, the performance scoring forms do not account for them. In addition, any video-based capture provides a biplanar representation of motion. In other words, the person who scores the performance does not have perspective of concurrent movements that may be taking place in the third (eg, transverse) plane of motion.[3] Moreover, the evaluation of the videotaped performance does not allow accurate quantification of the ROM used

by the patient to accomplish a task. Consequently, Davids and collaborators[26] have expressed the need for quantification of the dynamic positioning of the UE segments during SHUEE testing through 3DMA and biomechanical modeling to improve accuracy, reliability, and objectivity. Finally, the SFA section of the SHUEE, which represents the patient's intent to move the involved UE to accomplish a task, may be inherently limited because it is based on observed motion. Typically, the lack of motion implies that the patient neglects the involved extremity. Similar to when evaluating strength, however, a patient may have a trace of activity of the muscle tested, but the segment involved may not move. As such, there is the need to augment this component of the SHUEE with a measure that can better capture the intent of movement and the quality of the neuromotor response.

In their CMA laboratory, the authors have selected the SHUEE as their primary instrument for assessing UE function in children with hemiplegia CP, but also augment the assessment with 3DMA. Of the 16 functional tasks performed in SHUEE, the authors have selected 5 for 3DMA: "unscrew the bottle cup" (UBC) and "pull the playdough apart" (PPA), assessing wrist and hand flexion/extension and radial/ulnar deviation; "accept coins/change" (AC); and "take hand to mouth" (HTM), which evaluate forearm pronation/supination; and "place sticker on ball" or "poke the ball" (PB) evaluating elbow flexion/extension. The authors concurrently collect synchronized electromyography (EMG) data from selected UE muscle groups using a 16-channel surface EMG system (Motion Labs Systems, Baton Rouge, LA, USA) with a bandwidth of 20 to 500 Hz, which is bandpass filtered from 20 to 250 Hz. The authors position surface electrodes on the skin over the muscle belly of the muscles of interest: biceps brachii, long head of the triceps, brachioradialis, flexor carpi ulnaris, and extensor carpi ulnaris. Crosstalk quality control is performed with every electrode placement, using manual muscle testing (MMT) principles.[21] The kinematic information can augment the DPA section of the SHUEE, whereas the EMG can augment the SFA component.

Another important question is whether the SHUEE can be used to evaluate UE function for pediatric neuromuscular conditions other than CP. There is evidence suggesting that it can be used to assess children with neonatal brachial plexus palsy (BPP),[27] although it has not been used to assess patients with spinal cord injury or stroke. **Table 1** shows results from a principal component analysis evaluating the SHUEE components used to assess UE function in children with BPP. Correlation coefficients were very low, and the

Table 1
The correlation matrix and the respective Eigenvalues from a principal components analysis comparing the Shriners Hospital Upper Extremity Evaluation output components for children with neonatal brachial plexus palsy

Parameter	Correlation Matrix			Eigenvalues of the Correlation Matrix			
	SFA, %	DPA, %	GRA, %	Eigenvalue	Difference	Proportion	Cumulative
SFA, %	1.0000	0.5687	0.3668	1.86276762	1.15612702	0.6209	0.6209
DPA, %	0.5687	1.0000	0.3454	0.70664060	0.27604882	0.2355	0.8565
GRA, %	0.3668	0.3454	1.0000	0.43059178	—	0.1435	1.0000

Abbreviations: DPA, dynamic positional analysis; GRA, grasp and release analysis; SFA, spontaneous functional analysis.

Eigenvalues of the correlation matrix were very different. The disassociation among the 3 components of the SHUEE suggests that each component measures a different aspect of UE function. Although more studies are needed to validate this finding, the authors' preliminary analysis indicates that it is reasonable to use the SHUEE to evaluate UE function of pediatric populations with neuromuscular conditions other than CP.

THREE-DIMENSIONAL MOTION ANALYSIS AND CLINICAL DECISION MAKING

One consequence of the lack of an established 3DMA protocol and of the variability in biomechanical approaches for UE functional analysis is the difficulty in interpretation and comparison of results across studies using 3DMA. Concurrently, the need to be able to objectively discriminate pathological from normal UE motion has led most researchers to develop their own 3DMA-based normative databases. This approach allows factoring their particular biomechanical approach and their tasks of interest and allows investigation of the functional effects of pathology on UE motion.[1,4,7,8] Consequently, from a predetermined task-specific starting position and the position of the joint or joints of interest at the point of task accomplishment (PTA), each UE joint ROM or functional ROM for each task of interest is determined. The patient's task-specific PTA is subsequently compared with the respective normative database in order to identify deficits that may need medical or surgical management.

The development of normative databases for functional tasks or ADLs has provided the opportunity to use kinematic variables from the collected data to construct indices that can objectively quantify and characterize different aspects of UE motor performance. For example, the ratio of the distance of the hand from the target at the starting position to the hand trajectory (ie, the Hand Path Ratio) is a kinematic index that can quantify the efficiency aspect of motor performance while reaching a target.[28,29] A comprehensive review on the kinematic indexes for UE function has been provided by others.[2,30]

In an effort to provide a potentially more accurate assessment of patient function, some investigators postulate the use of the uninvolved UE as reference for the performance of the involved UE.[5,7] Wang and colleagues[5] found this approach to be feasible in a cohort of patients with BPP. Conversely, Klotz and colleagues[7] suggest that this may not be appropriate in patients with hemiplegic CP. However, careful examination of their data suggests that, with the exception of shoulder extension and external rotation, the performance of all UE joints of the uninvolved UE was statistically the same as that of their healthy control group. Therefore, UE studies involving patients with hemiplegic CP can use the performance of the uninvolved UE for the elbow and wrist as reference.

The approach in the CMA laboratory involves a 3-step process: (a) the authors have augmented the 3DMA for the SHUEE tasks of interest with their own normative database for these tasks; (b) they superimpose the kinematic segment and joint excursions plots of the involved over the uninvolved extremities; and (c) they quantify movement coordination after developing a normative inter-joint coordination index (IJC), which is used to contrast the performance of their patients.

The authors' 3DMA normative database for the 3DMA-specific SHUEE tasks is based on 24 healthy individuals (6–17 years of age, 14 girls, 10 boys for a total of 48 UEs performing the selected tasks, except for the UBC). This age range was selected because it is representative of the patient population typically assessed in the CMA. All subjects underwent the full SHUEE protocol. Then, following anthropometric measurements, the placements of electrodes over the muscles of interest, the placements of markers and a calibration, 3D motion data were collected for the SHUEE tasks of interest. All subjects were given identical, standardized, instructions to perform the tasks, based on the training materials for the SHUEE. Subjects performed the tasks standing, at their own self-selected pace and manner, 3 times. Each task was performed with both UEs, except for the UBC, which is a bimanual task. The testing order of each UE (ie, dominant vs nondominant first) was randomized. The start and end position of each task was standardized, and movement initiation was determined from the movement of the marker on the hand. The transition from rest to movement was reproducibly identified by several technicians within 5 frames, representing 0.04 seconds from the initiation of motion. Data were collected during the entire movement, and these data were used to construct the authors' PTA-based normative database.[8] **Table 2** reflects the PTA values (ie, the ranges of joint mobility required for each task) concurrently, by all UE segments.

In addition, from the PTA values for each task, the authors computed the IJC[2] (**Table 3**). Results close to 1 suggest a high correlation, or coordination, between the joints when completing a task. The authors consider correlations greater than 0.75 strong. The IJC reflects the concurrent accessory movements used to accomplish a task; these accessory movements should not be ignored when formulating a treatment plan. Consequently,

the IJC itself and combined with the normative PTA values can be useful clinical tools with implications for management of UE deficits.

Table 3 suggests that the IJC is task-specific and that there is a strong relationship between the distal and more proximal UE segments. This relationship, especially during tasks focusing on the distal UE function (ie, UBC and PPA) may illustrate that the purpose of the UE is to position the hand and wrist such that they can perform their functions. Therefore, UE functional evaluation should include all UE segments concurrently. Furthermore, **Table 3** provides support to the position that proximal UE limitations in children with hemiplegia may be related to compensatory movement strategies, which can improve following treatment of distal UE impairments. Therefore, treatment of the proximal UE segments should occur after treatment of the distal segments.[12]

EXAMPLE CASE

A 13-year-old girl with left hemiplegia and developmental delay was referred to the authors' CMA laboratory for analysis. The mother reported that the patient requires assistance with ADLs, such as bathing, dressing, and tying her shoes. The patient was not receiving occupational or physical therapy. She had no other significant past medical history, but did undergo surgical intervention to address

Table 2
Average ranges of motion at the point of task achievement

Position at PTA	UBC	PPA	HTM	AC	PB
Wrist flexion	1.7 (2.9)	—	15.9 (8.3)	7.2 (1.4)	**5.2 (4.3)**
Wrist extension	**22.9 (8.7)**	**16.0 (11.7)**	10.9 (6.7)	6.7 (4.8)	8.2 (4.8)
Ulnar deviation	**10.7 (7.6)**	**13.8 (6.9)**	**8.5 (6.0)**	7.9 (11.9)	14.6 (1.5)
Radial deviation	5.9 (1.5)	12.6 (4.1)	6.3 (5.7)	**10.8 (4.4)**	**15.2 (7.2)**
Forearm pronation	**25.4 (18.2)**	**44.9 (17.4)**	**17.8 (10.3)**	—	**29.9 (3.4)**
Forearm supination	—	—	51 (15)	50.7 (17.8)	—
Elbow flexion/extension[a]	**93.5 (12.2)**	**83.4 (17.4)**	**138.3 (7.7)**	**91.2 (8.4)**	**28.0 (11.6)**
Shoulder horizontal abduction[b]	**26.4 (16.7)**	**24.6 (22.5)**	35.1 (18.3)	20.7 (12.1)	—
Shoulder horizontal adduction	12.8 (5.5)	—	28.9 (16.7)	—	**44.2 (12.1)**
Shoulder elevation[c]	**26.1 (6.4)**	**50.9 (28.6)**	**42.7 (5.0)**	16.1 (4.4)	**85.1 (5.5)**
Shoulder internal rotation	**35.1 (19.2)**	23.6 (15.7)	**43.7 (8.3)**	34.1 (15.3)	24.5 (10.4)
Shoulder external rotation	—	6.4 (4.2)	—	47.5 (1.6)	—

Standard deviations are in parentheses.
Bold indicates 80% of UE demonstrated that positional orientation.
[a] No upper extremities exhibited elbow hyperextension; in PB, the value shown represents the subject moving to elbow extension.
[b] Horizontal abduction/adduction can be thought of as abduction/adduction in the plane of the scapula.
[c] Elevation can be thought of as flexion in the plane of scapula.

Table 3
Interjoint correlation coefficients demonstrating the coordination across upper extremity segments while performing selected Shriners Hospital Upper Extremity Evaluation tasks

UBC	Wrist Ext	Rad Dev	Uln Dev	Elbow Flex	Pronation	Sh Abd	Sh Fl
Uln dev	**−0.96**	—	—	—	—	—	—
Elbow flex	−0.43	—	0.26	—	—	—	—
Pronation	−0.74	0.5	0.35	−0.17	—	—	—
Sh abd	−0.61	0.43	0.35	0.06	−0.01	—	—
Sh fl	0.38	−0.65	−0.46	−0.34	−0.15	0.42	—
Sh IR	0.07	0.11	**0.77**	0.39	−0.48	0.39	−0.37

PPA	Wrist Ext	Rad Dev	Uln Dev	Elbow Flex	Pronation	Sh Abd	Sh Fl
Rad dev	**−0.85**	—	—	—	—	—	—
Uln dev	−0.03	0.24	—	—	—	—	—
Elbow flex	**−0.79**	0.32	−0.34	—	—	—	—
Pronation	−0.38	0.74	**0.90**	−0.13	—	—	—
Sh abd	**0.83**	−0.34	−0.14	**−0.81**	−0.29	—	—
Sh fl	−0.21	**0.99**	**0.76**	0.05	0.70	−0.48	—
Sh IR	−0.69	0.30	**−0.85**	**0.94**	−0.40	**−0.80**	0.03

AC	Wrist Ext	Rad Dev	Elbow Flex	Supination	Sh Abd	Sh Fl
Rad dev	0.38	—	—	—	—	—
Elbow flex	0.10	**0.84**	—	—	—	—
Supination	−0.37	**0.95**	0.78	—	—	—
Sh abd	0.21	0.64	−0.35	−0.63	—	—
Sh fl	0.11	0.08	0.25	−0.12	0.67	—
Sh IR	−0.12	**0.75**	**0.80**	**−0.82**	**0.83**	0.54

HTM	Wrist Flex	Wrist Ext	Uln Dev	Elbow Flex	Supination	Sh Abd	Sh Add	Sh Fl
Uln dev	0.49	−0.52	—	—	—	—	—	—
Elbow flex	**−0.89**	−0.61	−0.25	—	—	—	—	—
Supination	−0.41	−0.41	0.45	0.54	—	—	—	—
Sh abd	0.46	0.54	0.60	−0.59	0.61	—	—	—
Sh add	−0.47	−0.17	0.02	0.72	0.55	0.43	—	—
Sh fl	0.55	−0.31	**0.94**	−0.38	0.21	0.47	−0.01	—
Sh ER	0.24	0.41	−0.32	0.16	−0.55	−0.38	0.32	−0.14

PB	Wrist Flex	Wrist Ext	Rad Dev	Uln Dev	Elbow Ext	Pronation	Supination	Sh Add	Sh Fl
Rad dev	−0.18	0.67	—	—	—	—	—	—	—
Uln dev	**0.94**	—	—	—	—	—	—	—	—
Elbow ext	0.09	0.315	**0.90**	−0.14	—	—	—	—	—
Pronation	0.52	**0.91**	0.71	**0.89**	0.49	—	—	—	—
Supination	−0.12	**0.99**	0.67	−0.27	−0.62	0.18	—	—	—
Sh add	−0.13	−0.72	0.65	−0.45	**0.81**	0.29	−0.46	—	—
Sh fl	−0.01	0.51	−0.71	0.60	−0.73	−0.52	0.17	**−0.93**	—
Sh IR	−0.20	**−0.89**	−0.10	**−0.77**	0.07	−0.29	−0.18	0.60	−0.55

Bold indicates correlation coefficients >0.75.
  Selected SHUEE tasks include: UBC, PPD, AC, HTM, PB.
  Parameters: Wrist extension (Wrist ext); radial deviation (Rad dev); ulnar deviation (Uln dev); elbow flexion (Elbow flex); elbow extension (Elbow ext); shoulder abduction, that is, horizontal shoulder abduction (Sh abd); shoulder adduction, that is, horizontal shoulder adduction (Sh add); shoulder flexion, that is, elevation (Sh fl); shoulder internal rotation (Sh IR); shoulder external rotation (Sh ER).

LE function. Physical examination findings include the following: elbow extension −30° active, −10° passive, arc of elbow motion from 30° to 140° active and 10° to 150° passive, full supination, pronation 75° active, and full passive pronation; wrist ulnar deviation to 30° active and passive; radial deviation 0° active and 30° passive. MMT showed significantly decreased strength in the left UE. SHUEE SFA score was 58%, reflecting moderate assistive use. DPA score was 58%, reflecting mild to moderate deformity, with distribution among all segments –the most affected segments were the wrist (17/24) and elbow (8/12). 3DMA indicated that left elbow extension was limited while performing tasks; forearm pronation was limited (contrary to ROM findings). The wrist remained in ulnar deviation, and muscle activity was phasic for all muscle groups (**Fig. 2**). Based on the findings, the procedures recommended were biceps and brachioradialis fractional lengthening and flexor carpi ulnaris transfer to extensor carpi radialis brevis tendon transfer. In summary, the 3DMA determined that there was no contracture, and functional forearm pronation was limited, and confirmed the elbow extension and radial deviation limitations were, indeed, functionally limiting.

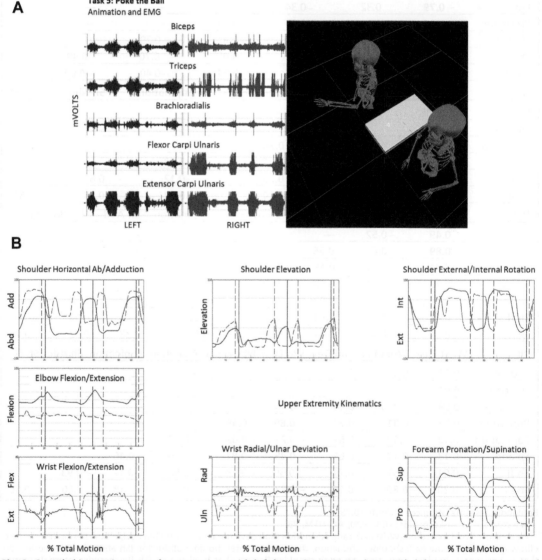

Fig. 2. Sample kinematic output from a patient with left hemiplegia. EMG along with (*A*) animation output, and (*B*) UE kinematic output while performing the PB functional task. The vertical lines represent the time the task was accomplished (*blue, left; red, right*).

SUMMARY

Current research challenges the validity of clinical decision-making based on 2-dimensional video-taped assessments alone.[3,8] In addition, the correlation of the typical clinical examination to the performance of functional tasks is debatable.[3,7] Although clinical scales are routinely used, there is a strong element of subjectivity when scoring a patient's performance, and the assessment cannot describe the overall motor strategies recruited by the patient to accomplish a task. Consequently, the usefulness of 3DMA for quantifying and assessing UE motion to identify functional limitations and, subsequently, facilitate clinical decision-making or assess treatment efficacy, is well supported in the literature.

The authors' experience suggests that the optimal approach to assess UE function is the combination of clinical examination, a diagnosis-specific clinical scale, the 3DMA with EMGs associated with the clinical scale-specific tasks to quantify motion and coordination patterns, and a 3DMA task-specific normative database. Importantly, the authors' work focuses on children with neuromuscular disorders that affect UE function. The clinical tool the authors have selected is the SHUEE. The authors' approach augments the SHUEE with EMG and 3DMA, which is not subjected to biomechanical limitations, such as the gimbal-lock,[4,8] by virtue of the tasks assessed and the focus of the evaluation. The PTA-specific ROM for selected SHUEE tasks, combined with the UE IJC data, can be used for preoperative and postoperative assessment in patients with UE spasticity.

REFERENCES

1. Aizawa J, Masuda T, Koyama T, et al. Three-dimensional motion of the upper extremity joints during various activities of daily living. J Biomech 2010; 43(15):2915–22.

2. de los Reyes-Guzman A, Dimbwadyo-Terrer I, Trincado-Alonso F, et al. Quantitative assessment based on kinematic measures of functional impairments during upper extremity movements: a review. Clin Biomech (Bristol, Avon) 2014;29(7):719–27.

3. Fitoussi F, Diop A, Maurel N, et al. Kinematic analysis of the upper limb: a useful tool in children with cerebral palsy. J Pediatr Orthop B 2006; 15(4):247–56.

4. van Andel CJ, Wolterbeek N, Doorenbosch CA, et al. Complete 3D kinematics of upper extremity functional tasks. Gait Posture 2008;27(1):120–7.

5. Wang JS, Petuskey K, Bagley AM, et al. The contralateral unimpaired arm as a control for upper extremity kinematic analysis in children with brachial plexus birth palsy. J Pediatr Orthop 2007;27(6):709–11.

6. Hingtgen B, McGuire JR, Wang M, et al. An upper extremity kinematic model for evaluation of hemiparetic stroke. J Biomech 2006;39(4):681–8.

7. Klotz MC, Kost L, Braatz F, et al. Motion capture of the upper extremity during activities of daily living in patients with spastic hemiplegic cerebral palsy. Gait Posture 2013;38(1):148–52.

8. Petuskey K, Bagley A, Abdala E, et al. Upper extremity kinematics during functional activities: three-dimensional studies in a normal pediatric population. Gait Posture 2007;25(4):573–9.

9. Rundquist PJ, Dumit M, Hartley J, et al. Three-dimensional shoulder complex kinematics in individuals with upper extremity impairment from chronic stroke. Disabil Rehabil 2012;34(5):402–7.

10. Murgia A, Kyberd PJ, Chappell PH, et al. Marker placement to describe the wrist movements during activities of daily living in cyclical tasks. Clin Biomech (Bristol, Avon) 2004;19(3):248–54.

11. Schmidt R, Disselhorst-Klug C, Silny J, et al. A marker-based measurement procedure for unconstrained wrist and elbow motions. J Biomech 1999; 32(6):615–21.

12. Fitoussi F, Diop A, Maurel N, et al. Upper limb motion analysis in children with hemiplegic cerebral palsy: proximal kinematic changes after distal botulinum toxin or surgical treatments. J Child Orthop 2011; 5(5):363–70.

13. Kreulen M, Smeulders MJ, Veeger HE, et al. Movement patterns of the upper extremity and trunk before and after corrective surgery of impaired forearm rotation in patients with cerebral palsy. Dev Med Child Neurol 2006;48(6):436–41.

14. Kreulen M, Smeulders MJ, Veeger HE, et al. Movement patterns of the upper extremity and trunk associated with impaired forearm rotation in patients with hemiplegic cerebral palsy compared to healthy controls. Gait Posture 2007;25(3):485–92.

15. Rab G, Petuskey K, Bagley A. A method for determination of upper extremity kinematics. Gait Posture 2002;15(2):113–9.

16. Wu G, van der Helm FC, Veeger HE, et al. ISB recommendation on definitions of joint coordinate systems of various joints for the reporting of human joint motion–part II: shoulder, elbow, wrist and hand. J Biomech 2005;38(5):981–92.

17. Jobe CM, Iannotti JP. Limits imposed on glenohumeral motion by joint geometry. J Shoulder Elbow Surg 1995;4(4):281–5.

18. Neumann DA. Kinesiology of the musculoskeletal system: foundations for physical rehabilitation. 1st edition. St Louis (MO): Mosby Inc; 2002.

19. Norkin CC, White JD. Measurement of joint motion: a guide to goniometry. Philadelphia: F.A. Davis Company; 2003.

20. Goldstein H. Classical mechanics. 2nd edition. New York: Addison-Wesley; 1960.

21. Kendall-Peterson F, McCreary-Kendall E, Provance-Geise P, et al. Muscles: testing and function with posture and pain. 5th edition. Baltimore (MD): Lippincott Williams & Wilkins; 2005.

22. Jebsen RH, Taylor N, Trieschmann RB, et al. An objective and standardized test of hand function. Arch Phys Med Rehabil 1969;50(6):311–9.

23. Ottenbacher KJ, Msall ME, Lyon NR, et al. Interrater agreement and stability of the Functional Independence Measure for Children (WeeFIM): use in children with developmental disabilities. Arch Phys Med Rehabil 1997;78(12):1309–15.

24. Sperle PA, Ottenbacher KJ, Braun SL, et al. Equivalence reliability of the functional independence measure for children (WeeFIM) administration methods. Am J Occup Ther 1997;51(1):35–41.

25. Keith RA, Granger CV, Hamilton BB, et al. The functional independence measure: a new tool for rehabilitation. Adv Clin Rehabil 1987;1:6–18.

26. Davids JR, Peace LC, Wagner LV, et al. Validation of the Shriners Hospital for Children Upper Extremity Evaluation (SHUEE) for children with hemiplegic cerebral palsy. J Bone Joint Surg Am 2006;88(2):326–33.

27. Karakostas T, King E, Hsiang S. Constrained induced movement therapy for children with brachial plexus injury: upper and lower extremity immediate and long term changes. Arch Phys Med Rehabil 2016;97(10):e8–9.

28. Karakostas T, Nichols D, Quesada PM, et al. Reach time responses of patients with hemiparesis following different rehabilitation protocols Third World Conference on Integrated Design and Process Technology. Berlin, Germany, July 5–9, 1998.

29. Nichols D, Karakostas T, Quesada PM, et al. Contextual interference effects on reach time in patients with hemiparesis. Los Angeles (CA): Society for Neuroscience; 1998.

30. Zollo L, Rossini L, Bravi M, et al. Quantitative evaluation of upper-limb motor control in robot-aided rehabilitation. Med Biol Eng Comput 2011;49(10):1131–44.

Nonsurgical Treatment Options for Upper Limb Spasticity

Laura Black, MD, MPH[a],*, Deborah Gaebler-Spira, MD[b]

KEYWORDS

- Rehabilitation • Upper extremity • Muscle spasticity • Muscle hypertonia • Cerebral palsy • Stroke
- Brain injuries • Occupational therapy

KEY POINTS

- The International Classification of Functioning, Disability, and Health is a valuable framework for setting functional goals in rehabilitation.
- Recent research in constraint-induced movement therapy and bimanual therapy shows promising results for upper extremity functional improvement.
- Reduction of spasticity using medications and chemodenervation procedures can maximize upper limb function.
- Technological advances, including robotics and virtual reality platforms, can enhance traditional therapies.
- Coordination of rehabilitation interventions with the surgical team ensures optimal outcomes.

INTRODUCTION

Many nonsurgical options exist for the rehabilitation of upper limb spasticity (ULS). The central focus of rehabilitation is to identify functional goals across multiple domains and develop a comprehensive plan that meets each goal. Age, cause of spasticity, severity, baseline and current functional status, cognitive impairment, family/environmental support, and medical comorbidities are important to consider when setting functional goals. The decision-making process involves the individual, caregivers, occupational therapist, rehabilitation, and the medical and surgical teams. The International Classification of Functioning, Disability, and Health (ICF) is a useful framework to guide management that incorporates an individual's body structure and function, including strength, spasticity, range of motion (ROM), activities of daily living (ADLs), participation in vocational/community settings, and intrapersonal and environmental factors[1] (**Fig. 1**).

Spasticity, defined as a velocity-dependent resistance to muscle stretch, is a positive symptom of the upper motor neuron syndrome, which commonly occurs in central nervous system (CNS) disorders, including stroke, spinal cord injury, and cerebral palsy (CP). Muscles that cross 2 joints tend to be disproportionately affected by ULS. The typical pattern of ULS involves the shoulder adductors and internal rotators, forearm pronators, and elbow and wrist flexors. Involvement of the fingers and thumb depends on timing of brain injury. Children with antenatal brain injury may be more likely to retain distal muscle movements, such as grasp and release of the fingers,

Disclosure Statement: Dr D. Gaebler-Spira is a consultant for Rehabtek and receives research funding from Merz (maker of Xeomin) and Allergan (maker of Botox).
[a] Shirley Ryan AbilityLab, Department of Physical Medicine and Rehabilitation, Northwestern University Feinberg School of Medicine, 355 East Erie Street, 21st Floor, Suite 2127, Chicago, IL 60601, USA; [b] Shirley Ryan AbilityLab, Department of Physical Medicine and Rehabilitation, Northwestern University Feinberg School of Medicine, 355 East Erie Street, Chicago, IL 60601, USA
* Corresponding author.
E-mail address: lblack@sralab.org

hand.theclinics.com

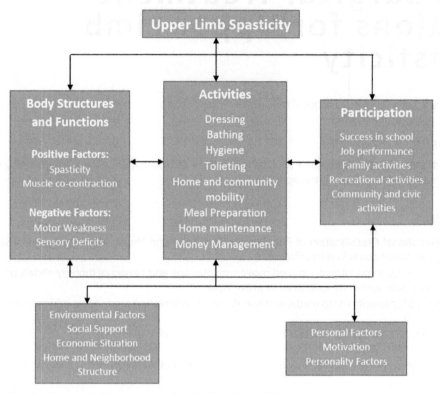

Fig. 1. The functional impact of ULS portrayed using the ICF model.

whereas adults and children with postnatal brain injury occurring after the pruning of corticospinal input during early infancy tend to have distal muscle involvement.[2,3]

ULS impairs function by limiting active movement and passive ROM of the arm and hand, resulting in a cascade of secondary impairments, including pain and contracture (see **Fig. 1**).[4–6] The rehabilitation plan incorporates prevention of these secondary impairments. Oral medications and neurolytic injections can successfully reduce muscle tone; however, spasticity management must include targeted interventions to address secondary impairments, such as weakness and reduced selective motor control.

This article presents an algorithmic approach to the management of ULS, encompassing evidence-based rehabilitation therapies, medications, and insight into innovations in orthotics and robotics that hold promise in expanding rehabilitation efforts (**Fig. 2**).

THERAPY INTERVENTIONS

- Patients with ULS should have an assessment with a therapist experienced in upper limb management.

- Constraint-induced movement therapy (CIMT) encourages use of the paretic hand in activities by restraining the opposite hand.
- Bimanual therapy (BMT) facilitates acquisition of skills that use both hands.
- Electrical stimulation (E-Stim) of spastic muscles may improve spasticity and muscle strength.

All children and adults with ULS should be referred to therapy for a functional assessment. This assessment may be provided by an occupational therapist, a physical therapist, or a hand specialist. The therapist provides an assessment of ULS and its secondary symptoms and creates a therapeutic plan to address ROM, stretching, strengthening, and functional goals.

One of the most extensively studied therapies for the paretic upper limb in both adults and children is CIMT, which encourages one-handed activity of the paretic hand and arm by constraining the unaffected upper extremity using a cast or mitt. Multiple systematic reviews have showed that CIMT is more effective than other upper extremity therapies in adults with stroke.[7–9] CIMT has also shown benefits in children with hemiplegic CP.[10,11] Traditional CIMT requires 6 hours per day of cast use for 10 days in a 2-week period.

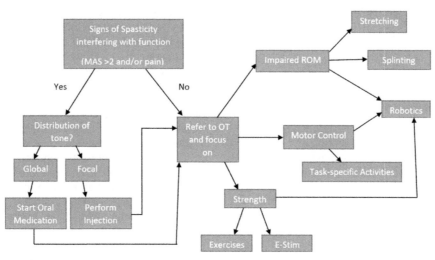

Fig. 2. An algorithmic approach to spasticity management. OT, occupational therapy.

Because these lengthy schedules can increase the likelihood of fatigue and eventual attrition from the program, modified CIMT regimens with shorter periods of cast wear have been used. These adapted regimens have shown similar improvements in upper extremity function.[10,12]

BMT uses the symmetric movement of both hands to facilitate movement of the affected hand. BMT activates both cerebral cortices, and activation of the unaffected cortex may enable the activation of the injured cortex.[13,14] Compared with CIMT, BMT better simulates ADLs that are typically performed using both hands.[14,15] CIMT, however, may be more effective in reducing upper limb impairment.[15]

Variability in intensity, frequency, and approaches of therapy regimens complicates research of therapeutic interventions.[16] The development and use of appropriate outcomes measures to assess upper limb function after therapeutic intervention complement recent research advances. In children, the quality of unimanual movement can be measured using the Melbourne Assessment of Unilateral Upper Limb function and the Quality of Upper Extremity Skills Test, whereas the Assisting Hands Assessment focuses on bimanual tasks.[15,17] Speed of upper extremity tasks can be evaluated using the Jebsen-Taylor test in both children with CP and adults with stroke.[17,18] Additional outcome measures used in adults with stroke include the Nine-Hole Peg Test, the Motor Assessment Scale, the Chedoke-McMaster Stroke Assessment, the Fugl-Meyer Assessment, and the Action Research Arm Test.[18,19] The Test of Selective Arm Control is a quick clinical tool that evaluates upper extremity selective motor control.[20] Measuring sensory impairments of the hand is difficult but can be evaluated

using 2-point discrimination testing and stereognosis.[21,22] Upper-extremity surgeons use the Shriners Hospital Upper Extremity Evaluation to characterize ULS using precise video analysis to aid surgical decision making.[23]

Animal studies show that significant reorganization of the motor cortex occurs in primates undergoing motor task-specific retraining after a focal infarct.[24,25] This reorganization is not seen in animals with spontaneous recovery after an infarct.[26] Learning specific motor tasks is a crucial part of the rehabilitation process that may influence CNS plasticity and postinfarct cortical reorganization.[24–26] Motor learning involves focused attention and repetition of a desired task, and therapies involving repetitive movements of the upper extremity can improve outcomes in ULS caused by stroke.[24]

E-Stim of the muscles affected by ULS may strengthen muscles, reduce spasticity, and improve ROM. A small study of adults with hemiparetic stroke showed that E-Stim via implantable Radio Frequency Microstimulator applied near motor points in the upper extremity was associated with improvement in upper extremity motor function compared with a control group.[27] E-stim may also improve shoulder subluxation after stroke.[28,29] The impact of E-stim on ADL performance, however, is less clear.[27] In children with CP, treatment with E-stim may temporarily improve upper limb function; however, these improvements diminish with cessation of the therapy.[30] In order to improve attention and motivation in both children and adults, these evidence-based therapies can be integrated into a rehabilitation program that can be used in the home environment or into play activities.

PHARMACOLOGIC MANAGEMENT

- Oral medications used to manage global spasticity include baclofen, diazepam, dantrolene, and tizanidine.
- Chemodenervation agents, such as botulinum toxin (BoNT) and phenol, can be used for focal management of ULS.

Selection of an appropriate pharmacologic treatment depends on the distribution and severity of spasticity. Painful or severe spasticity, defined as a Modified Ashworth Scale Score greater than 2, may warrant treatment with antispasmodic medications. Oral medications are appropriate for global spasticity affecting multiple limbs, whereas focal spasticity is best managed with a chemodenervation agent that targets the affected muscle group. Tone-reducing medications are used in tandem with other treatments, such as splinting or therapy regimens.

Oral antispasticity medications are typically used as first-line agents because of their ease of administration and effect on pain. Baclofen is a commonly used medication in children and adults with spasticity and functions by inhibiting release of excitatory neurotransmitters and substance P via γ-aminobutyric acid-B (GABA-B) receptor activation at the spinal cord.[31–33] Despite common use, little evidence exists to support the efficacy of baclofen.[32,34,35] The main side effects of baclofen include drowsiness and cognitive impairment; drowsiness can be minimized by a slow uptitration of the dose.[32,34]

Benzodiazepines, such as diazepam, act on GABA-A receptors at the spinal and supraspinal levels.[33,34] Sedation is the most common side effect with diazepam, and the medication is often dosed at night to facilitate sleep. Other side effects include problems with cognition and behavior, urinary retention, ataxia, and constipation.[36] Diazepam has a similar efficacy profile to baclofen.[34] Both baclofen and diazepam are associated with withdrawal syndromes, and care must be taken to taper off of these medications slowly, because withdrawal can cause seizure and agitation.[32,36]

Dantrolene blocks the release of calcium from the sarcoplasmic reticulum and has fewer CNS side effects.[36,37] Dantrolene improves function and reduces spasm and athetoid movements in children with athetoid CP.[36] In adults, dantrolene is less effective in reducing resistance to stretch, has not been shown to improve function, and is associated with muscle weakness.[37] Furthermore, liver function should be monitored during treatment with dantrolene, because liver injury is a rare adverse effect.[36] The potential for hepatotoxicity may limit its use in children.

Tizanidine, an alpha-2 adrenergic agonist, is used in adult spasticity management.[33–35,37] The medication reduces tone by hyperpolarization of motor neurons, and it may have an antinociceptive effect by regulating substance P release from the spinal cord.[36] Side effects include nausea and vomiting, and liver function should be monitored because of potential hepatotoxicity.[36,37] In adults, tizanidine is one of the only medications to show improvement in spasticity; however, there is little evidence that it improves function.[34] Tizanidine has not been studied in children with CP.[36] Individuals with ULS may be sensitive to oral antispasmodics, so it is essential to start at a low dose and increase the medication slowly. Medically reducing spasticity may uncover weakness of the target muscle groups as well as in other muscle groups.[34]

If focal ULS limits function, chemodenervation of affected nerves or muscles is an appropriate treatment. Alcohol or phenol nerve blocks have been used in spasticity management for many years. Phenol injection initially produces an anesthetic nerve block, followed by demyelination and axonal degeneration of the target nerve via protein denaturation, resulting in atrophy of the involved muscles.[38–40] Paresthesias after phenol injection are uncommon, particularly in nerves with a greater percentage of motor rather than sensory fascicles.[40,41] Nerve localization and injection require sedation in children and can be technically difficult. However, the medication is inexpensive and has an immediate onset, and its effects can last for 6 to 9 months. Alcohol injections for the musculocutaneous nerve have shown improvement in elbow ROM in adults with elbow flexor spasticity.[41–43]

BoNT, produced by *Clostridium botulinum*, is more commonly used for focal spasticity management. BoNT reduces acetylcholine release from cholinergic neurons at the neuromuscular junction, resulting in impaired impulse transmission to the target muscle.[44] BoNT may be used in conjunction with phenol injections. The reduction in spasticity from BoNT typically lasts for up to 12 weeks in children and adults, but the course can be variable.[39,45] The peak effect of the injections occurs between 2 and 6 weeks.[39,46] The most common effects include transient muscle weakness from local diffusion of the toxin and pain at the injection site.[44,47] There have been case reports of systemic effects of BoNT, including respiratory compromise and dysphagia, in children with CP and preexisting bulbar dysfunction.[48] Larger clinical trials have found these adverse events to be rare in both children and adults.[48,49] Concomitant oral medications should be considered for painful ULS because BoNT has a delayed onset of action.

BoNT to the upper limb has been shown to reduce spasticity and improve function in systematic reviews of adults with stroke.[44,50–52] In children, BoNT injections for ULS improve spasticity and hand function, but reports of improvement in overall function have been mixed.[47,53] Functional improvement in the upper extremity is an appropriate therapeutic goal for BoNT injections in children with mild to moderate upper extremity hypertonia, some active upper extremity movement, adequate grip strength, social support, and for those who can tolerate intensive therapy after injections. For children with moderate to severe spasticity and muscle contractures, the goals of injection focus on symptom relief rather than functional improvement.[45] Oral medications and chemodenervation procedures can be used in combination if both global and focal spasticity inhibit function or cause pain.

REFERRAL FOR SURGICAL INTERVENTION

BoNT and phenol injections provide temporary results. Conversely, surgery to address ULS may provide a durable improvement in posture and function. The primary goals of surgical intervention are to improve function and the ability to perform self-care. A secondary, although important, goal is an improvement in the appearance of the arm and hand. Open discussion of functional goals with collaborating upper extremity surgeons ensures the best outcomes. Surgical management is considered when nonoperative modalities do not improve function, when upper extremity contractures limit function, or when the patient requires repeated injections over time. The patient and family should have an appropriate understanding of the goals of surgery. Although it is ideal for the patient to possess the cognitive capacity to comply with postoperative restrictions and therapy regimens, many patients and their caregivers benefit from postural improvements that result from a well-planned surgery in a cognitively impaired patient. It is important to reiterate that referral for surgical management is not a failure of medical management, but an adjunct in ULS management.

ORTHOTICS

- Orthotics can decrease deformity and improve function.
- Serial casting increases joint ROM through slow, progressive stretching.

Orthotics are used to decrease the risk of deformity and to improve function. They can maintain ROM gained after stretching exercises and other nonoperative interventions. ULS and muscle weakness contribute to the dysfunctional posture of the upper extremity; these deformities cause discomfort, impede function, pose problems for hygiene, and place stress on the affected joints. Orthotic options include casts of fiberglass or plaster and splints made of molded plastic, soft neoprene, or Lycra. Orthotics may be used to place the affected extremity in a desired position to prevent development of contractures and are thought to reduce spasticity by reducing excitatory input on muscle spindles.[54,55]

Serial casting provides a stepwise opposing force against joint deformity. In the upper limb, most of the published literature focuses on the elbow. However, casting of the wrist and metacarpophalangeal joints has been described.[54] Once serial casting is complete, additional therapies and less restrictive orthotics are used to preserve any newly acquired ROM. Case reports and case series in children with CP suggest improvement in passive ROM and spasticity after serial casting, and similar effects have been seen in adults with stroke.[54,56] Prefabricated dynamic splints, including Ultraflex (Ultraflex Systems, Inc, Pottstown, PA, USA) and Dynasplint (Dynasplint Systems, Inc, Severna Park, MD, USA), are available with adjustable joints that provide a continuous active stretch to promote tissue lengthening.[57,58] Inhibitory casts and orthotics are typically used to encourage shoulder abduction, elbow extension, or forearm supination. Less restrictive options include dropout casts, which encourage movement in the desired direction and limit movement in the direction of potential contracture, and bivalve casts, that allow for removal of parts to allow access for hygiene.[56]

Some orthoses enable the patient to perform specific functional tasks or strengthening exercises.[59] Patients with C4-C5 tetraplegia due to spinal cord injury have successfully used mobile arm supports to facilitate tasks such as feeding and power wheelchair mobility.[60] A dynamic wrist orthosis, known as the Saeboflex (Saebo, Inc, Charlotte, NC, USA), enables patients to actively flex their fingers and wrist, and a spring mechanism enables extension. The Saeboflex has allowed for increased repetition of grasp and release exercises compared with conventional therapy alone.[61] Splints made from softer materials, such as Lycra or neoprene, may also be used to facilitate muscle strength and proprioceptive feedback.[62] Case series reporting use of Second Skin Lycra upper limb splints showed variable results in children with CP and acquired brain injury.[63] In adults with stroke, the Second Skin Lycra splints showed improvement in wrist and finger flexor spasticity and reduced edema.[64] Neoprene thumb opponens splints, or McKie splints (McKie Splints, LLC, Duluth, MN, USA) and wrist-hand orthoses improve upper extremity function.[65,66] Therapists may also incorporate kinesiotaping as a means to provide sensory feedback. Improvements in self-care and dexterity are reported in studies comparing kinesiotape to matched controls.[67]

NEW REHABILITATION TECHNOLOGIES

- Robotic therapy (RT) favors increased task repetition.
- Virtual reality (VR) augments motor experiences with sensory feedback.
- Transcranial magnetic stimulation (TMS) may impact cortical reorganization that occurs after an injury.
- Brain-Computer Interface (BCI) systems can be paired with other emerging technologies to enhance sensory feedback to the recovering cortex.

Innovative technology can optimize efforts at early mobilization, task-specific and ADL training, and outcome assessments. RT enables task-specific practice, whereas VR provides engaging sensory information to the cerebral cortex to facilitate recovery.[68,69] The MIT-Manus (Interactive Motion Technologies, Cambridge, MA, USA) was the first robot that facilitated supported movement of the shoulder and elbow and could record data on position, velocity, and forces applied to the arm.[70,71] More complex upper extremity robotics with increased degrees of freedom allows for the manipulation of multiple joints, including the hand and wrist.[72]

RT has the potential to increase repetition of motor tasks compared with conventional therapies, which rarely support more than 40 repetitions per task.[73] RT also uses a consistent and engaging format to provide additional sensory feedback during therapies.[74] Outcomes of robot-based therapies correlate with established upper extremity functional outcomes measures in stroke patients and are measured in real time.[75] RT is more expensive than more conventional therapies. However, it has the potential to reduce long-term costs by enabling more therapy with less supervision.[76,77] Portable robotic devices also can enhance home exercise programs and provide high-quality therapies to patients in remote areas. Nonetheless, there is limited research comparing RT to conventional therapies.[77]

Current studies comparing RT to conventional therapies are limited by the variability of types of robots and therapy regimens used in the research. Upper extremity robotics is more complicated than those in the lower extremity because of the complexity of arm placement and hand positions.[78] Therefore, it is not surprising that the studies comparing RT to conventional therapies of comparable intensity show mixed results.[79,80] VR uses computer interfaces with interactive simulated games and activities. Children show improvements in upper extremity motor function when using VR.[81] More research needs to be done in adults with stroke to compare VR therapy to conventional therapies.[69,82] Nonetheless, an interactive gaming interface has the potential to encourage participation in rehabilitation[77] (**Fig. 3**).

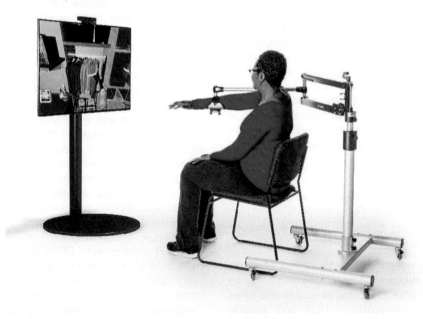

Fig. 3. SaeboVR VR program for ULS. (*Courtesy of* Saebo, Inc, Charlotte, NC.)

Noninvasive cortical stimulation techniques, including TMS, have also been studied in ULS, particularly in adults with stroke. TMS is thought to impact the significant cortical reorganization that occurs after neurologic injury, which can impact neurologic recovery.[83,84] TMS may improve finger and hand function, dexterity, and spasticity. However, current studies are limited by methodological flaws, including the concurrent administration of other therapies, such as CIMT. There is also variability in TMS techniques, locations, and dosing used in these studies.[84–89] In both children and adults, TMS may have an additive benefit when combined with other therapies.[84,90]

BCI systems detect activity in specific regions of the brain using electroencephalography or functional MRI. BCI can provide sensory feedback using other modalities, including E-stim or robotic locomotion, which is thought to promote neuroplasticity by reinforcing synaptic connections. A few small studies have shown improvement in upper limb function in stroke patients after therapy with BCI. However, study limitations are similar to those found in the TMS literature.[91] New technologies in rehabilitation have the potential to improve outcomes for patients with ULS, but improvements in portability, usability, and cost are needed for widespread adoption of these innovations.[77]

SUMMARY

A multidisciplinary team approach to ULS management is necessary to optimize function and prevent deformity. Medications and chemodenervation can improve baseline control of muscle tone, enabling therapists to maximize muscle strengthening, maintain joint integrity, and increase task-specific training. The explosion of new technology presents many options for creative task-specific learning for patients with ULS.

REFERENCES

1. World Health Organization. International classification of functioning, disability and health: ICF. Geneva (Switzerland): World Health Organization; 2001.
2. Sukal-Moulton T, Krosschell KJ, Gaebler-Spira DJ, et al. Motor impairments related to brain injury timing in early hemiparesis. Part II. Neurorehabil Neural Repair 2014;28(1):24–35.
3. Sukal-Moulton T, Krosschell KJ, Gaebler-Spira DJ, et al. Motor impairment factors related to brain injury timing in early hemiparesis Part I: expression of upper extremity weakness. Neurorehabil Neural Repair 2014;28(1):13–23.
4. Sheean G, McGuire JR. Spastic hypertonia and movement disorders: pathophysiology, clinical presentation, and quantification. PM R 2009;1(9): 827–33.
5. Sanger TD, Delgado MR, Gaebler-Spira D, et al. Classification and definition of disorders causing hypertonia in childhood. Pediatrics 2003;111(1). e89–97.
6. Graham HK, Selber P. Musculoskeletal aspects of cerebral palsy. Bone Joint J 2003;85(2):157–66.
7. Peurala SH, Kantanen MP, Sjogren T, et al. Effectiveness of constraint-induced movement therapy on activity and participation after stroke: a systematic review and meta-analysis of randomized controlled trials. Clin Rehabil 2012;26(3):209–23.
8. Shi YX, Tian JH, Yang KH, et al. Modified constraint-induced movement therapy versus traditional rehabilitation in patients with upper-extremity dysfunction after stroke: a systematic review and meta-analysis. Arch Phys Med Rehabil 2011;92(6):972–82.
9. Stevenson T, Thalman L, Christie H, et al. Constraint-induced movement therapy compared to dose-matched interventions for upper-limb dysfunction in adult survivors of stroke: a systematic review with meta-analysis. Physiother Can 2012;64(4):397–413.
10. Hoare BJ, Wasiak J, Imms C, et al. Constraint-induced movement therapy in the treatment of the upper limb in children with hemiplegic cerebral palsy. Cochrane Database Syst Rev 2007;(2):CD004149.
11. Huang HH, Fetters L, Hale J, et al. Bound for success: a systematic review of constraint-induced movement therapy in children with cerebral palsy supports improved arm and hand use. Phys Ther 2009;89(11):1126–41.
12. Page SJ, Boe S, Levine P. What are the "ingredients" of modified constraint-induced therapy? An evidence-based review, recipe, and recommendations. Restor Neurol Neurosci 2013;31(3):299–309.
13. Stewart KC, Cauraugh JH, Summers JJ. Bilateral movement training and stroke rehabilitation: a systematic review and meta-analysis. J Neurol Sci 2006;244(1–2):89–95.
14. Stoykov ME, Corcos DM. A review of bilateral training for upper extremity hemiparesis. Occup Ther Int 2009;16(3–4):190–203.
15. Dong VA, Tung IH, Siu HW, et al. Studies comparing the efficacy of constraint-induced movement therapy and bimanual training in children with unilateral cerebral palsy: a systematic review. Dev Neurorehabil 2013;16(2):133–43.
16. Van Peppen RP, Kwakkel G, Wood-Dauphinee S, et al. The impact of physical therapy on functional outcomes after stroke: what's the evidence? Clin Rehabil 2004;18(8):833–62.
17. Klingels K, Jaspers E, Van de Winckel A, et al. A systematic review of arm activity measures for children with hemiplegic cerebral palsy. Clin Rehabil 2010;24(10):887–900.
18. Velstra IM, Ballert CS, Cieza A. A systematic literature review of outcome measures for upper extremity

function using the international classification of functioning, disability, and health as reference. PM R 2011;3(9):846–60.

19. Croarkin E, Danoff J, Barnes C. Evidence-based rating of upper-extremity motor function tests used for people following a stroke. Phys Ther 2004;84(1): 62–74.

20. Sukal-Moulton T, Gaebler-Spira D, Krosschell KJ. The validity and reliability of the Test of Arm Selective Control for children with cerebral palsy: a prospective cross-sectional study. Dev Med Child Neurol 2018;60(4):374–81.

21. Auld ML, Ware RS, Boyd RN, et al. Reproducibility of tactile assessments for children with unilateral cerebral palsy. Phys Occup Ther Pediatr 2012;32(2):151–66.

22. Krumlinde-Sundholm L, Eliasson AC. Comparing tests of tactile sensibility: aspects relevant to testing children with spastic hemiplegia. Dev Med Child Neurol 2002;44(9):604–12.

23. Tedesco AP, Nicolini-Panisson RDA, de Jesus A. SHUEE on the evaluation of upper limb in cerebral palsy. Acta Ortop Bras 2015;23(4):219–22.

24. Daly JJ, Ruff RL. Construction of efficacious gait and upper limb functional interventions based on brain plasticity evidence and model-based measures for stroke patients. ScientificWorldJournal 2007;7: 2031–45.

25. Dimyan MA, Cohen LG. Neuroplasticity in the context of motor rehabilitation after stroke. Nat Rev Neurol 2011;7(2):76–85.

26. Nudo RJ, Wise BM, SiFuentes F, et al. Neural substrates for the effects of rehabilitative training on motor recovery after ischemic infarct. Science 1996; 272:1791–4.

27. Mann GE, Burridge JH, Malone LJ, et al. A pilot study to investigate the effects of electrical stimulation on recovery of hand function and sensation in subacute stroke patients. Neuromodulation 2005; 8(3):193–202.

28. Vafadar AK, Cote JN, Archambault PS. Effectiveness of functional electrical stimulation in improving clinical outcomes in the upper arm following stroke: a systematic review and meta-analysis. Biomed Research International 2015;2015:729768.

29. Barreca S, Wolf SL, Fasoli S, et al. Treatment interventions for the paretic upper limb of stroke survivors: a critical review. Neurorehabil Neural Repair 2003;17(4):220–6.

30. Ozer K, Chesher SP, Scheker LR. Neuromuscular electrical stimulation and dynamic bracing for the management of upper-extremity spasticity in children with cerebral palsy. Dev Med Child Neurol 2006;48(7):559–63.

31. Sommerfeld DK, Gripenstedt U, Welmer A-K. Spasticity after stroke: an overview of prevalence, test instruments, and treatments. Am J Phys Med Rehabil 2012;91(9):814–20.

32. Navarrete-Opazo AA, Gonzalez W, Nahuelhual P. Effectiveness of oral baclofen in the treatment of spasticity in children and adolescents with cerebral palsy. Arch Phys Med Rehabil 2016;97(4):604–18.

33. Bakheit AM. The pharmacological management of post-stroke muscle spasticity. Drugs Aging 2012; 29(12):941–7.

34. Nair K, Marsden J. The management of spasticity in adults. BMJ 2014;349:g4737.

35. Montane E, Vallano A, Laporte J. Oral antispastic drugs in nonprogressive neurologic diseases A systematic review. Neurology 2004;63(8):1357–63.

36. Verrotti A, Greco R, Spalice A, et al. Pharmacotherapy of spasticity in children with cerebral palsy. Pediatr Neurol 2006;34(1):1–6.

37. Marciniak C. Poststroke hypertonicity: upper limb assessment and treatment. Top stroke Rehabil 2011;18:179–94.

38. Kolaski K, Ajizian SJ, Passmore L, et al. Safety profile of multilevel chemical denervation procedures using phenol or botulinum toxin or both in a pediatric population. Am J Phys Med Rehabil 2008;87(7):556–66.

39. van Kuijk AA, Geurts AC, Bevaart BJ, et al. Treatment of upper extremity spasticity in stroke patients by focal neuronal or neuromuscular blockade: a systematic review of the literature. J Rehabil Med 2002; 34(2):51–61.

40. Wood KM. The use of phenol as a neurolytic agent: a review. Pain 1978;5(3):205–29.

41. Kong KH, Chua KS. Neurolysis of the musculocutaneous nerve with alcohol to treat poststroke elbow flexor spasticity. Arch Phys Med Rehabil 1999; 80(10):1234–6.

42. Keenan MA, Tomas ES, Stone L, et al. Percutaneous phenol block of the musculocutaneous nerve to control elbow flexor spasticity. J Hand Surg 1990;15(2): 340–6.

43. McCrea PH, Eng JJ, Willms R. Phenol reduces hypertonia and enhances strength: a longitudinal case study. Neurorehabil Neural Repair 2004;18(2):112.

44. Shaw L, Rodgers H, Price C, et al. BoTULS: a multicentre randomised controlled trial to evaluate the clinical effectiveness and cost-effectiveness of treating upper limb spasticity due to stroke with botulinum toxin type A. Health Technol Assess 2010; 14(26):1–113, iii–iv.

45. Fehlings D, Novak I, Berweck S, et al. Botulinum toxin assessment, intervention and follow-up for paediatric upper limb hypertonicity: international consensus statement. Eur J Neurol 2010;17(Suppl 2):38–56.

46. Lee HM, Chen JJ, Wu YN, et al. Time course analysis of the effects of botulinum toxin type a on elbow spasticity based on biomechanic and electromyographic parameters. Arch Phys Med Rehabil 2008; 89(4):692–9.

47. Lukban MB, Rosales RL, Dressler D. Effectiveness of botulinum toxin A for upper and lower limb

spasticity in children with cerebral palsy: a summary of evidence. J Neural Transm (Vienna) 2009;116(3): 319–31.

48. Hoare BJ, Wallen MA, Imms C, et al. Botulinum toxin A as an adjunct to treatment in the management of the upper limb in children with spastic cerebral palsy (UPDATE). Cochrane Database Syst Rev 2010;(1):CD003469.

49. Olvey EL, Armstrong EP, Grizzle AJ. Contemporary pharmacologic treatments for spasticity of the upper limb after stroke: a systematic review. Clin Ther 2010;32(14):2282–303.

50. Foley N, Pereira S, Salter K, et al. Treatment with botulinum toxin improves upper-extremity function post stroke: a systematic review and meta-analysis. Arch Phys Med Rehabil 2013;94(5):977–89.

51. Dashtipour K, Chen JJ, Walker HW, et al. Systematic literature review of abobotulinumtoxinA in clinical trials for adult upper limb spasticity. Am J Phys Med Rehabil 2015;94(3):229–38.

52. Baker JA, Pereira G. The efficacy of Botulinum Toxin A on improving ease of care in the upper and lower limbs: a systematic review and meta-analysis using the Grades of Recommendation, Assessment, Development and Evaluation approach. Clin Rehabil 2015;29(8):731–40.

53. Reeuwijk A, van Schie PE, Becher JG, et al. Effects of botulinum toxin type A on upper limb function in children with cerebral palsy: a systematic review. Clin Rehabil 2006;20(5):375–87.

54. Lannin NA, Novak I, Cusick A. A systematic review of upper extremity casting for children and adults with central nervous system motor disorders. Clin Rehabil 2007;21(11):963–76.

55. Tyson SF, Kent RM. The effect of upper limb orthotics after stroke: a systematic review. NeuroRehabilitation 2011;28(1):29–36.

56. Flinn SR, Craven K. Upper limb casting in stroke rehabilitation: rationale, options, and techniques. Top stroke Rehabil 2014;21(4):296–302.

57. Yasukawa A, Lulinski J, Thornton L, et al. Improving elbow and wrist range of motion using a dynamic and static combination orthosis. J Prosthet Orthot 2008;20(2):41.

58. Lai JM, Francisco GE, Willis FB. Dynamic splinting after treatment with botulinum toxin type-A: a randomized controlled pilot study. Adv Ther 2009; 26(2):241–8.

59. Jackman M, Novak I, Lannin N. Effectiveness of hand splints in children with cerebral palsy: a systematic review with meta-analysis. Dev Med Child Neurol 2014;56(2):138–47.

60. Atkins MS, Baumgarten JM, Yasuda YL, et al. Mobile arm supports: evidence-based benefits and criteria for use. J Spinal Cord Med 2008;31(4):388–93.

61. Barry JG, Ross SA, Woehrle J. Therapy incorporating a dynamic wrist-hand orthosis versus manual assistance in chronic stroke: a pilot study. J Neurol Phys Ther 2012;36(1):17–24.

62. Samson-Fang L, Darrah J, McLaughlin J, et al. A systematic review of the effects of soft splinting on upper limb function in people with cerebral palsy An AACPDM Evidence Report Initial Publication In Database. 2006. Available at: https://www.aacpdm.org/education/systematic-reviews.

63. Corn K, Imms C, Timewell G, et al. Impact of second skin lycra splinting on the quality of upper limb movement in children. Br J Occup Ther 2003;66(10):464.

64. Gracies J-M, Marosszeky JE, Renton R, et al. Short-term effects of dynamic Lycra splints on upper limb in hemiplegic patients. Arch Phys Med Rehabil 2000;81(12):1547–55.

65. Ten Berge SR, Boonstra AM, Dijkstra PU, et al. A systematic evaluation of the effect of thumb opponens splints on hand function in children with unilateral spastic cerebral palsy. Clin Rehabil 2011;26(4):362–71.

66. Louwers A, Meester-Delver A, Folmer K, et al. Immediate effect of a wrist and thumb brace on bimanual activities in children with hemiplegic cerebral palsy. Dev Med Child Neurol 2011;53(4):321.

67. Kaya Kara O, Atasavun Uysal S, Turker D, et al. The effects of Kinesio Taping on body functions and activity in unilateral spastic cerebral palsy: a single-blind randomized controlled trial. Dev Med Child Neurol 2015;57(1):81.

68. Mehrholz J, Pohl M, Platz T, et al. Electromechanical and robot-assisted arm training for improving activities of daily living, arm function, and arm muscle strength after stroke. Cochrane Database Syst Rev 2015;(11):CD006876.

69. Mumford N, Wilson PH. Virtual reality in acquired brain injury upper limb rehabilitation: evidence-based evaluation of clinical research. Brain Inj 2009;23(3):179–91.

70. Riener R, Nef T, Colombo G. Robot-aided neurorehabilitation of the upper extremities. Med Biol Eng Comput 2005;43(1):2–10.

71. Krebs HI, Ferraro M, Buerger SP, et al. Rehabilitation robotics: pilot trial of a spatial extension for MIT-Manus. J Neuroeng Rehabil 2004;1(1):5.

72. Balasubramanian S, Klein J, Burdet E. Robot-assisted rehabilitation of hand function. Curr Opin Neurol 2010;23(6):661–70.

73. Lang CE, MacDonald JR, Gnip C. Counting repetitions: an observational study of outpatient therapy for people with hemiparesis post-stroke. J Neurol Phys Ther 2007;31(1):3–10.

74. Hochstenbach-Waelen A, Seelen HA. Embracing change: practical and theoretical considerations for successful implementation of technology assisting upper limb training in stroke. J Neuroeng Rehabil 2012;9:52.

75. McKenzie A, Dodakian L, See J, et al. Validity of robot-based assessments of upper extremity

function. Arch Phys Med Rehabil 2017;98(10):1969–76.e2.

76. Zhang C, Li-Tsang CW, Au RK. Robotic approaches for the rehabilitation of upper limb recovery after stroke: a systematic review and meta-analysis. Int J Rehabil Res 2017;40(1):19–28.

77. Caramenti M, Bartenbach V, Gasperotti L, et al. Challenges in neurorehabilitation and neural engineering. In: Emerging therapies in neurorehabilitation II. Springer; 2016. p. 1–27.

78. Basteris A, Nijenhuis SM, Stienen AH, et al. Training modalities in robot-mediated upper limb rehabilitation in stroke: a framework for classification based on a systematic review. J Neuroeng Rehabil 2014; 11:111.

79. Mehrholz J, Hadrich A, Platz T, et al. Electromechanical and robot-assisted arm training for improving generic activities of daily living, arm function, and arm muscle strength after stroke. Cochrane Database Syst Rev 2012;(6):CD006876.

80. Norouzi-Gheidari N, Archambault PS, Fung J. Effects of robot-assisted therapy on stroke rehabilitation in upper limbs: systematic review and meta-analysis of the literature. J Rehabil Res Dev 2012; 49(4):479–96.

81. Galvin J, McDonald R, Catroppa C, et al. Does intervention using virtual reality improve upper limb function in children with neurological impairment: a systematic review of the evidence. Brain Inj 2011; 25(5):435–42.

82. Henderson A, Korner-Bitensky N, Levin M. Virtual reality in stroke rehabilitation: a systematic review of its effectiveness for upper limb motor recovery. Top stroke Rehabil 2007;14(2):52–61.

83. Ludemann-Podubecka J, Bosl K, Nowak DA. Repetitive transcranial magnetic stimulation for motor recovery of the upper limb after stroke. Prog Brain Res 2015;218:281–311.

84. Leo A, Naro A, Molonia F, et al. Spasticity management: the current state of transcranial neuromodulation. PM R 2017;9(10):1020–9.

85. Corti M, Patten C, Triggs W. Repetitive transcranial magnetic stimulation of motor cortex after stroke: a focused review. Am J Phys Med Rehabil 2012; 91(3):254–70.

86. Tedesco Triccas L, Burridge JH, Hughes AM, et al. Multiple sessions of transcranial direct current stimulation and upper extremity rehabilitation in stroke: a review and meta-analysis. Clin Neurophysiol 2016; 127(1):946–55.

87. Le Q, Qu Y, Tao Y, et al. Effects of repetitive transcranial magnetic stimulation on hand function recovery and excitability of the motor cortex after stroke: a meta-analysis. Am J Phys Med Rehabil 2014;93(5): 422–30.

88. Butler AJ, Shuster M, O'Hara E, et al. A meta-analysis of the efficacy of anodal transcranial direct current stimulation for upper limb motor recovery in stroke survivors. J Hand Ther 2013;26(2):162–70 [quiz: 171].

89. Chhatbar PY, Ramakrishnan V, Kautz S, et al. Transcranial direct current stimulation post-stroke upper extremity motor recovery studies exhibit a dose-response relationship. Brain Stimul 2016;9(1):16–26.

90. Kirton A, Andersen J, Herrero M, et al. Brain stimulation and constraint for perinatal stroke hemiparesis: the PLASTIC CHAMPS trial. Neurology 2016; 86(18):1659–67.

91. Monge-Pereira E, Ibanez-Pereda J, Alguacil-Diego IM, et al. Use of Electroencephalography Brain Computer Interface systems as a rehabilitative approach for upper limb function after a stroke. A systematic review. PM R 2017;9(9):918–32.

Considerations in the Management of Upper Extremity Spasticity

Michael S. Gart, MD[a], Joshua M. Adkinson, MD[b],*

KEYWORDS

- Spasticity • Surgical management • Management considerations • Cerebral palsy
- Spinal cord injury • Stroke

KEY POINTS

- Spasticity is a movement disorder characterized by a velocity-dependent increase in muscle tone and a hyperexcitable stretch reflex.
- Treatment plans for spasticity depend on several patient and disease-specific considerations.
- Patient characteristics include goals of treatment, age, intellect, resources/support system, and associated neurologic conditions.
- Spasticity characteristics include duration, severity, and pattern of motor involvement.
- The underlying cause of spasticity has implications for its treatment.

INTRODUCTION

Spasticity is as a motor disorder characterized by a velocity-dependent increase in muscle tone with exaggerated tendon jerks, resulting from a hyperexcitable stretch reflex.[1–4] These characteristics limit the functional use of the upper extremity in patients with central nervous system (CNS) disorders or injury. Spasticity is a common, but not inevitable, component of the upper motor neuron (UMN) syndrome: a collection of positive and negative signs that occur following a CNS injury (eg, cerebral hypoxia, trauma, spinal cord injury [SCI]).[1,5] It is characterized by muscle overactivity and hypertonicity, which, if left untreated, lead to muscle and soft tissue contractures.[3,6] Impaired intraspinal processing of primary afferent signals is responsible for the clinical manifestations of spasticity and the UMN syndrome.[7] Spasticity alone can lead to significant disability but may be exacerbated by coexisting features of the UMN syndrome. The clinical picture of the UMN syndrome depends on the characteristics of the injury, such as location, onset, and size. Spasticity is a positive sign, which, along with hyperreflexia, spastic dystonia, and clonus, creates a clinical picture of increased muscle activity. Negative signs include paresis, early hypotonia, loss of dexterity, and fatigability.[8]

For the hand surgeon, the most commonly encountered causes of spasticity include cerebral palsy (CP), SCI, and cerebrovascular accident (or stroke). Spasticity is estimated to affect 17% to 38% of patients following stroke, 34% of patients with traumatic brain injury, and up to 78% of patients with spinal cord injury.[8–17] These patients are at risk for development of soft tissue contractures and painful deformities of the upper limb. The muscle imbalances that develop often lead to characteristic postures, such as the flexed elbow and clenched fist, which hinder functional

Disclosure Statement: The authors have no commercial or financial conflicts of interest regarding the content of this article.
[a] Plastic & Reconstructive Surgery, Hand and Upper Extremity Surgery, OrthoCarolina Hand Center, 1915 Randolph Road, Charlotte, NC 28207, USA; [b] Division of Plastic Surgery, Department of Surgery, Indiana University School of Medicine, 545 Barnhill Drive, Emerson Hall 232, Indianapolis, IN 46202, USA
* Corresponding author.
E-mail address: jadkinso@iu.edu

hand.theclinics.com

use of the upper extremity. The impairments of a patient suffering from the UMN syndrome contribute to their baseline functional limitations in posture, hygiene, mobility, and other activities of daily living.

In this article, the authors discuss the pathophysiology of spasticity as well as general considerations regarding surgical management. Specific considerations for common causes of spasticity, namely, SCI/tetraplegia, CP, stroke, and traumatic brain injury (TBI), are presented.

PATHOPHYSIOLOGY OF SPASTICITY

Patients with spasticity are affected by impaired motor function (paresis), muscle overactivity (hypertonia), and, eventually, soft tissue contractures.[3,6] Immediately following a neurologic injury, paresis (or paralysis) occurs. Paresis is defined by the inability to voluntarily recruit skeletal muscles to generate movement. If the paretic limb is immobilized in a shortened position and not stretched sufficiently, myo-static shortening and muscle fibrosis occur alongside loss of functional muscle units.[1] Furthermore, poor posturing in conjunction with myofibrosis leads to joint contractures and disuse atrophy, further exacerbating the paresis. Over time, these shortened and stiff muscles develop increased tone (hypertonia) and abnormal responses to stretch, including velocity-dependent resistance to stretch. The hypertonia further exacerbates soft tissue contracture, which, in turn, worsens the spasticity.

Spasticity affects muscles of the upper extremity in characteristic patterns,[18] predominantly the flexor and adductor muscles, resulting in the characteristic flexion-pronation deformity of the upper limb. Furthermore, spasticity is typically more pronounced in the distal extremity. In the shoulder, adduction and internal rotation predominate; in the elbow, the biceps, brachialis, and brachioradialis contribute to the flexion deformity.[19] The wrist flexors are the most commonly involved muscles in upper limb spasticity; spasticity of the flexor carpi ulnaris is common and leads to a wrist flexion and ulnar deviation deformity. Hand and finger involvement varies depending on which muscles are predominantly affected but most often appear clenched into a fist. The thumb typically assumes an adducted posture because of increased adductor pollicis activity; but the flexor pollicis longus may also be affected, leading to metacarpophalangeal and interphalangeal joint flexion. As discussed later, the optimal treatment of spasticity depends on several factors and requires a highly individualized approach to patient management.

CONSIDERATIONS IN SPASTICITY MANAGEMENT

There are several guiding principles when considering how and when to manage patients with spasticity. In all patients, therapy to prevent soft tissue contractures and combat spasticity is critical. Therapists can work with patients on strengthening weakened muscles, maintaining proper joint alignment, and preventing soft tissue contractures. Weakening of a spastic muscle alone, without appropriate strengthening or alignment, is of little functional benefit.[20] Patients who fail conservative management or are inadequately managed early in the course of their disease often present to the hand surgeon for assistance. The most important, and occasionally most difficult, decision is whether or not patients are indeed surgical candidates. Patients with spasticity needing surgery require a comprehensive approach to treatment planning. Further, as with most upper extremity surgeries, a well-planned postoperative rehabilitation program will improve outcomes.

Defining Goals of Treatment

Before a discussion of surgical intervention, the priorities and needs of patients and caregivers must be assessed in the context of the patients' baseline function. Often, the underlying cause of spasticity can help guide preoperative discussions and define the goals of treatment. It is essential to clearly outline the treatment goals and surgical plan before intervention. Failure to set reasonable expectations before surgery will result in an unhappy patient and surgeon.

Although spasticity is often considered a hindrance to function, its mere presence is not an indication to operate. Spasticity should only be treated if there is a reasonable expectation of improvement in mobility, self-care, hygiene, or relief from painful contractures. Some patients adapt well to increased motor tone and depend on spastic muscle groups to assist with transfers or other activities. In such patients, a reduction in muscle tone would be detrimental to overall function. Other patients may lack the voluntary motor control necessary to achieve a substantial functional benefit after reconstruction. It is, therefore, essential to observe patients performing tasks of daily living to ensure that function is not lost by a well-intentioned surgery.

Patterns of Motor Involvement

In order to develop a treatment plan, the surgeon must first be able to correctly identify which spastic muscles are adversely affecting motor function.

Patients with UMN syndrome can exhibit cocontractions of agonist and antagonist muscle pairs, which limit muscle movements. Patients may also have synergistic contractions of multiple flexor or extensor muscles with poor individual muscle control. They may also exhibit inappropriate activation of agonists, antagonists, or both. Furthermore, muscle tone may vary at rest compared with active motion. Accurately identifying the muscles causing spasticity can be difficult by physical examination alone, and adjunctive methods are often used. Common methods of assessment in patients with spasticity include physical examination, motion analysis, and electromyography/nerve conduction studies.

Motivation and Resources/Support

Motivation on the part of patients and caregivers is essential. In general, patients must understand the benefits (and risks) of surgery and have sufficient motivation to be an active participant in postoperative rehabilitation. Many of the surgical interventions for spasticity management require extensive postoperative rehabilitation. Patients must have the appropriate support to enable them to attend regular therapy sessions as well as the resources to fund therapy. Patients who are unable to attend therapy or complete a prescribed home therapy regimen will not benefit fully from surgery. An exception to these considerations is for patients/caregivers who are seeking surgery for improvement in posture alone, without a possibility of functional improvement. Regardless, patients will often need a substantial amount of help at home to assist with range-of-motion exercises following surgery and to prevent the development of soft tissue contractures.

Spasticity Characteristics

The clinical presentations of patients with spasticity vary based on cause. Therefore, the decisions regarding whether, when, and how to intervene is different for each patient. Although some patients benefit from early surgical intervention, others can be significantly worsened by slight alterations in their physiology. The distribution of the underlying neurologic deficit has implications for treatment. Global neurologic problems must be treated more proximal or centrally, whereas focal problems can be treated peripherally at the individual muscle or joint level. Botulinum toxin (Botox) injections, for example, will be far more effective in patients who have had a stroke with a very focal deficit than patients with global palsy resulting from severe CP-related hemiplegia. In addition, the location of the neurologic injury may affect the efficacy of various treatment methods.

For example, certain medications, such as oral baclofen, are more effective in treating spinal spasticity than cerebral-origin spasticity.[2]

The duration and severity of spasticity are also important considerations. Patients with acute spasticity following an injury may demonstrate a degree of neurologic recovery over the following 1 to 2 years. Treatment of spasticity in these patients should, therefore, be delayed for at least 1 year or until the neurologic examination has stabilized for several months. During the recovery period, short-term treatments for isolated spasticity, such as Botox injections, may be useful to improve function. Further, patients with acute spasticity tend to have less severe manifestations and are more responsive to nonsurgical treatments, such as stretching, orthotics, and therapy.

Patients with long-standing spasticity tend to suffer more from soft tissue and joint contractures. Severe spasticity is also less likely to respond to conservative management and will more often require surgical intervention. Some patients, however, may have developed functional adaptations; it is imperative not to inadvertently compromise one function in an effort to improve another.

Patient Characteristics

The patients' age, intellect, and other associated neurologic conditions affect treatment decisions. The age of patients—and, hence, the length of time living with disability—must be considered in the treatment plan. Early surgery is typically deferred in the absence of a severe, progressive deformity. In adults with long-standing spasticity, the surgeon must evaluate for adaptive mechanisms that may obviate surgery and ensure that surgical intervention does not reduce function.[18] Ideally, patients must have sufficient intellect and the ability to effectively communicate in order to optimize postsurgical outcomes. Patients with severe cognitive deficits, behavioral problems, or an inability to communicate may be unable to comply or participate with therapy. In general, surgery requiring significant active rehabilitation is not considered with IQ scores less than 70, although this should be considered on a case-by-case basis. However, procedures aimed at improving hygiene, cosmesis, or comfort are indicated regardless of patient intellectual ability.[21]

Other Neurologic Impairments

Other neurologic impairments must also be considered when evaluating patients for treatment. In the absence of discriminatory sensation, visual guidance is mandatory for voluntary limb control; visual acuity must be sufficient to guide positioning. Patients without adequate sensation and visual acuity should not be considered for functional surgery; however, they remain candidates for surgery aimed at improving hygiene and/or comfort. Additionally, many patients with CP, TBI, or SCI will also have lower extremity and mobility impairments, which are often addressed before upper extremity surgery.

Another essential determination is the degree of preoperative voluntary motor control. Patients with poor control may have little functional improvement with surgery, and stronger consideration should be given to techniques that prioritize care and comfort. As a general rule, voluntary motor control is inversely related to the severity of spasticity. In addition to the more common manifestations of upper limb paresis, patients with a CNS injury may have syndromes of excessive limb motion. These symptoms are attributed to disorders of the extrapyramidal system, which plays an important role in initiating and maintaining movement, postural control, and resting muscle tone. Common extrapyramidal symptoms are summarized in **Table 1**. If these symptoms are present, but mild, surgery can be considered to improve hygiene or comfort. For patients with severe disorders of movement, selective arthrodesis may be the only reliable technique, as their underlying movement disorders will overcome soft tissue rebalancing alone.

SPECIFIC CAUSES OF UPPER LIMB SPASTICITY
Cerebral Palsy

CP is a functionally limiting, nonprogressive disorder of movement and posture that occurs as a result of disturbed brain development in the fetus or infant.[22] Approximately 1.5 to 4.0 per 1000 live births are affected, making CP the most common motor disability of childhood.[23] Several causes have been identified, including fetal stroke or anoxia, infection, teratogens, CNS malformations, prematurity, and metabolic diseases. Epidemiologic studies have demonstrated that the predominant cause is metabolic and not neonatal ischemia, as previously thought. The timing of

the CNS insult varies, with 75% occurring in utero, 5% during delivery, and 15% to 20% post partum. CP also occurs with much greater frequency in premature infants.[24]

Specific considerations for patients with cerebral palsy

The presentation of spasticity in CP will vary based on age at onset, severity, location and extent of the brain injury, presence of associated neurologic disorders, and baseline function. Because CP is a nonprogressive disorder, early surgical intervention can be considered; however, elective interventions should be delayed until the child can cooperate with a rehabilitation program. Adults with long-standing spasticity from CP should be approached cautiously, as they may already have established compensatory functions.[18] For elderly patients with poor voluntary motor control, surgery for hygiene and improved posture is often indicated.

The brain injury in CP can be widespread and may be associated with severe cognitive impairment, impaired sensibility, and extrapyramidal symptoms, including athetosis. These impairments will all affect the patients' ability to comply with a therapy program as well as their degree of voluntary motor control. Furthermore, because CP affects newborns, these patients particularly depend on their support system for routine and postoperative care. A robust social support system and, ideally, a school program that has experience working with children with CP are associated with successful outcomes. Children with severe cognitive impairment, poor motor control, or severe spasticity are good candidates for procedures that assist caregivers in hygiene and prevent or eliminate painful contractures.

Spinal Cord Injury

Approximately 12,000 new cases of SCI occur in the United States each year, a number that does not account for the approximately 20% who die before reaching a hospital. Young adult males are the most commonly affected demographic,

---

Table 1
Common extrapyramidal symptoms

Chorea	Athetosis	Dystonia
• Rapid, nonpurposeful, involuntary movements of variable amplitude • Affects the limbs and/or axial musculature as well as the head and neck	• Slow, involuntary oscillation of the limbs and trunk • Varies with emotional state and wakefulness • May have associated choreiform movements (choreoathetosis)	• Torsion spasms of the limbs, trunk, and neck • May be static or progressive

with trauma representing the most common mechanism for injury.[25–27] The terms *tetraplegia*, *quadriplegia*, and *paraplegia* are often used incorrectly when describing patients with SCI. Tetraplegia (or quadriplegia) refers to an injury in one of the 8 cervical segments of the spinal cord, which, by definition, will result in a neurologic deficit in the upper and lower extremities; paraplegia refers to an injury in the thoracic or lumbar spine with preserved upper extremity function. Here, the authors focus their discussion on patients with tetraplegia and considerations in the management of related upper extremity manifestations.

The level of injury within the spinal cord is referred to as the injured metamere and can vary in size depending on the mechanism of injury. Above the injured metamere, neurologic function is intact and muscles innervated by this spinal level have normal strength. Below the injured metamere, neurologic function may be stimulated in the absence of lower motor neuron injury[28] and muscles may demonstrate flaccid paralysis or characteristics of spasticity. At the level of the injury, neurologic function is absent, although partial recovery is possible, typically within one to 2 years after injury.[29,30]

Specific considerations for patients with spinal cord injuries

Upper extremity function is critical for patients with tetraplegia to assist in mobility/transfers, eating, hygiene, and self-catheterization. Not surprisingly, most tetraplegic patients equate improved upper extremity function with a significant improvement in quality of life.[31] The goal of spasticity surgery in tetraplegic patients is to promote independent function. Therefore, the patients must have limitations that can be reasonably expected to improve with surgery, and a discussion of realistic expectations must take place before surgery. Ideal patients will have a strong support system and be motivated to improve their function through surgery and an intensive postoperative rehabilitation program. Unrealistic expectations and/or poor support systems should be considered relative contraindications to surgery. However, as most SCI occur in young patients, appropriate functional reconstruction can provide significant, long-term benefits.

All patients with an SCI should have physical therapy initiated early and maintained throughout the period of neurologic recovery to prevent or treat any soft tissue contractures. Uncontrolled spasticity is strongly linked to poor outcomes and should be considered a contraindication to surgery.[32–34] Avoiding spasticity and soft tissue contractures maintains options for patients who have incomplete recovery after SCI.

Traditional teaching states that surgical reconstruction is deferred for at least 18 months following injury because of the potential for recovery and is only considered in patients with stable neurologic examinations. In complete SCI, some advocate for earlier intervention in patients with a stable examination for at least 3 months, as the prognosis for further recovery is poor.[35,36] The theoretic advantage of this early approach is an easier and more rapid reintegration into society and return to independent functioning. There is still consensus that reconstruction be deferred in incomplete injuries, which demonstrate highly variable patterns of recovery; any signs of ongoing recovery should delay surgery until the motor examination has stabilized for several months.

Additionally, patients with tetraplegia often have significant medical comorbidities, including autonomic dysreflexia or hypotension, recurrent urinary tract infections, and pressure ulcers. Patients should be medically optimized before elective upper extremity reconstruction. SCI is also strongly associated with posttraumatic stress disorder and depression.[37,38] Before surgery, patients should be evaluated by a psychiatrist and deemed mentally fit to undergo both surgery and the rigorous postoperative rehabilitation that is requisite for a good result.

Stroke

Strokes are a major cause of morbidity and mortality worldwide. Globally, stroke ranks as the second-leading cause of death behind ischemic heart disease; nearly 800,000 new strokes are reported annually in the United States.[39] Spasticity is estimated to affect up to 38% of patients following a stroke.[8,11,15,17] The neurologic deficits present in patients who have had a stroke will depend on the area of the brain affected. Strokes in the vascular territory of the anterior cerebral artery will predominantly affect the lower extremity, whereas strokes of the middle cerebral artery, the most commonly affected territory, will result in the more classic clinical picture of hemiplegia predominantly affecting the upper extremity, facial palsy, and speech difficulties. The motor function in the upper extremity is commonly compromised following a stroke, with up to 76% of patients demonstrating some loss of function in one or both arms.[40] Because the sensory cortex is also affected, patients may have deficits in touch, proprioception, and awareness of the affected limbs, which portend a poor functional prognosis. Furthermore, visual disturbances can occur following stroke and are important to consider, as visual input contributes to upper extremity function, particularly in the presence of sensory impairments.

Specific considerations for patients with stroke

When considering surgical management for post-stroke spasticity, the most critical determination is whether or not patients have a functional extremity that has adequate sensation, proprioception, and volitional motor control. In patients who meet this condition, the specific type of deformity present will dictate the most appropriate treatment strategy. For patients who do not have a functional upper extremity, surgery to improve ease of care can be considered.

The typical pattern of motor recovery following stroke is flaccid paralysis in the acute phase, followed by muscle rigidity for several weeks to months. During the subacute phase, occupational therapy is important to maintain joint mobility and prevent contractures as paresis transitions into spasticity. At approximately 3 months following a stroke, motor recovery progresses in a proximal to distal direction and typically plateaus around 6 months. Once patients have stabilized, a hand surgeon may be consulted to help manage spasticity. Before this time, there is little intervention by the surgeon. As with other forms of spasticity, the patients' baseline function, associated neurologic deficits, age, degree of spasticity, and expectations must be considered before surgery.

SUMMARY

When devising a treatment plan for patients with spasticity, consideration must be given to multiple patient and disease-specific factors. The goals of care must be discussed with patients and caregivers before embarking on any intervention, and a careful assessment of the patients' overall function must be made. Surgical intervention is only indicated when it will reasonably improve function in patients with adequate voluntary motor control or to improve hygiene and self-care in patients with poor motor control. Characteristics of the spasticity, including the duration and severity, will have implications on treatment decisions, as will the patients' age, intellect, and support system. Associated neurologic disorders, specifically disorders of movement, must be carefully evaluated to ensure patients will benefit from surgical management. For all patients, care must be individualized in order to optimize functional outcomes and patient satisfaction.

REFERENCES

1. Balakrishnan S, Ward AB. The diagnosis and management of adults with spasticity. Handb Clin Neurol 2013;110:145–60.
2. Gormley ME Jr, O'Brien CF, Yablon SA. A clinical overview of treatment decisions in the management of spasticity. Muscle Nerve Suppl 1997;6:S14–20.
3. Gracies JM. Pathophysiology of spastic paresis. I: paresis and soft tissue changes. Muscle Nerve 2005;31(5):535–51.
4. Sheean G. The pathophysiology of spasticity. Eur J Neurol 2002;9(Suppl 1):3–9 [discussion: 53–61].
5. Thibaut FA, Chatelle C, Wannez S, et al. Spasticity in disorders of consciousness: a behavioral study. Eur J Phys Rehabil Med 2015;51(4):389–97.
6. Gracies JM. Pathophysiology of spastic paresis. II: emergence of muscle overactivity. Muscle Nerve 2005;31(5):552–71.
7. Pandyan AD, Gregoric M, Barnes MP, et al. Spasticity: clinical perceptions, neurological realities and meaningful measurement. Disabil Rehabil 2005;27(1–2):2–6.
8. Sommerfeld DK, Eek EU, Svensson AK, et al. Spasticity after stroke: its occurrence and association with motor impairments and activity limitations. Stroke 2004;35(1):134–9.
9. Anson CA, Shepherd C. Incidence of secondary complications in spinal cord injury. Int J Rehabil Res 1996;19(1):55–66.
10. Johnson RL, Gerhart KA, McCray J, et al. Secondary conditions following spinal cord injury in a population-based sample. Spinal Cord 1998;36(1):45–50.
11. Lundstrom E, Terent A, Borg J. Prevalence of disabling spasticity 1 year after first-ever stroke. Eur J Neurol 2008;15(6):533–9.
12. Maynard FM, Karunas RS, Waring WP 3rd. Epidemiology of spasticity following traumatic spinal cord injury. Arch Phys Med Rehabil 1990;71(8):566–9.
13. Noreau L, Proulx P, Gagnon L, et al. Secondary impairments after spinal cord injury: a population-based study. Am J Phys Med Rehabil 2000;79(6):526–35.
14. Skold C, Levi R, Seiger A. Spasticity after traumatic spinal cord injury: nature, severity, and location. Arch Phys Med Rehabil 1999;80(12):1548–57.
15. Watkins CL, Leathley MJ, Gregson JM, et al. Prevalence of spasticity post stroke. Clin Rehabil 2002;16(5):515–22.
16. Wedekind C, Lippert-Gruner M. Long-term outcome in severe traumatic brain injury is significantly influenced by brainstem involvement. Brain Inj 2005;19(9):681–4.
17. Welmer AK, von Arbin M, Widén Holmqvist L, et al. Spasticity and its association with functioning and health-related quality of life 18 months after stroke. Cerebrovasc Dis 2006;21(4):247–53.
18. Leclercq C. General assessment of the upper limb. Hand Clin 2003;19(4):557–64.
19. Keenan MA, Haider TT, Stone LR. Dynamic electromyography to assess elbow spasticity. J Hand Surg Am 1990;15(4):607–14.

20. Childers MK, Brashear A, Jozefczyk P, et al. Dose-dependent response to intramuscular botulinum toxin type A for upper-limb spasticity in patients after a stroke. Arch Phys Med Rehabil 2004;85(7):1063–9.

21. Mital MA, Sakellarides HT. Surgery of the upper extremity in the retarded individual with spastic cerebral palsy. Orthop Clin North Am 1981;12(1):127–41.

22. Bax M, Goldstein M, Rosenbaum P, et al. Proposed definition and classification of cerebral palsy, April 2005. Dev Med Child Neurol 2005;47(8):571–6.

23. Winter S, Autry A, Boyle C, et al. Trends in the prevalence of cerebral palsy in a population-based study. Pediatrics 2002;110(6):1220–5.

24. Evans K, Rigby AS, Hamilton P, et al. The relationships between neonatal encephalopathy and cerebral palsy: a cohort study. J Obstet Gynaecol 2001;21(2):114–20.

25. National Spinal Cord Injury Statistical Center. Spinal cord injury facts and figures at a glance. J Spinal Cord Med 2013;36(1):1–2.

26. Bernhard M, Gries A, Kremer P, et al. Spinal cord injury (SCI)–prehospital management. Resuscitation 2005;66(2):127–39.

27. Sekhon LH, Fehlings MG. Epidemiology, demographics, and pathophysiology of acute spinal cord injury. Spine (Phila Pa 1976) 2001;26(24 Suppl):S2–12.

28. Coulet B, Allieu Y, Chammas M. Injured metamere and functional surgery of the tetraplegic upper limb. Hand Clin 2002;18(3):399–412, vi.

29. Ditunno JF Jr, Stover SL, Freed MM, et al. Motor recovery of the upper extremities in traumatic quadriplegia: a multicenter study. Arch Phys Med Rehabil 1992;73(5):431–6.

30. Waters RL, Adkins RH, Yakura JS, et al. Motor and sensory recovery following complete tetraplegia. Arch Phys Med Rehabil 1993;74(3):242–7.

31. Snoek GJ, IJzerman MJ, Hermens HJ, et al. Survey of the needs of patients with spinal cord injury: impact and priority for improvement in hand function in tetraplegics. Spinal Cord 2004; 42(9):526–32.

32. Freehafer AA, Kelly CM, Peckham PH. Tendon transfer for the restoration of upper limb function after a cervical spinal cord injury. J Hand Surg Am 1984; 9(6):887–93.

33. Freehafer AA, Vonhaam E, Allen V. Tendon transfers to improve grasp after injuries of the cervical spinal cord. J Bone Joint Surg Am 1974;56(5): 951–9.

34. Moberg E. Surgical treatment for absent single-hand grip and elbow extension in quadriplegia. Principles and preliminary experience. J Bone Joint Surg Am 1975;57(2):196–206.

35. Kozin SH. Tetraplegia. J Hand Surg Am 2002;2(3): 141–52.

36. Friden J, Gohritz A. Tetraplegia management update. J Hand Surg Am 2015;40(12):2489–500.

37. Cao Y, Li C, Newman S, et al. Posttraumatic stress disorder after spinal cord injury. Rehabil Psychol 2017;62(2):178–85.

38. Schonenberg M, Reimitz M, Jusyte A, et al. Depression, posttraumatic stress, and risk factors following spinal cord injury. Int J Behav Med 2014; 21(1):169–76.

39. Benjamin EJ, Blaha MJ, Chiuve SE, et al. Heart disease and stroke statistics-2017 update: a report from the American Heart Association. Circulation 2017;135(10):e146–603.

40. Rathore SS, Hinn AR, Cooper LS, et al. Characterization of incident stroke signs and symptoms: findings from the atherosclerosis risk in communities study. Stroke 2002;33(11):2718–21.

Surgical Management of Spasticity of the Thumb and Fingers

Jennifer F. Waljee, MD, MPH*, Kevin C. Chung, MD, MS

KEYWORDS

• Spasticity • Surgery • Hand • Cerebral palsy

KEY POINTS

• Hand spasticity prevents prehension and grasp, which are critical for activities of daily living and hand hygiene.
• Surgical management is elective and should be tailored to patient cognitive and physical functioning.
• Assessing active and passive digital flexion and extension should be assessed to identify spasticity and determine the need for additional tendon transfers to augment wrist and digital extensors and flexors.

INTRODUCTION

Spasticity of the hand and upper extremity often occurs secondary to central nervous pathologic condition, including cerebral palsy (CP), stroke, traumatic brain injury (TBI), and spinal cord injury. Spasticity of the hand is particularly debilitating because it prevents prehension and grasp, which are critical for independently performing activities of daily living (ADLs). Furthermore, hand postural deformities resulting from spasticity can result in poor hygiene and hand appearance. In this review, the authors describe surgical options for spastic conditions of the hand, specifically, wrist and digital flexion deformities, thumb-in-palm deformities, and swan-neck deformities caused by intrinsic and extrinsic spasticity.

PATIENT EVALUATION

For many patients, surgical intervention can improve hand function, effective grip and release, hand appearance and posture, hand hygiene, and ultimately, quality of life.[1] Surgical options for spasticity can be undertaken in an elective fashion, underscoring the importance of careful preoperative evaluation to tailor the treatment plan according to the patient's abilities, preferences, and needs. The indications for surgery differ based on cognitive ability, function, and sensation. For patients with cognitive challenges such as little voluntary hand control and poor sensation, hand hygiene is the primary indication for surgery. In contrast, patients with greater cognitive ability, normal sensation, and some degree of voluntary upper extremity control can derive more functional benefit from surgery.

Physical examination is often challenging in the setting of spasticity. It is, nonetheless, important to identify the muscles involved, weakness of antagonist muscles, and degree of joint and muscle contracture. In contrast to contracture, patients with isolated spasticity will have full range of motion with relaxation (eg, with botulinum toxin A injection or selective nerve blockade), and

Disclosure Statement: No disclosures.
Department of Surgery, Section of Plastic Surgery, Michigan Medicine, 2131 Taubman Center, 1500 East Medical Center Drive, Ann Arbor, MI 48109, USA
* Corresponding author.
E-mail address: filip@med.umich.edu

Hand Clin 34 (2018) 473–485
https://doi.org/10.1016/j.hcl.2018.06.005

increased muscle tone can often be overcome with gentle counterpressure/resistance in the opposite direction. Observing patients performing common ADLs can be useful in surgical planning. In addition, surgical decision making may also be impacted by patient and caregiver input regarding activities that are challenging and those that can be accomplished with ease. Recent evidence also supports the role of videotaping clinic evaluations and multiple preoperative assessments to get an accurate assessment of upper extremity function.[2] Finally, sensation should be assessed, including stereognosis, 2-point discrimination, and proprioception.

Selective nerve blocks can be used to sequentially assess spasticity and contracture of muscle groups.[3,4] For example, the ulnar nerve can be blocked either above the elbow (for spasticity of the flexor digitorum profundus [FDP] of the ring and small fingers or the flexor carpi ulnaris [FCU]) or at the wrist (to assess intrinsic muscle spasticity). In addition, the median nerve can be blocked above the elbow to determine the contribution of spasticity of the flexor digitorum superficialis (FDS), flexor carpi radialis (FCR), median-innervated FDP, and palmaris longus (PL). Similarly, muscle groups can be blocked sequentially to assess individual muscles after removing spasticity of the antagonists or co-contractions of adjacent muscles. For example, injection of spastic pronator teres can differentiate spasticity from contracture of the interosseous membrane. In this way, selective nerve blocks can be used to differentiate spasticity from contracture.

Various classification systems exist to describe upper extremity function, and these can be useful for both preoperative planning and postoperative assessment, primarily in the context of CP.[5] Classification systems largely focus on active and passive use of the hand as it relates to the ability to complete ADLs. The classification system described by House categorizes upper extremity function into 9 groups based on active and passive motion, grip, and assistance from the contralateral hand[6] (**Table 1**). The Manual Abilities Classification System is briefer and evaluates hand function across 5 simple categories:

- Handles objects with ease,
- Handles objects but with reduced speed and ability,
- Handles objects with difficulty requiring modification,
- Handles objects only in adapted situations, and
- Does not handle objects.[7]

Table 1
House classification of hand function for patients with cerebral palsy

Class	Description	Activity
0	No use	Patient does not use hand for activities
1	Poor passive assist	Patient uses hand to stabilize
2	Fair passive assist	Patient is able to hold object placed in hand
3	Good passive assist	Can hold object in hand for use by contralateral hand
4	Poor active assist	Weak active grasp and hold
5	Fair active assist	Active grasp and stability
6	Good active assist	Active grasp with stability and manipulation against other hand
7	Partial spontaneous use	Bimanual activities performed and occasional spontaneous use
9	Full spontaneous use	Independent use of hand

From House JH, Gwathmey FW, Fidler MO. A dynamic approach to the thumb-in palm deformity in cerebral palsy. J Bone Joint Surg Am 1981;63(2):222; with permission.

Finally, the Shriners Hospital for Children Upper Extremity Evaluation integrates video assessment to describe spontaneous function, position, and grasp. Overall, measures focused solely on impairment, such as range of motion or stereognosis, are less predictive than measures that focus on activity limitations, and defining ability in the context of ADLs is likely more sensitive when considering surgical planning.[8]

NONOPERATIVE MANAGEMENT

Surgical intervention for spasticity of the hand and upper extremity is elective. It is essential to coordinate surgical planning in a multidisciplinary fashion to integrate physical medicine and rehabilitation, occupational and physical therapy, neurology, and primary care as indicated to ensure readiness for surgery, compliance with postoperative protocols, and smooth transitions of care. Among adult patients with acquired central nervous system injuries (eg, TBI or stroke), definitive surgical procedures are typically delayed until recovery has plateaued, often at 6 months among patients who have suffered a stroke and up to 18 months among patients with a TBI.

Conservative measures to prevent contracture and alleviate spasticity include splinting, occupational therapy, including therapist directed and home-based programs, and serial casting.[9] Pharmacologic options include both peripheral, such as botulinum toxin A, and central, such as baclofen, and are directed toward minimizing muscle spasticity. Centrally directed pharmacologic agents have deleterious side effects, however, and peripherally directed medical treatments have transient effectiveness, which requires repeated intervention.[10] Therefore, when possible, surgical intervention can provide durable improvements in overall quality of life and upper extremity function in appropriately selected patients.[1]

Wrist and Digital Flexion Deformities

Wrist and digital flexion deformities are common among patients with spasticity attributed to central nervous system conditions and impair function by limiting hand grasp and release. Wrist flexion deformities occur due to spasticity of the wrist flexors and often occur in conjunction with poor active wrist extension resulting from weakness of the extensors and/or tightness of the volar wrist capsule (**Fig. 1**). Wrist flexion deformities also weaken grip, by functionally shortening the length and mechanical advantage of the digital flexors, and prevent visualization of the hand and digits. For patients who suffer acquired central nervous system conditions, such as stroke or TBI, clenched-fist deformities can occur as an unmasking of the primitive grasp reflex. As a result, the hand assumes the posture of a clenched fist, resulting in poor hand hygiene, skin injury, and maceration (**Fig. 2**). These deformities may be a combination of spasticity and contracture of the digital flexors, exacerbated by concomitant spasticity and flexion of the wrist.

Evaluation

When considering surgical intervention, it is critical to assess the degree of voluntary hand control for each patient. For patients with voluntary hand control and wrist or digital flexion deformities, fractional myotendinous lengthening is preferred to maintain grip strength, with or without proximal row carpectomy (PRC). For patients with poor upper extremity volition and more severe deformities, the wrist flexors can be released in conjunction with superficialis to profundus (STP) tendon transfer to alleviate spastic flexion. Although these procedures effectively improve hand and wrist position, STP transfer diminishes grip strength and is reserved for patients with poor voluntary function and severe deformities (**Fig. 3**).

Active and passive wrist and digital extension is assessed to tailor surgical planning, identify spasticity, determine the need for additional tendon transfers to augment the motor function of weak wrist and digital extensors, and evaluate the extent

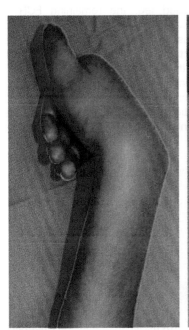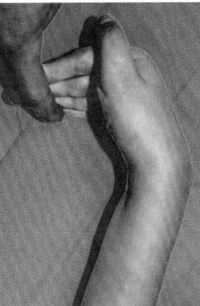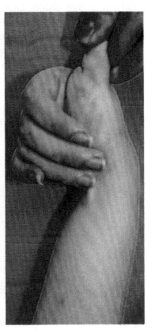

Fig. 1. Wrist and digital flexion deformities.

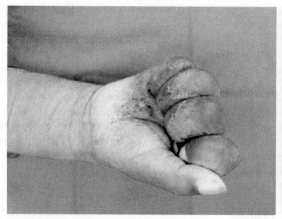
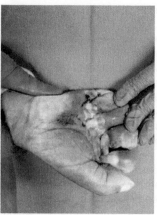

Fig. 2. Clasped hand deformity following stroke.

to which patients rely on tenodesis for hand function. Zancolli[11] has classified spasticity for patients with CP, which can guide treatment planning (**Table 2**). Active digital extension is determined by holding the wrist in neutral and asking the patient to grasp an object. For patients with full passive, but not active, digital extension with the wrist held in neutral, tendon transfers are indicated to augment digital extension (most commonly FCU to extensor digitorum communis [EDC]). Given that full passive motion in this position is possible, lengthening of the digital flexors is not necessary. However, when passive digital extension is limited with the wrist in extension, spasticity of the digital flexors is present and needs to be addressed with lengthening. Simultaneous tendon transfers to augment active digital extension should also be considered. For patients with weak active extension and limited passive wrist flexion, lengthening of the digital flexors in conjunction with tendon transfers can improve active extension.

In addition to digital motion, the wrist should be examined for static contracture. For patients with a full active and passive arc of motion, but spasticity of the wrist flexors with activity, fractional

lengthening of the wrist flexors is indicated. For patients without static contracture and full passive extension of the wrist, but poor active extension, tendon transfers to augment wrist extension can be performed; this allows the spastic force of another tendon to be redirected to wrist extension. In patients with CP, for example, the FCU is transferred to extensor carpi radialis longus (ECRL) in the setting of weak wrist extension. Because the wrist is flexed in ulnar deviation, transferring FCU to ECRL releases this ulnarly directed force and rebalances the wrist via radial pull. Numerous alternative tendon transfers have also been described, including extensor carpi ulnaris (ECU) to ECRB, FCU to ECRL, pronator teres (PT) to ECRB, and brachioradialis (BR) to ECRB if FCU is contraindicated (eg, the remaining FCR is weak) or unavailable (eg, FCU previously used for digit extensors) (**Fig. 4**). The FCU to ECRL transfer predictably corrects flexible wrist flexion deformities in the setting of spasticity due to CP, but late deformities can occur, including hyperextension, supination, and recurrent flexion deformities, particularly with age.[12] The authors advocate setting the tension of transfer such that

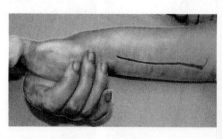
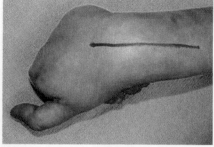

Fig. 3. Surgical incision placement for PRC with STP transfer for digital and wrist flexion deformities in a nonfunctional hand.

Table 2
Zancolli classification of upper extremity spasticity

1	Minimal flexion spasticity	Complete finger extension with the wrist in neutral	Procedures for functional improvement: conservative management or tenotomy of FCU
2		Active extension of fingers with wrist flexed >20°	Procedures for functional improvement: fractional lengthening of flexors, tenotomy of FCU
A	Moderate flexion spasticity	Can actively extend wrist with fingers flexed	Procedures for functional improvement: FCU to ECRB transfer and fractional lengthening of flexors
B		Cannot actively extend wrist due to weakness of extensors	Procedures for hand hygiene and appearance: STP transfer, wrist fusion
3	Severe flexion spasticity	Cannot extend digits with maximal wrist flexion	

Data from Zancolli EA. Surgical management of the hand in infantile spastic hemiplegia. Hand Clin 2003;19(4):609–29.

the wrist is held in slight flexion at 30°, as the digital extensors are often weak. By maintaining slight wrist flexion, tenodesis can be used by the patient to accomplish finger extension. However, placing the wrist at neutral or in extension will predictably limit finger extension. As a result, the patient will not be able to accomplish the release phase of grip, but will instead be limited to the grasp phase only. For patients with fixed contractures, PRC can alleviate tension in the spastic flexors secondary to a relative lengthening that occurs with wrist shortening (**Fig. 5**).

FRACTIONAL LENGTHENING OF THE WRIST AND DIGITAL FLEXORS

Fractional lengthening of the extrinsic digital flexors and wrist flexors can be performed to alleviate spasticity of the extrinsic flexor muscle bellies and is indicated for patients with volitional control of the upper extremity. Fractional lengthening can provide lengthening of up to 15% to 20% of the muscle for patients in whom the fingers cannot be passively extended with the wrist placed in flexion. Keenan and colleagues[13] reported that approximately 2 cm of length can be gained from fractional lengthening, and the musculotendinous junction will generally accommodate 2 incisions for lengthening. Lengthening is performed through a longitudinal incision across the volar forearm. After identifying and protecting the median nerve, the PL is divided distally so it can used for tendon transfer to augment extensor pollicis longus (EPL) tendon extension, if necessary. Fractional lengthening of the FCU and/or FCR is performed by incising the tendinous aspect of the myotendinous junction of the muscle belly, without incising the muscle belly (**Fig. 6**). The wrist and fingers are then passively extended, and care is taken to ensure that the musculotendinous junction is not torn or detached during this maneuver (**Fig. 7**). Similarly, lengthening along the

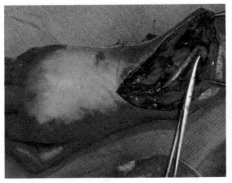 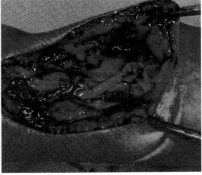

Fig. 4. FCU to ECRL tendon transfer.

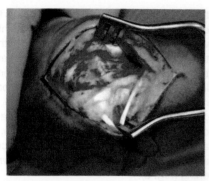
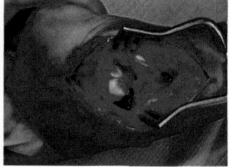

Fig. 5. PRC for wrist flexion deformities in a nonfunctional hand.

musculotendinous junctions of FDS, FDP, and flexor pollicis longus (FPL) can be performed, as needed.

For patients in whom greater release is needed, step-cut lengthening can be performed (**Fig. 8**). A stair-step incision is created in the tendon. The tendon is divided longitudinally and then woven to itself. The tension is set in order release the flexion deformity, but maintains the digital cascade and accommodates 3 tendon weaves in the repair[14] (**Fig. 9**). Following fractional lengthening, the hand is typically immobilized in a resting position with the interphalangeal (IP) joints of the fingers extended for 3 weeks. Overall, this procedure can be applied to both patients with functional and patients with nonfunctional hands with good results, including improved hand position and function, with the advantage of it being a relatively simple procedure compared with the flexor-pronator origin slide procedure, as described in later discussion.[13]

FLEXOR-PRONATOR ORIGIN SLIDE

The flexor-pronator slide procedure is an alternative to fractional lengthening for patients with functionally limiting spastic contracture of the wrist and

digits who have volitional hand control and sensation.[15] The advantages include the ability to alleviate spastic deformities of forearm pronation and lengthening of the wrist and finger flexors. Selective lengthening of the digits is not possible, because the muscle bellies are released as a unit from their origins. The forearm is approached at the medial epicondyle. The muscle belly of FDP is detached from the ulna and interosseous membrane, and the FDS and FCR are detached from the medial epicondyle. FPL is released from the radius, and care is taken to protect the median nerve, ulnar nerve, radial artery, and brachial artery. Fractional or z-lengthening of the FCU can be performed if residual muscle contracture is noted. A PT release can be performed simultaneously to address any residual pronation deformity. Although this procedure can effectively alleviate wrist and digital flexion deformities, it requires a technically challenging dissection and can result in a supination deformity of the forearm.

SUPERFICIALIS TO PROFUNDUS TRANSFER

STP transfer is indicated to improve hand hygiene for patients with spastic clenched-fist deformities

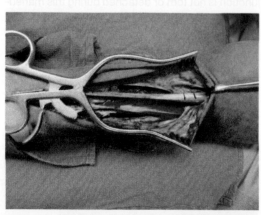

Fig. 6. Fractional lengthening of wrist flexors for wrist flexion deformity.

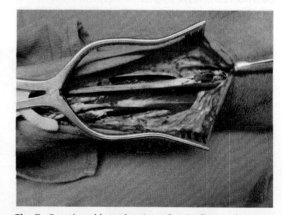

Fig. 7. Fractional lengthening of wrist flexors for wrist flexion deformity.

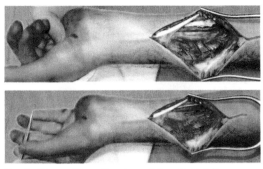

Fig. 8. Step-cut lengthening of the digital flexors.

of the hand without volitional control.[13,16] To achieve full release of a wrist flexion deformity accompanied by metacarpophalangeal (MCP) and IP joint flexion deformities (ie, clenched-fist deformity), up to 4.5 cm of digital tendon excursion is needed; this cannot be accomplished with fractional lengthening alone.[13] Although greater lengthening can be achieved by opening the carpal tunnel to divide the FDS tendons, this is seldom required to achieve an adequate release of the digits. The tendon transfer simply maintains the hand posture rather than causing a flaccid hand by transecting the tendons alone. STP transfer may also be performed in conjunction with intrinsic release or procedures to correct wrist flexion deformities. The volar forearm is approached through a longitudinal incision to identify PL, FDS, and FDP. The median nerve is identified and protected, and PL is transected. The tendons of the FDS are identified and divided as distally as possible, whereas the FDP tendons are transected as proximally as possible, to provide adequate length for finger extension (**Fig. 10**). The fingers are extended, and the tendons are woven together either en masse or individually by ensuring that restoration of the normal digital cascade is accomplished (**Fig. 11**). If spastic, the FPL tendon may be lengthened or divided as well. The wrist is splinted until the incision is healed, and then night-time splinting and passive range of motion exercises are initiated. Overall,

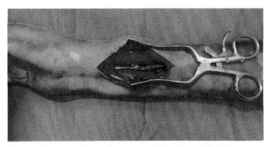

Fig. 9. Step-cut lengthening of flexor pollicis longus.

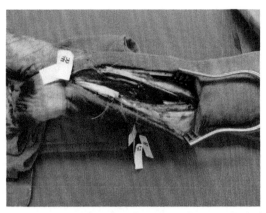

Fig. 10. STP transfer. Note the FDS tendons are divided as distally as possible, and the FDP tendons are divided as proximally as possible to achieve length.

STP transfer is effective in alleviating spastic clenched-fist deformities, but it can unmask intrinsic spasticity resulting in swan-neck and MCP joint flexion deformities in some patients.[17]

WRIST ARTHRODESIS

For skeletally mature patients with fixed capsular contractures or no volitional control of the upper extremity, wrist arthrodesis with PRC can be performed to correct wrist flexion deformities. Wrist arthrodesis is advantageous to provide extension for hygiene and appearance, but should be avoided in patients who may rely on tenodesis for hand opening. For this reason, the authors primarily rely on PRC to release wrist flexion deformities without adding wrist arthrodesis. Nonetheless, results of dorsal plating are favorable, with high rates of bony union and improvement in patient satisfaction. Before fusion, the FCR, PL, and FCU are transected, and the wrist fusion is performed through a dorsal approach between the second and fourth compartments. Incorporating a PRC can provide a local option for bone graft to achieve fusion without the need for iliac crest harvest, reduce the number of fusion sites needed to heal, and shorten the length of the wrist to alleviate the flexion contracture. Overall, wrist arthrodesis is well tolerated in both adults and children with few complications, although similar to other procedures, it can unmask intrinsic spasticity and thumb-in-palm deformities.[18] Wrist fusion rates are high through a dorsal approach with few hardware complications and a low incidence of nonunion.[19]

Thumb-in-Palm Deformity

Thumb-in-palm deformities commonly occur in the setting of CP, but may also occur from stroke

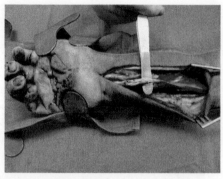
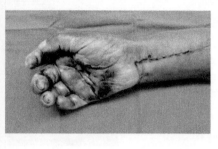

Fig. 11. STP transfer. The tendons are woven to achieve length, to re-create the digital cascade, and to open the palm for wound care and hygiene.

and traumatic brain injuries. These deformities limit the ability for tripod or key pinch, as well as grasp, and can cause poor hand hygiene and skin maceration in severe cases. The thumb-in-palm deformity may result from a combination of muscle spasticity (FPL, adductor pollicis, FPB, and first dorsal interosseous), weakness of the thumb extensors (EPL, extensor pollicis brevis [EPB]) and abductors (abductor pollicis longus [APL], abductor pollicis brevis [APB]), laxity of the MCP joint, and skin and soft tissue contracture of the first web space[20] **(Fig. 12)**. Treatment options focus on alleviating spasticity of the involved flexors, augmenting the weakness of the extensors and abductors, stabilizing the MCP joint, and recontouring the first web space, and can be considered by the type of deformity **(Table 3)**.[6,21,22]

A type 1 deformity describes an adduction contracture of the thumb metacarpal due to spasticity of the adductor pollicis and first dorsal interosseous muscle. If the MCP joint is flexed, spasticity of FPB may also contribute to the deformity (type 2). Treatment includes release of the adductor pollicis and first dorsal interosseous, and FPB if needed. The adductor pollicis is released from its origin along the long finger metacarpal. The origin is approached volarly in the interval between the index and long finger through a curvilinear incision along the crease of the thenar eminence **(Fig. 13)**. The dissection proceeds

between the flexor tendon sheaths of the index and middle finger metacarpal, after identifying and protecting the neurovascular bundles to the index and long finger. The deep palmar arch and the motor branch of the ulnar nerve are identified between the oblique and transverse heads of the adductor pollicis, and protected as the muscle is released off of the metacarpal distally to proximally. The first dorsal interosseous is approached dorsally through an incision along the ulnar aspect of the thumb metacarpal, or through an extension of the incision used to release the adductor **(Fig. 14)**. The muscle is released from the base of the thumb metacarpal, taking care to protect the princeps pollicis artery. Finally, if spastic, FPB is released from its origin proximally along the transverse carpal ligament, taking care to identify and protect the motor branch of the median nerve. Intrinsic spasticity of the adductor and first dorsal interosseous may also be accompanied by laxity of the MCP joint (type 3 deformity). For patients with laxity greater than 20°, additional stabilization of the joint should be considered to improve thumb posture and stability for pinch via either an MCP joint capsulodesis or arthrodesis.

In addition to intrinsic spasticity, extrinsic spasticity may contribute to the thumb-in-palm deformity if the FPL is spastic (type 4 deformity). Extrinsic spasticity of the FPL may be tested by examining the position of the IP and MCP joint

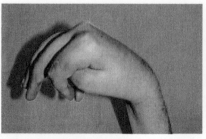
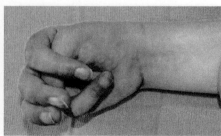

Fig. 12. Thumb in palm deformity.

Table 3
Classification of thumb in palm deformities

	Classification	Cause	Treatment
Type 1	Adduction of the first metacarpal	Spasticity of the adductor pollicis and first dorsal interosseous muscle	Release of the adductor pollicis and first dorsal interosseous
Type 2	Adduction of the first metacarpal with MCP joint flexion	Spasticity of adductor pollicis, first dorsal interosseous, and flexor pollicis brevis	Release of the adductor pollicis, first dorsal interosseous, and flexor pollicis brevis
Type 3	Adduction of the first metacarpal with an MCP joint extension >20°	Spasticity of the adductor pollicis, first dorsal interosseous, and extensor pollicis brevis muscles in the setting of MCP joint laxity	Release of the adductor pollicis, first dorsal interosseous, and extensor pollicis brevis with stabilization of the MCP joint via capsulorrhaphy or arthrodesis
Type 4	Adduction of first metacarpal adduction with MCP joint and IP joint flexion	Spasticity of the adductor pollicis, first dorsal interosseous, FPB, flexor pollicis longus	Release of adductor pollicis, first dorsal interosseous, FPB, flexor pollicis longus
Type 5	IP joint flexion	Spasticity of FPL and weakness of EPL	Fractional lengthening of FPL with augmentation of EPL
Type 6	Weak extension and abduction	Weakness of EPL, EPB, APL	Augmentation of thumb extensors

Adapted from Bhardwaj P, Sabapathy SR. Assessment of the hand in cerebral palsy. Indian J Plast Surg 2011;44(2):348–56; with permission.

with the wrist in flexion and extension. Patients with extrinsic spasticity of FPL will have pronounced IP flexion with the wrist in neutral. In these cases, FPL fractional lengthening can be performed through a limited incision in the volar forearm. The tendon is divided transversely at the musculotendinous junction and allowed to slide approximately 1 cm. Alternatively, step-cut lengthening can be performed for more pronounced flexion (**Fig. 15**).[22] As with other fractional lengthening procedures, care is taken not to excessively extend the thumb and overlengthen the musculotendinous junction, which may cause weakening.

Finally, weakness of the thumb extensors and abductors can exacerbate the flexed posture of the thumb. Numerous tendon transfers have been described to augment thumb extension, including brachioradialis to EPL, brachioradialis to APL, PL to EPL, or FCR to EPL.[23] Although EIP is commonly used as a donor tendon for EPL, it can be diminutive, and local wrist extensors, specifically ECRL, can provide sufficient

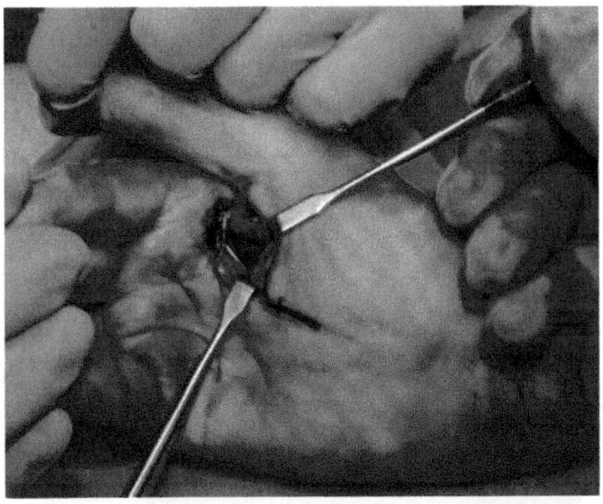

Fig. 13. Adductor pollicis release performed through a curvilinear incision in the palm.

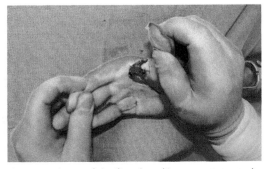

Fig. 14. Release of the first dorsal interosseous muscle.

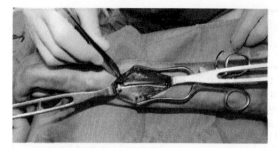

Fig. 15. Step-cut lengthening of flexor pollicis longus.

power, length, and excursion to EPL in this setting (see **Fig. 15**; **Figs. 16–18**). Finally, APL tenodesis and EPL rerouting to EPB can be performed to augment thumb extension, which obviates a donor tendon. When tendon transfers are considered, it is important to evaluate MCP joint stability, because tendon transfers will worsen MCP joint hyperextension in the setting of laxity. As mentioned previously, if the MCP joint can be passively extended by 20° or more, capsulodesis or arthrodesis should be considered in conjunction with the tendon transfer to prevent hyperextension. For all patients with thumb-in-palm deformities, skin coverage should be considered following release, and the need for local flaps is common. Options include a 4-flap z-plasty or a variety of flap options based off of the dorsal index finger.[24,25]

SWAN-NECK DEFORMITIES

Swan-neck deformities describe the hyperextension posture of the proximal interphalangeal (PIP) joint and extension lag of the distal interphalangeal (DIP) joint. In addition to aesthetic concerns, swan-neck deformities also impair grip due to the difficulty of flexing the PIP joint from a hyperextension position. Swan-neck deformities can result from spasticity of the either extrinsic finger flexors, intrinsic spasticity, or both. Extrinsic extensor

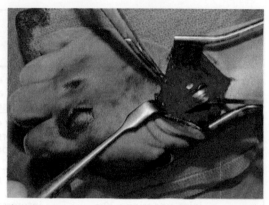

Fig. 16. ECRL transfer to EPL to augment extension for thumb-in-palm deformity.

spasticity results in attenuation and laxity of the volar plate, particularly in the setting of wrist flexion which exacerbates the deformity.

For patients with intrinsic spasticity, MCP joint flexion is pronounced, and PIP joint hyperextension occurs with active finger extension. Spasticity of the intrinsic muscles increases the force directed through the lateral bands, leading to extension of the PIP joint. Over time, the transverse retinacular ligament and volar plate attenuate, resulting in dorsal translation of the lateral bands. In some settings, alleviating spasticity of the extrinsic digital flexors, such as that which occurs following STP transfer, will exacerbate swan-neck deformities because the spasticity of the intrinsic muscles is no longer counterbalanced by extrinsic spasticity. Intrinsic spasticity can be assessed using the Bunnell test, and patients with intrinsic muscle spasticity will have greater passive PIP joint flexion with the MCP joints placed in flexion compared with PIP flexion when the MCP joints are placed in extension (**Fig. 19**).

Initial conservative treatment includes figure-of-8 digital splinting to correct the hyperextension, and this will ensure that correction of the

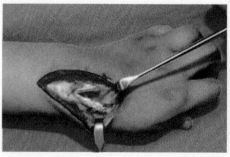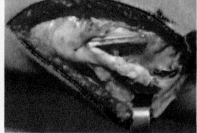

Fig. 17. ECRL transfer to EPL to augment extension.

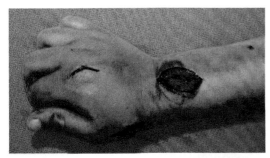

Fig. 18. ECRL transfer to EPL to augment extension.

deformity results in improved digital flexion. For deformities that are pronounced (ie, >20° of PIP joint hyperextension), aesthetically concerning, or functionally limiting, surgical options can alleviate the deformity and improve digital flexion. However, it is critical to distinguish between fixed and flexible deformities, because arthrodesis is indicated for patients with fixed deformities or arthrosis.

For patients with flexible deformities due to extrinsic spasticity, FDS tenodesis, lateral band translocation, or central slip tenotomy can be considered. Although FDS tenodesis has largely been described in the context of rheumatoid arthritis, it can be applied for patients with extrinsic spasticity resulting in a swan-neck deformity.[26] A slip of the FDS is mobilized with its distal attachment left intact and then secured to the proximal phalanx and the flexor tendon sheath. In addition, the lateral band can be rerouted volar to the PIP joint axis for correction of flexible swan-neck deformities; typically the radial lateral band is selected because it includes the lumbrical.[27,28] This is accomplished through a midlateral approach, taking care to protect the neurovascular bundle volarly and the dorsal sensory branches. The volar dissection is continued to expose the A3 pulley. The lateral band is kept in continuity and mobilized from the central slip to the middle of the middle phalanx. The A3 pulley is opened, and the lateral band is then secured within the flexor tendon sheath by closing the A3 pulley over the lateral band (or alternatively creating a sling from the volar plate or slip of FDS). The tensioning is adjusted such that the PIP joint is flexed to approximately 20 to 30°. Finally, central slip tenotomy is appealing given the technical simplicity and alleviation of the spastic force transmitted through the extensor mechanism at the central slip. The procedure is performed through a dorsal approach, where the central slip is transected at the level of the PIP joint, and the joint is mobilized and temporarily pinned in slight flexion following the procedure.[29]

For patients with intrinsic tightness, intrinsic release can be performed either palmarly or dorsally. Before release, extrinsic flexor strength should be evaluated to ensure that it is adequate to achieve MCP joint flexion once the intrinsic muscles are released. A dorsal approach over both the second and the fourth metacarpals offers direct access to all of the dorsal interossei. In an intrinsic slide procedure, the muscles are released from the metacarpals to promote distal translation of the muscle (**Fig. 20**). A volar approach is performed through a transverse incision at the distal palmar crease.[30] The neurovascular bundles are identified and protected, and the lumbricals and interossei are visualized. The lumbricals, followed by the palmar and dorsal interossei, are released sequentially through tenotomies at the musculotendinous junction (single for lumbricals, 2 tenotomies for interossei).

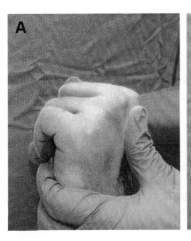

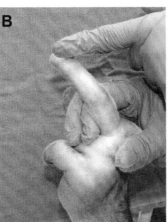

Fig. 19. Physical examination to assess intrinsic tightness. Among patients with intrinsic tightness, the PIP joint has (*A*) full passive flexion with the MP joint in flexion, but (*B*) limited flexion with MP joint extension.

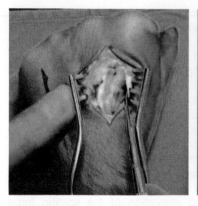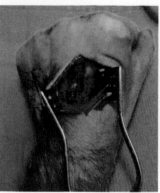

Fig. 20. Intrinsic muscle release from the metacarpals.

SUMMARY

Spasticity of the hand from central nervous system injury can profoundly limit the ability to accomplish self-care and ADLs independently by preventing simple grasp and release. Fortunately, multiple surgical procedures are available to address the spastic hand, but these must be specifically tailored to patient need. Patients with severe cognitive injuries and poor upper extremity function may also benefit from surgery to improve appearance and hygiene. Careful preoperative examination and planning are needed, and consideration is given to the potential unintended detrimental effect of a surgical procedure on hand function, such as the loss of tenodesis or exacerbation of an unstable thumb MCP joint with extensor tendon transfers. However, when selected appropriately, surgical intervention for hand spasticity can greatly enhance hand function, appearance, and overall quality of life.

REFERENCES

1. Van Heest AE, Bagley A, Molitor F, et al. Tendon transfer surgery in upper-extremity cerebral palsy is more effective than botulinum toxin injections or regular, ongoing therapy. J Bone Joint Surg Am 2015;97(7):529–36.

2. Carlson MG, Spincola LJ, Lewin J, et al. Impact of video review on surgical procedure determination for patients with cerebral palsy. J Hand Surg Am 2009;34(7):1225–31.

3. Viel EJ. Neurophysiological approach in the peripheral anesthetic blocks as a diagnosis and prognosis tool for spasticity. Clin Neurophysiol 2005;116(7): 1491–2.

4. Kozin SH, Keenan MA. Using dynamic electromyography to guide surgical treatment of the spastic upper extremity in the brain-injured patient. Clin Orthop Relat Res 1993;(288):109–17.

5. Gong HS, Chung CY, Park MS, et al. Functional outcomes after upper extremity surgery for cerebral palsy: comparison of high and low manual ability classification system levels. J Hand Surg Am 2010; 35(2):277–83.e1-3.

6. House JH, Gwathmey FW, Fidler MO. A dynamic approach to the thumb-in palm deformity in cerebral palsy. J Bone Joint Surg Am 1981;63(2):216–25.

7. Arner M, Eliasson AC, Nicklasson S, et al. Hand function in cerebral palsy. Report of 367 children in a population-based longitudinal health care program. J Hand Surg Am 2008;33(8):1337–47.

8. James MA, Bagley A, Vogler JB 4th, et al. Correlation between standard upper extremity impairment measures and activity-based function testing in upper extremity cerebral palsy. J Pediatr Orthop 2017;37(2):102–6.

9. Lomita C, Ezaki M, Oishi S. Upper extremity surgery in children with cerebral palsy. J Am Acad Orthop Surg 2010;18(3):160–8.

10. Koman LA, Smith BP, Williams R, et al. Upper extremity spasticity in children with cerebral palsy: a randomized, double-blind, placebo-controlled study of the short-term outcomes of treatment with botulinum A toxin. J Hand Surg Am 2013;38(3): 435–46.e1.

11. Zancolli EA. Surgical management of the hand in infantile spastic hemiplegia. Hand Clin 2003;19(4): 609–29.

12. Patterson JM, Wang AA, Hutchinson DT. Late deformities following the transfer of the flexor carpi ulnaris to the extensor carpi radialis brevis in children with cerebral palsy. J Hand Surg Am 2010;35(11): 1774–8.

13. Keenan MA, Abrams RA, Garland DE, et al. Results of fractional lengthening of the finger flexors in adults with upper extremity spasticity. J Hand Surg Am 1987;12(4):575–81.

14. Hashimoto K, Kuniyoshi K, Suzuki T, et al. Biomechanical study of the digital flexor tendon sliding lengthening technique. J Hand Surg Am 2015; 40(10):1981–5.

15. Thevenin-Lemoine C, Denormandie P, Schnitzler A, et al. Flexor origin slide for contracture of spastic finger flexor muscles: a retrospective study. J Bone Joint Surg Am 2013;95(5):446–53.

16. Pomerance JF, Keenan MA. Correction of severe spastic flexion contractures in the nonfunctional hand. J Hand Surg Am 1996;21(5):828–33.

17. Peraut E, Taïeb L, Jourdan C, et al. Results and complications of superficialis-to-profundus tendon transfer in brain-damaged patients, a series of 26 patients. Orthop Traumatol Surg Res 2018;104(1): 121–6.

18. Neuhaus V, Kadzielski JJ, Mudgal CS. The role of arthrodesis of the wrist in spastic disorders. J Hand Surg Eur Vol 2015;40(5):512–7.

19. Van Heest AE, Strothman D. Wrist arthrodesis in cerebral palsy. J Hand Surg Am 2009;34(7):1216–24.

20. Van Heest AE. Surgical technique for thumb-in-palm deformity in cerebral palsy. J Hand Surg Am 2011; 36(9):1526–31.

21. Bhardwaj P, Sabapathy SR. Assessment of the hand in cerebral palsy. Indian J Plast Surg 2011;44(2): 348–56.

22. Tonkin MA, Hatrick NC, Eckersley JR, et al. Surgery for cerebral palsy part 3: classification and operative procedures for thumb deformity. J Hand Surg Br 2001;26(5):465–70.

23. Sakellarides HT, Mital MA, Matza RA, et al. Classification and surgical treatment of the thumb-in-palm deformity in cerebral palsy and spastic paralysis. J Hand Surg Am 1995;20(3):428–31.

24. Ezaki M, Oishi SN. Index rotation flap for palmar thumb release in arthrogryposis. Tech Hand Up Extrem Surg 2010;14(1):38–40.

25. Mahmoud M, Abdel-Ghani H, Elfar JC. New flap for widening of the web space and correction of palmar contracture in complex clasped thumb. J Hand Surg Am 2013;38(11):2251–6.

26. Wei DH, Terrono AL. Superficialis sling (flexor digitorum superficialis tenodesis) for swan neck reconstruction. J Hand Surg Am 2015;40(10): 2068–74.

27. Van Heest AE, House JH. Lateral band rerouting in the treatment of swan neck deformities due to cerebral palsy. Tech Hand Up Extrem Surg 1997;1(3): 189–94.

28. Charruau B, Laulan J, Saint-Cast Y. Lateral band translocation for swan-neck deformity: outcomes of 41 digits after a mean follow-up of eight years. Orthop Traumatol Surg Res 2016;102(4 Suppl): S221–4.

29. Carlson MG, Gallagher K, Spirtos M. Surgical treatment of swan-neck deformity in hemiplegic cerebral palsy. J Hand Surg Am 2007;32(9):1418–22.

30. Matsuo T, Matsuo A, Hajime T, et al. Release of flexors and intrinsic muscles for finger spasticity in cerebral palsy. Clin Orthop Relat Res 2001;(384): 162–8.

Surgical Management of Spasticity of the Forearm and Wrist

Stephen P. Duquette, MD, Joshua M. Adkinson, MD*

KEYWORDS

- Forearm spasticity • Wrist spasticity • Cerebral palsy • Traumatic brain injury • Stroke
- Upper extremity spasticity surgery • Tendon transfer

KEY POINTS

- Upper extremity spasticity manifestations can range from mild to profoundly debilitating and may result from cerebral palsy, traumatic brain injury, or stroke.
- Careful examination in a multidisciplinary setting is necessary to formulate the best treatment plan.
- Nonsurgical options for treatment include serial casting, orthotics, therapy, baclofen, valium, and botulinum toxin A.
- In specific cases, forearm and wrist deformities are addressed by surgery directed at the involved joints and tendons.
- The most commonly used procedures include FCU to ECRB transfer, PT release/rerouting, flexor tendon lengthening, and wrist arthrodesis.

INTRODUCTION

Upper extremity spasticity manifestations range from mild to profoundly debilitating. Spasticity is a frequent sequelae of cerebral palsy (CP),[1] traumatic brain injury, and stroke.[2] Taken together, these conditions comprise a substantial number of patients. The commonality among these diagnoses is that of an upper motor neuron syndrome, in which a supraspinal central nervous system lesion disrupts the balance of inhibitory and excitatory input into the spinal reflex arch.[3]

After the initial insult to the central nervous system, there is flaccid paralysis followed by the return of reflexes and the eventual development of spasticity.[4] Physiologic and structural changes subsequently occur in an attempt to mitigate functional compromise resulting from the pathologic insult.[5] These rearrangements contribute to subcortical hyperexcitability, which leads to increased muscle activity and exaggerated spinal reflex responses to peripheral stimulation.[6] Furthermore, there is a velocity-dependent increase in the resistance of a passively stretched muscle or muscle group.[3] Joints become restricted in the direction of action of the strongest crossing muscle. Digital, wrist, and elbow flexors tend to overpower their antagonists because of a larger cross-sectional area (**Fig. 1**).[7]

Upper extremity spasticity can affect all ages and sociodemographics and is a complex clinical problem with a variety of treatment options depending on the patient, the underlying disease process, and postoperative expectations. The goal of this review is to discuss indications for surgery, preoperative work-up, surgical techniques,

Disclosure Statement: The authors have no commercial or financial conflicts of interest regarding the content of this article.
Division of Plastic Surgery, Department of Surgery, Indiana University School of Medicine, 545 Barnhill Drive, Emerson Hall 232, Indianapolis, IN 46202, USA
* Corresponding author.
E-mail address: jadkinso@iu.edu

hand.theclinics.com

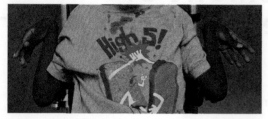

Fig. 1. Common examination findings in upper extremity spasticity. Note the flexed posture of the wrist and pronated forearm.

postoperative care, and outcomes for patients with forearm and wrist spasticity.

WORK-UP

Before surgical intervention, one should assess the patient's overall cognitive and functional status. After obtaining a relevant history from the patient or caregiver, the surgeon must complete a thorough upper extremity functional evaluation. The examination should focus on passive range of motion, active range of motion, degree of spasticity or joint contracture, and the presence of dystonia. Sensibility should be assessed using a two-point discriminator. Skin creases over contracted joints are examined for hygiene and skin breakdown. More than one preoperative functional evaluation is recommended to confirm any proposed surgical plan.

Further work-up may include plain radiographs of the involved extremity, dynamic electromyography, and motion analysis studies. Dynamic electromyography records muscle activity with certain movements, such as grasp, release, wrist flexion and extension, elbow flexion and extension, and forearm supination and pronation.[8] Muscle recordings are obtained from the spastic muscles and their antagonists to guide decision making regarding tendon transfers.[8]

Three-dimensional motion analysis has become an increasingly used quantitative measurement of upper extremity function.[9] Motion analysis records movements using reflective markers and specialized cameras while patients complete standardized tasks. Although labor- and time-intensive, this analysis is recommended in all but the most functional patients, because the results of motion analysis may change the surgical plan.

NONSURGICAL TREATMENT

Nonsurgical treatment of spasticity of the wrist and forearm ranges from serial casting, orthotics, and therapy, to oral drug therapy, intrathecal baclofen, and injection of phenol or botulinum toxin type A.[10]

Serial casting has been shown to have a positive short-term effect on the spasticity of the wrist in adults and children. By maintaining muscle fiber length, casting provides a static impediment to joint contracture. However, casts require frequent changes and adverse events, such pain and skin breakdown, may occur.[11] Oral medications, such as baclofen, valium, and clonidine, are used to treat spasticity. However, effectiveness must be balanced against the side effects of drowsiness, dizziness, and generalized weakness.[2] Continuous infusion of intrathecal baclofen is effective in decreasing spasticity.[2] Because small concentrations of the medication are administered directly into the intrathecal space, systemic side effects are minimal. Phenol is a neurolytic agent that is useful for temporary treatment (3–5 months) of spasticity. It is injected into or adjacent to a nerve controlling the muscles of interest. Botulinum toxin type A inhibits the release of acetylcholine at the neuromuscular junction and is injected directly into spastic upper extremity musculature. A total of 400 units may be injected in one setting and this may be repeated every 12 weeks, as needed. The reduction in forearm, wrist, and finger spasticity with administration of botulinum toxin type A has been shown to increase upper extremity function,[10,12] but like phenol results are temporary.

SURGICAL TREATMENT

Tendon transfers, releases, reroutings, and lengthenings are the mainstays of surgical treatment of the spastic forearm and wrist (**Table 1**).[2] Additional surgical treatments include selective peripheral neurotomy[13] and adjunctive surgeries for secondary symptoms, such as carpal tunnel release in the

Table 1
Surgical options for the treatment of wrist and forearm spasticity

Forearm pronation deformity	PT release, PT rerouting
Forearm supination deformity	Biceps rerouting
Wrist flexion deformity	FCU to ECRB, PT to ECRB, BR to ECRB, wrist arthrodesis, flexor-pronator slide, tendon lengthening
Wrist extension deformity	Extensor lengthening or release

Abbreviations: BR, brachioradialis; ECRB, extensor carpi radialis brevis; FCU, flexor carpi ulnaris; PT, pronator teres.

setting of marked wrist flexion causing median nerve compression.[14] The goals of surgery must be practical and understood by the patient (when possible), caregivers, therapists, support staff, and surgical team.[2]

FOREARM SPASTICITY
Pronation Deformity

A pronation deformity is caused by spasticity of the pronator teres (PT) and pronator quadratus (PQ) muscles (**Fig. 2**). This deformity makes it difficult to transfer objects between hands, because the palms are unable to face each other. Furthermore, self-feeding and grooming are dependent on forearm supination and these tasks are compromised in many patients with upper extremity spasticity. In extreme cases, ulnar-sided grasping is used because patients are unable to present the radial side of the hand.[15] Caution should be used, however, when addressing a pronation deformity, because overcorrection into a supinated posture may compromise assistive device and computer use.

Release of pronator insertion

Release of the PT insertion can address a pronation deformity of the forearm. This procedure may be contraindicated in patients without active supination, because the forearm may remain in a pronated position after surgery. Regardless, PT release may decrease resistance against passive forearm supination and complement the supination moment imparted by a simultaneous flexor carpi ulnaris (FCU) to extensor carpi radialis brevis (ECRB) transfer.

The procedure is simple and effective in the correct patient and is typically combined with additional upper extremity procedures. A 3-cm longitudinal incision is made on the radial aspect of the midforearm centered over the insertion of the PT tendon onto the radius. The interval between the brachioradialis (BR) and the extensor carpi radialis muscles is developed, while protecting the radial sensory nerve and radial artery. The PT insertion onto the radius is exposed and transected, allowing it to retract. Care should be taken to ensure that the entire tendinous insertion is taken down from the radius and the arm should be placed through full pronation and supination for verification (**Fig. 3**). A long-arm splint or cast is applied with 90° of elbow flexion and 60° of forearm supination.[16]

Pronator teres rerouting

PT rerouting has been shown to improve active supination and dynamic forearm positioning in children with CP.[17] As a result, it may have an advantage over PT release. Patient selection is important for this procedure. In patients with inadequate remaining PQ function, PT rerouting can lead to fixed supination deformity that may actually worsen position and function in these patients.[18]

The initial approach is similar to a PT release. However, after the PT insertion on the radius is exposed, it is released with a 3-cm-long extension of periosteum to provide extra length for rerouting and suture application. Rarely, if the distal periosteal or tendon extension is attenuated and unable to reliably hold sutures, a palmaris longus (PL) tendon graft may be used to assist with rerouting. After release of the insertion, the muscle is mobilized into the proximal forearm to ensure adequate excursion. Next, a window in the interosseous membrane is made and the tendon is passed from palmar to dorsal. The tendon is then inserted into the radius near the original insertion using transosseous sutures (in young children) or a single bone anchor, while maintaining the forearm in 50° to 60° of supination (**Fig. 4**). At times, tendon length or distal tendon integrity is not adequate for insertion into exactly the same position. Transposing the reinsertion site 1 cm more proximally

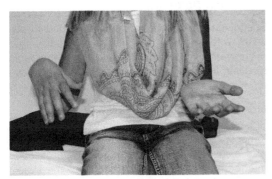

Fig. 2. Attempted bilateral forearm supination. Minimal active supination on the right; full active supination on the left.

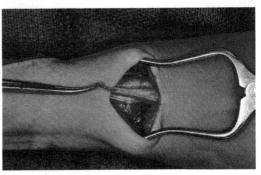

Fig. 3. The PT tendon is released from the radius in preparation for rerouting.

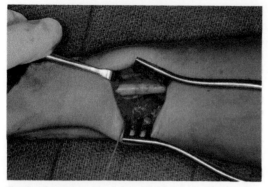

Fig. 4. The PT tendon is fixed to the radius with transosseous sutures.

has been shown to have an equivalent biomechanical effect.[18] After wound closure, the extremity is placed in a long-arm or sugar-tong splint or cast to protect the supinated position of the forearm (**Fig. 5**).[18]

Flexor-pronator muscle slide

The entire flexor/pronator origin on the ulnar side of the forearm is released to correct a forearm pronation and wrist flexion deformity. This procedure also addresses any concomitant digital flexion deformity. This was first described by Page[19] and Scaglietti[20] as a treatment of Volkmann ischemic contracture. The technique was later adapted for upper extremity spasticity by Inglis and colleagues.[21,22] This procedure is less commonly used because of the limited ability to make individual adjustments in tendon tension. Furthermore, appropriately selected patients must have some level of voluntary control of forearm and wrist function.

An anteromedial longitudinal incision is made over the elbow at the level of the medial epicondyle. Thick skin flaps are elevated and care is

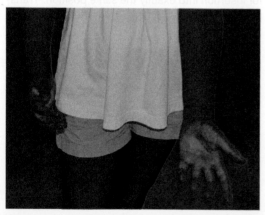

Fig. 5. Postoperative appearance of PT rerouting with improved active supination.

taken to preserve crossing branches of the medial antebrachial cutaneous nerve. The median nerve, ulnar nerve, and brachial vessels are identified and protected. The ulnar nerve is decompressed and the median nerve is freed of any adhesions to the flexor-pronator muscles. After confirming the location of the neurovascular structures and protecting the medial collateral ligament of the elbow, the entire flexor-pronator mass is elevated from the medial epicondyle. The radial border of the flexor digitorum superficialis (FDS), PL, and flexor carpi radialis (FCR) are elevated from the interosseous membrane while protecting branches of the median nerve. The flexor pollicis longus (FPL) is subsequently released from the radius. The wrist and digits are then passively extended, which translates the entire flexor-pronator mass distally. An ulnar nerve transposition is typically performed before closure. If the wrist extensors are unable to extend the wrist to neutral, wrist balance is restored by means of an ECRB tenodesis or a transfer of the FCU to the ECRB.[21]

After surgery, an above-elbow splint or cast is used to immobilize the wrist and fingers in full extension for 4 weeks with the elbow in 45° of flexion and the forearm in full supination. This is followed by therapy and static splinting of the wrist and fingers in full extension for another month, while leaving the elbow free. The patient is gradually transitioned to nighttime splinting only and unrestricted activities resume between 3 and 4 months postoperatively.

Some authors have described fractional lengthening of the PT and PQ, and although conceptually valid, we have no experience with this technique. Outcomes after surgical correction of forearm pronation deformities are generally good (**Table 2**).[16,17,23] Biomechanical studies comparing PT rerouting with other techniques show improvements in passive and active supination.[24]

Supination Deformity

Supination deformity has been described in patients with neonatal brachial plexus palsy and poliomyelitis, and less commonly from tetraplegia resulting from a loss of neurologic function above the fifth cervical nerve root.[25]

Biceps rerouting

Biceps rerouting was first published in 1967 by Zancolli[26] to provide active forearm pronation. It was also suggested to divide the interosseous membrane to assist in correction of the deformity,[25] although this is less commonly done. The technique is performed through an S-shaped incision over the antecubital fossa, beginning

Table 2
Surgical outcomes for pronation deformity

Technique	Study Type/ Authors	Study Population	Outcomes	Complications
PT release	Strecker et al,[16] 1988	Retrospective review comparing 41 PT rerouting with 16 PT release	Gain in supination was 78° for rerouting and 54° for tenotomy	No complications, no loss of function
PT rerouting	Roth et al,[23] 1993	Retrospective review of several tendon transfers in 17 children with CP	Preoperative arc of motion was from 90° to 38° of pronation Postoperative arc of motion improved to 56° of pronation to 11° of supination Forearm position improved from 64° of pronation before surgery to 22° of pronation after surgery	None reported
	Bunata,[17] 2006	Retrospective review of 31 patients with CP	Active supination increased 65°, and the dynamic positioning changed from 26° of pronation to 7° of pronation	9 patients overcorrected
	Cheema et al,[24] 2006	10 cadaver forearms underwent FCU to ECRB, PT rerouting, or BR rerouting to compare supination	FCU transfer: forearm reached its neutral position at a load of 9 N; continued to rotate to up to 84° of supination with 36 N BR transfer: reached its neutral position at 13 N rotated to up to 33° of supination with 36 N PT transfer: forearm never reached neutral position Under a maximum load of 36 N, only 55° of rotation from full pronation was achieved	not applicable

medially at the distal part of the humerus and ending laterally over the proximal part of the forearm. The lateral antebrachial cutaneous nerve is identified in the subcutaneous plane and is protected. The lacertus fibrosis is skeletonized and sharply released. Next, the brachial artery and median nerve are identified and protected. The interval between the BR and the brachialis is developed proximally; this allows for identification of the radial nerve and the dissection of its branches.

Distally, the interval between the BR and the PT is developed, which exposes the distal portion of the biceps tendon. The recurrent radial artery, passing anteriorly, is carefully ligated and divided to improve exposure. The biceps tendon is marked for lengthening in a Z-fashion, leaving the distal stump of the tendon attached to the radial tuberosity and the proximal stump to the biceps muscle (**Fig. 6**). The distal segment is then rerouted dorsally and laterally around the radial

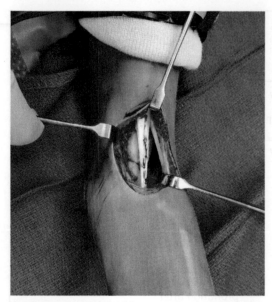

Fig. 6. Exposure of the biceps tendon in preparation for rerouting.

neck, while carefully avoiding the posterior interosseous nerve; a curved clamp that can sit directly against the radius is useful for this step. If desired, a counterincision may be made on the dorsoradial aspect of the proximal forearm to identify and protect the posterior interosseous nerve during rerouting. At this point, a minimum of 45° of passive pronation and supination should be possible. The biceps tendon is repaired with a Krakow stitch or, if length permits, a side-to-side technique using 2–0 nonabsorbable suture, with the elbow at 30° of flexion and the forearm in as much pronation as possible (45°–90°). Securing the tendon at 30° of elbow flexion decreases tension at the repair site, yet reduces the possibility of a postoperative elbow flexion contracture more commonly seen with immobilization at greater amounts of elbow flexion.[25] After wound closure, the limb is immobilized in an above-elbow splint or cast for 4 weeks. Biceps rerouting results in a mean increase in pronation of 75° (**Table 3**).[25,27]

Table 3
Surgical outcomes for supination deformity

Technique	Study Type	Study Population	Outcomes	Complications
Biceps rerouting	Gellman et al,[25] 1994	Retrospective review of 6 patients (8 forearms) with supination deformity caused by trauma	Preoperatively, the mean range of supination was 85°, with 14° of pronation After rerouting, pronation increased a mean of 75°, without affecting elbow motion Functional gains were made in patient ability to feed and groom themselves	Fixed flexion contracture of the elbow of 90° developed in 1 patient, less predictable results with nondominant extremity
	Metsaars et al,[27] 2014	13 study meta-analysis of correction of brachial plexus supination deformity with corrective osteotomy or biceps rerouting 238 patients (157 osteotomies and 71 biceps rerouting)	75° increase in pronation at rest and a 65° gain in passive pronation for the osteotomy group, 79° increase in pronation at rest for the biceps rerouting group, passive pronation not reported Recurrence in the osteotomy group was 20%–40%, vs 0% in the soft tissue group	1 patient had a biceps tendon rupture, 2 had scar formation No cases of nerve palsy or compartment syndrome

WRIST EXTENSOR SPASTICITY

Extensor spasticity of the wrist is rare. This deformity may cause hygiene problems because digital release is impaired. Median nerve compression has also been described and carpal tunnel release is indicated in this situation. In these unusual cases, extensor lengthening or release are potential options.

In the setting of dyssynergic wrist extensors, the extensor carpi ulnaris (ECU), ECRB, and extensor carpi radialis longus (ECRL) may be addressed with myotendinous lengthenings. The ECU is approached through an incision at the junction of the middle and distal third of the dorsoulnar forearm. The myotendinous junction is released and the muscle is stretched. Through a separate approach on the radial aspect of the dorsal forearm, the ECRL and ECRB muscles are lengthened. The wrist is gently passively flexed. Digital flexor tightness is reliably improved with an improvement in wrist posture.

Wrist extensor release may be performed for patients without volitional control of the wrist extensor muscles. The tendons are approached through a longitudinal dorsal wrist incision and are completely transected. In this situation, wrist arthrodesis with or without simultaneous proximal row carpectomy (PRC) is often necessary to address the deformity and to provide wrist stability. Given the rarity of the condition, evidence for treatment is limited.

WRIST FLEXOR SPASTICITY

The affected wrist in CP or stroke usually assumes a flexed position, which may or may not be passively correctable. Examination typically confirms spasticity of the extrinsic flexors acting on or crossing the wrist, including the FCR/FCU, FDS/flexor digitorum profundus (FDP), and FPL. Prolonged delays in evaluation, which are not uncommon in this population, may result in the additional challenges of skin or soft tissue deficiency, neurovascular shortening, and capsular contracture.[28] Severe wrist flexion may also lead to median nerve compression and this should be treated simultaneously with other procedures to address the deformity.

Flexor Carpi Ulnaris to Extensor Carpi Radialis Brevis

Transfer of the FCU to the ECRB (or ECRL), eponymously known as the Green transfer,[29] was first described in 1942 and has since become the first-line tendon transfer to address the wrist flexion and ulnar deviation deformity commonly found in patients with upper extremity spasticity.[30] One should ensure the presence of a functional FCR before tendon transfer to avoid a postoperative wrist extension deformity. If the FCR is nonfunctional, a BR or PT to ECRB transfer is indicated.

Because this transfer is typically performed in combination with other procedures to address digital flexion spasticity, the FCU is approached through a longitudinal 10-cm incision on the volar mid or ulnar forearm (**Fig. 7**). The FCU tendon is dissected distally to the pisiform and proximally toward the musculotendinous junction while protecting the ulnar neurovascular bundle. The FCU is then transected at the insertion on the pisiform and completely elevated off of the ulna. Small perforating vessels from the ulnar artery should be addressed with cautery. A wide subcutaneous tunnel is created connecting the ulnar volar forearm and the dorsal distal forearm. The hand is turned and a longitudinal incision is made over the ECRB tendon. The subcutaneous tunnel is completed through the dorsal incision. The tunnel should be as direct a line as possible, otherwise the tendon transfer pulls through the soft tissues over time and tension is lost. A Pulvertaft[31] weave of the FCU to the ECRB is performed with 2–0 nonabsorbable sutures. The weave is done with the wrist in neutral, and should be allowed to assume a position of 20° of flexion against gravity. After closure, the wrist is immobilized in 30° of extension for 4 weeks. A removable splint is applied for an additional 4 weeks with initiation of

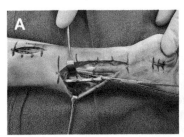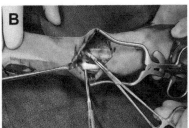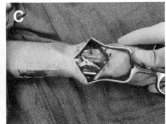

Fig. 7. (*A*) The FCU tendon is released from the distal insertion (held in clamp). (*B*) The FCU tendon (held in clamp) is transferred to the ECRB (under elevator). (*C*) Pulvertaft weave is used to secure the tendons.

range of motion exercises. Splinting is discontinued after 8 weeks.[15]

Evidence shows that the Green transfer consistently corrects the flexion, pronation, and ulnar deviation deformities common to patients with upper extremity spasticity.[30,32,33] A more recent review of postsurgical outcomes confirms that some patients develop a late extension deformity.[34] This complication seems to be more common in younger patients where ongoing limb growth causes an increase in tension within the transfer. Although the transfer is typically to the ECRB, a cadaveric study found no major difference in wrist extension or forearm supination when comparing transfer to the ECRB or the ECRL.[35] Additionally, a large series found no difference in functional use score between transferring the FCU, BR, or ECU to the ECRL/ECRB.[36]

Pronator Teres to Extensor Carpi Radialis Brevis

Transferring the PT to the ECRB was initially described by Colton and colleagues[37] in 1976. The procedure is most appropriate for patients with effective grip, but weak wrist extension and is commonly performed for patients with radial nerve palsy (Fig. 8).

The PT insertion is exposed through a 5-cm longitudinal incision over the middle-third of the radial forearm; a longer incision may be necessary if combined with other procedures to address spasticity. While protecting the radial sensory nerve and radial artery, the PT is elevated from the radius with a 3-cm sleeve of periosteum. The ECRB tendon is identified and separated from the adherent ECRL tendon through the same incision. The PT is transferred to the ECRB tendon with a Pulvertaft weave and secured in place with multiple 2–0 nonabsorbable suture with the wrist in

neutral. Postoperatively, the transfer is managed as with an FCU to ECRB transfer.

A cadaveric study by Abrams and colleagues[38] showed that PT was a suitable donor for restoration of wrist extension based on length, excursion, and cross-sectional area. Bisneto Ede and colleagues[39] compared PT to ECRB versus FCU to ECRB transfers in patients with CP with a wrist flexion deformity (Table 4). They found no significant difference in the functional hand test, but there was a statistically higher grip strength after the FCU transfer. Furthermore, the limited excursion of the PT compared with the FCU may limit postoperative wrist range of motion.

Brachioradialis to Extensor Carpi Radialis Brevis

The BR to ECRB transfer is an alternative option to restore active wrist extension.[40] This is not a first-line transfer, but is a potential donor when the FCU or PT transfers are unavailable or otherwise contraindicated.

A longitudinal incision is made over the radial aspect of the mid to distal forearm. The BR insertion is elevated from the distal radius while protecting the adjacent neurovascular structures. The BR is then mobilized proximally from adjacent soft tissues while protecting muscle perforators from the radial artery. The ECRB is prepared as previously described and the BR is secured to the ECRB with a Pulvertaft weave. The arm is splinted with the elbow at 90° of flexion, maximal supination, and 30° wrist extension for 4 weeks. A removable splint is applied for an additional 4 weeks with initiation of range of motion exercises. Splinting is discontinued after 8 weeks unless there is concern for recurrent deformity.

In a more recent cadaver study, it was shown that elbow position can affect tension of the transfer. The authors suggest that tensioning the transfer while the elbow is flexed may lead to better results, but the ultimate outcome depends on strength of the BR.[41]

Wrist Arthrodesis

Soft tissue procedures alone may not achieve adequate correction or a durable result in patients with severe deformities and little or no motor control.[42] In these patients, wrist arthrodesis is a more reliable option. A simultaneous PRC may be necessary in the most severe deformities to allow for passive wrist extension into neutral position.[43] Wrist arthrodesis are performed in adults and children with good results[44]; however, the technique differs depending on the age of the patient.

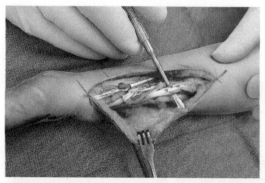

Fig. 8. PT to ECRB transfer placed on gentle traction. This patient also underwent PL to extensor pollicis longus and FCR to EDC transfers. EDC, extensor digitorum communis.

Table 4
Surgical outcomes for wrist flexion deformity

Technique	Study Type	Study Population	Outcomes	Complications
FCU to ECRB	Thometz & Tachdjian,[33] 1988	Retrospective review of 25 patients with CP	Average follow-up was 8 y, 7 mo The average active wrist dorsiflexion was 44.2°, palmar flexion was 19°, supination was 40.2°, and pronation was 53.4°	3 patients required additional future releases
	Beach et al,[30] 1991	17-y review of 43 patients with CP	Consistently corrected the flexion, pronation, and ulnar deviation deformities Shown to be more effective in children <12 y old and improved function and cosmesis	No infections or nerve injuries, 1 patient with supination contracture, 1 patient with stiffness requiring capsular release
	Wolf et al,[32] 1998	Retrospective review of 16 patients undergoing FCU transfer to ECRB, ECRL, or EDC	Resting position improved, center of the arc of motion averaged 6° pronation and 9° extension 14 of 16 parents believed there was an improvement in function, 16 of 16 believed that cosmesis was improved, 14 of 16 would recommend the procedure to others, and 15 of 16 were satisfied overall	None reported
	Van Heest et al,[35] 1999	Cadaveric study evaluating FCU to ECRB vs FCU to ECRL	Transfer of the FCU into the ECRB or ECRL provided similar supination and freeing the distal two-thirds of the FCU ulnar origin provided significantly more supination than freeing only the distal one-third	not applicable
	Van Heest et al,[36] 1999	Retrospective review of 718 procedures in 134 patients, including soft tissue releases, tendon transfers, and joint stabilization procedures	120 patients underwent wrist tendon transfers to ECRL/ECRB (50 BR, 42 ECU, and 28 FCU) All transfers gained an average of 2.5 points in functional use score (range, +1 to +5)	No operative complications noted
	Patterson et al,[34] 2010	Retrospective review of 24 patients with CP	12 patients developed a late deformity between 10 and 105 mo postoperatively These included extension deformities (8), supination deformities (1), and recurrent flexion deformities (3)	9 out of 12 patients with late deformities required revision surgery

(continued on next page)

Table 4
(continued)

Technique	Study Type	Study Population	Outcomes	Complications
PT to ECRB	Colton et al,[37] 1976	Retrospective review of 9 transfers	Results classified by surgeon as excellent, good, fair, and poor 3 patients classified as excellent had improved grip strength with the wrist extended beyond neutral and had active supination Patients classified as good had improved grip strength and wrist extension and lacked active supination	Not reported
	Abrams et al,[38] 2005	Cadaveric study of 10 specimens	PT is a suitable donor for restoration of wrist extension, based on length, excursion, and cross-sectional area	not applicable
	Bisneto Ede et al,[39] 2015	Retrospective cohort review (37 patients, 22 PT to ECRB/L, 15 FCU to ECRB/L)	No statistical difference in the functional hand test between groups, statistically higher grip strength with the FCU transfer	No complications
BR to ECRB	Freehafer & Mast,[40] 1967	Case series of 6 transfers	4 of 6 hands with transfer of a good or normal BR to weak or absent radial wrist extensors gained effective grasp 2 had improved posture of their hands	Not reported
	Murray et al,[41] 2002	Biomechanical model of 8 wrists	Altering the surgical tension could improve wrist extension when the elbow is flexed Result depends on strength of the BR	not applicable
Wrist arthrodesis	Rayan & Young,[46] 1999	Retrospective review of 9 patients	A 17-task hand function questionnaire was given to patients and 8 of 9 patients (10 wrists) reported improved function after surgery Face washing, propelling a wheelchair, and picking up large and small objects were among the most frequently improved functions Radiographic fusion was present in all cases The average position of wrist fusion was 15° flexion and the average amount of wrist correction was 85°	No complications reported

	Study	Design	Outcomes	Complications
	Sodl et al,[44] 2002	Retrospective review of 5 patients	Improved limb stability. Improved use of the extremity was reported in 4 of the 5 patients, with 1 patient noting good stability, but no significant improvement in function	No hardware problems; 1 patient developed numbness and tingling after wrist fusion and required carpal tunnel release
	Donadio et al,[47] 2016	Retrospective review of 20 adolescent patients with CP treated with PRC and wrist arthodesis	Average follow-up, 22 mo. Average age, 16.2 y. Average flexion deformity improved from 66° to 10°. Bony union was achieved in all patients within 6 mo	4 patients required hardware removal
Flexor-pronator slide	Thevenin-Lemoine et al,[21] 2013	Retrospective review of 55 patients	Improved wrist and finger motion. Mean gain of wrist extension was 67° with the fingers extended	12 cases had at least a partial recurrence of the deformity and 7 patients required additional surgical intervention
Tendon lengthening	Keenan et al,[48] 1987	Retrospective review of 27 adult patients undergoing fractional lengthening	5 nonfunctional hands with no motor control, improved posture, and hygiene. 20 of the 22 patients with potentially functional hands (91%) improved their spastic hand function score a mean of 3.7 points	2 patients (9%) decreased their spastic hand function score as a result of overlengthening of the finger flexors, with loss of grip strength; no recurrence
	Hashimoto et al,[50] 2015	Biomechanical evaluation of 56 flexor tendons from 12 cadavers comparing SL with ZL and compared single with double mattress suturing	Tensile strengths: 23 N for the SL compared with 7 N for the ZL at 20-mm lengthening and single mattress suture. 25 N for the SL compared with 10 N for the ZL with double mattress suture. 15 N for the SL vs 8 N for the ZL with 30-mm lengthening and single mattress suture. 18 N for the SL and 10 N for the ZL at 30-mm lengthening and double mattress suture	not applicable

Abbreviations: SL, sliding lengthening; ZL, Z-lengthening.

Epiphyseal wrist arthrodesis is a technical modification used in the immature skeleton that allows for continued growth of the distal radius. In all cases, the procedure begins by complete release of the wrist flexors (PL, FCR, and FCU). The wrist is then assessed for passive extension, which may be further limited by capsular contracture and/or volar soft tissue contracture. A 6-cm longitudinal incision is then made over the dorsal wrist. The extensor pollicis longus tendon is released from the third compartment and radialized. The interval between the second and fourth compartment is entered and the wrist capsule is elevated off of the underlying carpus, exposing the radiocarpal joint. The proximal articular surfaces of the scaphoid and lunate are removed to cancellous bone using a burr. The articular surface of the distal radius is similarly removed, while sparing the physis. The radiocarpal joint is held in neutral to slight extension and two large Steinmann pins are placed across the fusion site and buried beneath the skin (**Fig. 9**). The wrist is immobilized for approximately 3 months and the pins are removed after confirmation of adequate fusion.[15]

A standard wrist arthrodesis is performed in skeletally mature individuals with a severe wrist flexion deformity and little to no voluntary control (**Fig. 10**). The procedure begins similarly to an epiphyseal arthrodesis, although a 10-cm incision is used to accommodate plate application. After the preliminary steps outlined previously, an oscillating saw or burr is used to remove the articular surface of the radius and to expose cancellous bone. Lister tubercle is also removed to allow plate apposition. If the wrist can be passively extended to neutral, then the proximal carpal row is decorticated to cancellous bone to accommodate fusion. If not, a PRC is performed and the distal carpus is decorticated to accommodate fusion. Full passive wrist extension to neutral should then be possible. Internal fixation is accomplished with a 3.5-mm wrist fusion plate extending from the distal radius to the third metacarpal (**Fig. 11**). Bone graft harvested from the previously resected bone is packed into the fusion sites. The wrist is immobilized in a short-arm splint to allow for swelling. At the first postoperative visit, the patient is converted to a custom splint to allow for wound cleaning and scar management. Immobilization is maintained until radiographic evidence of fusion,[15] which typically takes at least 3 months.

It is unusual to perform wrist arthrodesis alone in patients with upper extremity spasticity. In severe flexion deformities of the wrist and fingers, arthrodesis is combined with other procedures, such as FDS to FDP transfer; carpal tunnel release; FPL lengthening; wrist flexor release; and, rarely, an ulnar motor neurectomy for intrinsic spasticity.[45] The improved wrist posture typically

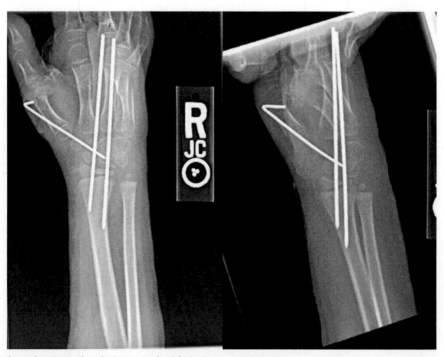

Fig. 9. Epiphyseal wrist arthrodesis secured with Steinmann pins.

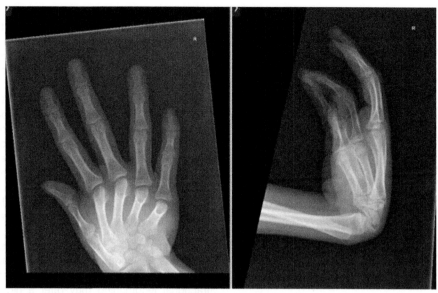

Fig. 10. Preoperative radiographs of severe flexion deformity at the wrist.

increases tone in the finger flexors, which must be addressed through lengthening in some fashion.

Wrist arthrodesis has been shown effective in treating severe wrist deformities secondary to spasticity. Authors report a stable and durable wrist position, improvements in object manipulation, and an improved ability to propel a wheelchair.[42,44,46,47]

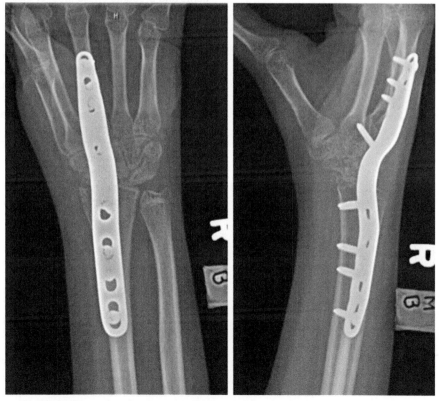

Fig. 11. Postoperative radiographs of wrist arthrodesis with 3.5-mm dorsal plate.

Flexor Tendon Lengthening

Fractional lengthening of the forearm and digital flexors has proven to effectively decrease the wrist flexion deformity in functional and nonfunctional extremities.[48] On occasion, a Z-lengthening of the tendons may be appropriate, particularly if greater lengthening is required (**Fig. 12**).[49]

Fractional lengthening is approached through a longitudinal incision over the volar forearm at the musculotendinous junction. A PL tenotomy is also routinely performed to assist with release and to improve exposure of the deeper digital flexors. Serial tenotomies are performed while placing gentle passive extension of the wrist or digits. The distal-most tenotomy must be at least 2 cm proximal to the distal-most aspect of the musculotendinous junction to prevent rupture.[15] For digital contractures contributing to wrist flexion, both the FDS and FDP are tight but one often contributes disproportionately to the deformity. As a result, it may be necessary to alternately lengthen the FDS and FDP for each finger to prevent overlengthening of the digital flexors. In severe contractures, passive extension of the wrist or digits after fractional lengthening may lead to avulsion of the tendon from the musculotendinous junction; in these cases, Z-lengthening is more appropriate.

If a greater release is required, one can proceed with Z-lengthening of the digital or wrist flexor tendons. As with a fractional lengthening, a longitudinal forearm incision is performed to expose the volar forearm. A longitudinal split is created in the midpoint of the tendon, and the tendon is divided ulnarly at one end and radially at the other end. The wrist and/or digits are extended to the desired length and the hemitendons are sutured end-to-end or side-to-side. After tendon lengthening, the patient is immobilized for 4 weeks, after which guided therapy is initiated. A removable splint is worn for an additional 4 weeks.[15]

Tendon lengthening procedures reliably improve posture and hygiene, but may decrease grip strength because of overcorrection.[48] Although the severity of flexion deformity dictates the best technique for lengthening, a biomechanical study by Hashimoto and colleagues[50] indicated that fractional lengthening may offer a higher tensile strength compared with Z-lengthening. Fractional lengthening, therefore, has the theoretic advantage of allowing earlier rehabilitation with a lower risk for rupture.

SUMMARY

Upper extremity spasticity is debilitating for patients and presents challenges for their caregivers. Although there are multiple surgical options to address the forearm and wrist deformity, it remains impossible to normalize upper extremity function using peripheral procedures in patients with CP, traumatic brain injury, and stroke. The upper extremity surgeon must carefully assess the patient in a multidisciplinary setting to formulate the best treatment plan; surgery is not always the first option, but is often the most reliable and durable. Standard procedures include the FCU to ECRB transfer; PT release/rerouting; and in severe cases, wrist arthrodesis. Using these procedures and their technical modifications and adjuncts leads to predictable and satisfactory outcomes.

REFERENCES

1. Arner M, Eliasson AC, Nicklasson S, et al. Hand function in cerebral palsy. Report of 367 children in a population-based longitudinal health care program. J Hand Surg Am 2008;33(8):1337–47.
2. Gharbaoui I, Kania K, Cole P. Spastic paralysis of the elbow and forearm. Semin Plast Surg 2016; 30(1):39–44.
3. Trompetto C, Marinelli L, Mori L, et al. Pathophysiology of spasticity: implications for neurorehabilitation. Biomed Res Int 2014;2014. https://doi.org/10.1155/2014/354906.

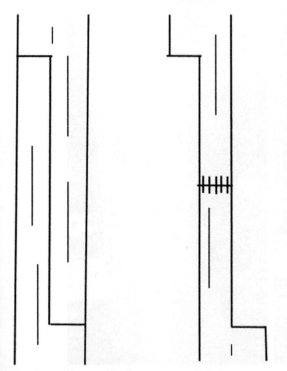

Fig. 12. Technique for tendon Z-lengthening.

4. Raghavan P. Upper limb motor impairment after stroke. Phys Med Rehabil Clin N Am 2015;26(4): 599–610.

5. Leafblad ND, Van Heest AE. Management of the spastic wrist and hand in cerebral palsy. J Hand Surg Am 2015;40(5):1035–40.

6. Naro A, Leo A, Russo M, et al. Breakthroughs in the spasticity management: are non-pharmacological treatments the future? J Clin Neurosci 2017;39: 16–27.

7. Pontén E, Fridén J, Thornell L-E, et al. Spastic wrist flexors are more severely affected than wrist extensors in children with cerebral palsy. Dev Med Child Neurol 2005;47(6):384–9.

8. Hoffer MM, Perry J, Melkonian GJ. Dynamic electromyography and decision-making for surgery in the upper extremity of patients with cerebral palsy. J Hand Surg Am 1979;4(5):424–31.

9. Mailleux L, Jaspers E, Simon-Martinez C, et al. Clinical assessment and three-dimensional movement analysis: an integrated approach for upper limb evaluation in children with unilateral cerebral palsy. Dev Med Child Neurol 2017;59(Suppl.2): 68–9.

10. Francis HP, Wade DT, Turner-Stokes L, et al. Does reducing spasticity translate into functional benefit? An exploratory meta-analysis. J Neurol Neurosurg Psychiatry 2004;75(11):1547–51.

11. Lannin NA, Novak I, Cusick A. A systematic review of upper extremity casting for children and adults with central nervous system motor disorders. Clin Rehabil 2007;21(11):963–76.

12. Brashear A, Gordon M, Elovic E, et al. Intramuscular injection of Botulinum toxin for the treatment of wrist and finger spasticity after a stroke. N Engl J Med 2002;347(6):395–400.

13. Maarrawi J, Mertens P, Luaute J, et al. Long-term functional results of selective peripheral neurotomy for the treatment of spastic upper limb: prospective study in 31 patients. J Neurosurg 2006;104(2): 215–25.

14. Orcutt SA, Kramer WG, Howard MW, et al. Carpal tunnel syndrome secondary to wrist and finger flexor spasticity. J Hand Surg Am 1990;15(6):940–4.

15. Carlson MG. Cerebral palsy. In: Wolfe SW, Hotchkiss RN, Pederson WC, et al, editors. Green's operative hand surgery, vol. 2, 6th edition. Philadelphia: Elsevier; 2011. p. 1139–72.

16. Strecker WB, Emanuel JP, Dailey L, et al. Comparison of pronator tenotomy and pronator rerouting in children with spastic cerebral palsy. J Hand Surg Am 1988;13(4):540–3.

17. Bunata RE. Pronator teres rerouting in children with cerebral palsy. J Hand Surg Am 2006;31(3):1–11.

18. Oishi S, Butler L. Technique of pronator teres rerouting in pediatric patients with spastic hemiparesis. J Hand Surg Am 2016;41(10):e389–92.

19. Page CM. An operation for the relief of flexion-contracture in the forearm. J Bone Joint Surg Am 1923;5(2):233–4.

20. Scaglietti O. Immediate and late clinical syndromes of vascular lesions in fractures of extremities. Riforma Med 1957;71(27):749–55.

21. Thevenin-Lemoine C, Denormandie P, Schnitzler A, et al. Flexor origin slide for contracture of spastic. J Bone Joint Surg Am 2013;95:446–53.

22. Inglis AE, Cooper W. Release of the flexor-pronator origin for flexion deformities of the hand and wrist in spastic paralysis. A study of eighteen cases. J Bone Joint Surg Am 1966;48(5):847–57.

23. Roth JH, Richards RS, Porte AM. Functional outcome of upper limb tendon transfers performed in children with spastic hemiplegia. J Hand Surg Eur Vol 1993;18B:299–303.

24. Cheema TA, Firoozbakhsh K, De Carvalho AF, et al. Biomechanic comparison of 3 tendon transfers for supination of the forearm. J Hand Surg Am 2006; 31(10):1640–4.

25. Gellman H, Kan D, Waters RL, et al. Rerouting of the biceps brachii for paralytic supination contracture of the forearm in tetraplegia due to trauma. J Bone Joint Surg Am 1994;76(3):398–402.

26. Zancolli EA. Paralytic supination contracture of the forearm. J Bone and Joint Surg 1967;49-A:1275–84.

27. Metsaars WP, Nagels J, Pijls BG, et al. Treatment of supination deformity for obstetric brachial plexus injury: a systematic review and meta-analysis. J Hand Surg Am 2014;39(10):1948–58.

28. Seruya M, Dickey RM, Fakhro A. Surgical treatment of pediatric upper limb spasticity: the wrist and hand. Semin Plast Surg 2016;30(1):29–38.

29. Green W. Tendon transplantation of the flexor carpi ulnaris for pronation-flexion deformity of the wrist. Surg Gynecol Obs 1942;75:337–42.

30. Beach WR, Strecker WB, Coe J, et al. Use of the Green transfer in treatment of patients with spastic cerebral palsy: 17-year experience. J Pediatr Orthop 1991;11(6):731–6. Available at: http://www.ncbi.nlm. nih.gov/pubmed/1960196.

31. Pulvertaft RG. Tendon grafts for flexor tendon injuries in the fingers and thumb. J Bone Joint Surg Br 1956;38:175–94.

32. Wolf TM, Clinkscales CM, Hamlin C. Flexor carpi ulnaris tendon transfers in cerebral palsy. J Hand Surg Eur Vol 1998;23(3):340–3.

33. Thometz JG, Tachdjian M. Long-term follow-up of the flexor carpi ulnaris transfer in spastic hemiplegic children. J Pediatr Orthop 1988;8(4): 407–12.

34. Patterson JMM, Wang AA, Hutchinson DT. Late deformities following the transfer of the flexor carpi ulnaris to the extensor carpi radialis brevis in children with cerebral palsy. J Hand Surg Am 2010;35(11):1774–8.

35. Van Heest AE, Murthy NS, Sathy MR, et al. The supination effect of tendon transfer of the flexor carpi ulnaris to the extensor carpi radialis brevis or longus: a cadaveric study. J Hand Surg Am 1999;24(5): 1091–6.

36. Van Heest AE, House JH, Cariello C. Upper extremity surgical treatment of cerebral palsy. J Hand Surg Am 1999;24(2):323–30.

37. Colton CL, Ransford AO, Lloyd-Roberts GC. Transposition of the tendon of pronator teres in cerebral palsy. J Bone Joint Surg Br 1976;58(2):220–3.

38. Abrams GD, Ward SR, Fridén J, et al. Pronator teres is an appropriate donor muscle for restoration of wrist and thumb extension. J Hand Surg Am 2005; 30(5):1068–73.

39. Bisneto Ede NF, Rizzi N, Setani EO, et al. Spastic wrist flexion in cerebral palsy. Pronator teres versus flexor carpi ulnaris transfer. Acta Ortop Bras 2015; 23(3):150–3.

40. Freehafer A, Mast W. Transfer of the brachioradialis to improve wrist extension in high spinal-cord injury. J Bone Joint Surg Am 1967;49:648–52.

41. Murray WM, Bryden AM, Kilgore KL, et al. The influence of elbow position on the range of motion of the wrist following transfer of the brachioradialis to the extensor carpi radialis brevis tendon. J Bone Joint Surg Am 2002;84-A:2203–10.

42. Gong HS, Kang JY, Lee JO, et al. Wrist arthrodesis with volar plate fixation in cerebral palsy. Tech Hand Up Extrem Surg 2010;14(2):69–72.

43. Pinzur MS. Carpectomy and fusion in adult-acquired hand spasticity. Orthopedics 1996;19(8):675–7.

44. Sodl JF, Kozin SH, Kaufmann RA. Development and use of a wrist fusion plate for children and adolescents. J Pediatr Orthop 2002;22(2):146–9.

45. Pomerance JF, Keenan MAE. Correction of severe spastic flexion contractures in the nonfunctional hand. J Hand Surg Am 1996; 21(5):828–33.

46. Rayan GM, Young BT. Arthrodesis of the spastic wrist. J Hand Surg Am 1999;24(5):944–52.

47. Donadio J, Upex P, Bachy M, et al. Wrist arthrodesis in adolescents with cerebral palsy. J Hand Surg Eur Vol 2016;41(7):758–62.

48. Keenan MAE, Abrams RA, Garland DE, et al. Results of fractional lengthening of the finger flexors in adults with upper extremity spasticity. J Hand Surg Am 1987;12(4):575–81.

49. Keenan MAE. Management of the spastic upper extremity in the neurologically impaired adult. Clin Orthop Relat Res 1988;(233):116–25.

50. Hashimoto K, Kuniyoshi K, Suzuki T, et al. Biomechanical study of the digital flexor tendon sliding lengthening technique. J Hand Surg Am 2015; 40(10):1981–5.

Surgical Management of Spasticity of the Elbow

Aaron Berger, MD, PhD[a],*, Saoussen Salhi, MD, FRCSC[a], Monica Payares-Lizano, MD[b]

KEYWORDS

- Elbow flexion contracture • Spastic elbow • Biceps release • Biceps Z-lengthening

KEY POINTS

- A spastic deformity is characterized by increased tone of the involved limb.
- Spastic elbow flexion contracture is a common deformity encountered in patients with upper motor neuron injuries.
- It results in functional limitation of the affected upper limb and is aesthetically displeasing.
- Surgery aims at improving both function and cosmesis through various surgical techniques tailored to the degree of elbow flexion contracture, presence or absence of joint contracture, and soft tissue deficit.

INTRODUCTION

A spastic limb has increased tone that results from disinhibition of reflex arcs following a neurologic injury that affects the upper motor neuron, pyramidal, or extrapyramidal structures. Affected patients exhibit muscle contractures, clonus, and hyperreflexia.[1] A number of neurologic conditions can lead to spasticity of the upper extremity, including cerebral palsy (CP), stroke, multiple sclerosis, and injuries or tumors of the brain and spinal cord.

The typical posture of the spastic elbow in patients with spasticity is one of flexion. The main muscles responsible for this typical flexion deformity are the biceps, brachialis, and brachioradialis muscles (**Fig. 1**).[1] The flexed position of the elbow interferes with functional use of the hand, which requires elbow extension for functional activities and is aesthetically displeasing. As the elbow contracture worsens, hygiene problems can develop within the antecubital fossa. Moreover, there is a belief among many laypeople that flexed posturing of the elbow is associated with impaired intelligence.[2]

Before initiating treatment, it is important to understand the goals of the patient and caregivers. Generally, treatment is aimed at improving hygiene, activities of daily living, pain, and appearance. The ability of the limb to function after spasticity reduction is not predictable. It must be discussed with the patient and family that treatment of the spastic limb will not necessarily result in the acquisition of previously undeveloped skills. In addition, the function of antagonistic muscles is unpredictable, and treatment of the agonists without treatment of the antagonists may create additional problems.

The initial treatment of spasticity includes conservative management, therapy and splinting, oral medications (eg, baclofen and dantrolene), and injectable neurolytic medications (eg, Botulinum toxin [BTX] and phenol). These techniques are usually attempted before surgical intervention. Surgical goals vary based on current and expected function and severity of the deformity. Children with spasticity present a unique challenge, as surgical intervention may be required to allow more normal bone, joint, and muscle development. For hemiplegia, the goal is

Disclosure Statement: No disclosures.
[a] Division of Plastic Surgery, Nicklaus Children's Hospital, 3100 Southwest 62 Avenue, Miami, FL 33155, USA;
[b] Department of Orthopaedic Surgery, Nicklaus Children's Hospital, 3100 Southwest 62nd Avenue, Miami, FL 33155, USA
* Corresponding author.
E-mail address: aaron.berger@mch.com

Hand Clin 34 (2018) 503–510
https://doi.org/10.1016/j.hcl.2018.06.007

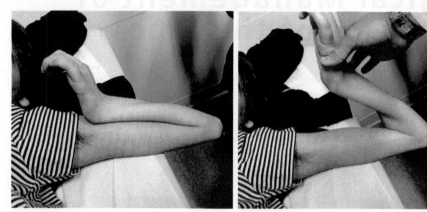

Fig. 1. Elbow flexion contracture seen in a patient with upper motor neuron disease. This is only partially passively correctable.

functional use as a helper hand. In quadriplegia, the goals are to improve access for hygiene, changing clothing, and positioning. Further, cosmesis (ie, the resting posture of the upper extremity) is also a significant factor. For more functional patients, it is important to ensure that the patient and family are aware that although surgical intervention can lead to improved function, it may lead to some loss of strength.

INDICATIONS/CONTRAINDICATIONS

The care of patients with elbow spasticity requires a team effort, with input from the patient, caregivers, and therapists. The decision to proceed with surgical intervention for elbow spasticity should not be entered hastily. Conservative measures, including therapy and medications, should be attempted first; if possible, during the acute phase of the underlying brain/spinal cord lesion. The primary goal of conservative measures is to prevent stiffness and joint contractures. Passive range of motion is required before restoring active motion. Splints and soft supports, as well as passive motion exercises and stretching, are critical to maximizing the patient's functional status and future surgical options (**Table 1**).

Barus and Kozin[3] have previously published a helpful treatment algorithm for initial treatment of elbow spasticity, used at Shriner's Hospital of Philadelphia. BTX is administered (50–100 units to each affected muscle), followed by immobilization in a cast with the elbow positioned at its end-range of extension. The cast is maintained for a few weeks to allow full effect of the BTX. The therapist then works with the patient to improve passive range of motion, and strengthen the antagonist elbow extensors. Serial splinting or casting is then performed until the contracture is less than 30°. Working closely with the patients and assessing function as the BTX wears off can help determine if lengthening of the flexors will offer the patient a long-term solution.

Table 1
Surgical options and indications

Surgical Options	Indications
1. Biceps step-lengthening	Mild hemiplegia, mild deformity
2. Biceps Z-lengthening	Functional upper extremity with more severe deformities
3. Brachialis fractional lengthening	Functional upper extremity with more severe deformities
4. Brachioradialis myofascial lengthening	Added to complete transection of biceps and brachialis in severe flexion deformities
5. Capsular release	Joint contracture >45°
6. Rotational flap	If inadequate soft tissue coverage in severe contractures after muscular lengthening
7. Musculocutaneous neurectomy	Spastic elbow with no joint contracture
8. Tendon transfer (posterior deltoid-to-triceps or biceps-to-triceps)	Supple elbow joint, corrected contracture and patient desires elbow extension

Surgical intervention is required when nonoperative treatment modalities have been exhausted. However, structural problems, such as previous concomitant trauma to the elbow joint or de novo heterotopic ossification, sometimes seen around the elbow joint after traumatic brain injury (TBI), can require operative intervention, as they preclude adequate stretching and splinting.

Elbow stiffness can be categorized as extrinsic, intrinsic, or mixed. Extrinsic (extra-articular) contractures can be caused by skin, subcutaneous tissue, neurovascular bundles, joint capsule, ligaments, muscle-tendon unit, or ectopic bone. Intrinsic contractures are due to problems within the joint, including intra-articular adhesions, articular cartilage loss, articular deformity, and internal hardware.[4] Surgical treatment directed at correcting a spastic elbow flexion deformity must take all of these factors into account. Generally, correction of the spastic elbow includes management of the skin and lengthening of the flexor tendons with release of ligaments and the joint capsule, as needed. The neurovascular bundles are often the limiting factor in correction of the deformity.

Surgical intervention is performed to restore elbow motion. Procedures include contracture release, resection of heterotopic bone, correction of fracture malunions, and lengthening or release of spastic muscles. When limited by spasticity alone, lengthening or release of the spastic elbow flexors is the procedure of choice. Occasionally, concomitant joint release is required. If the patient desires active elbow extension, tendon transfers may be considered.

We generally follow the guidelines described by Barus and Kozin,[3] with initial institution of passive stretch therapy and serial splinting or casting, as well as the use of BTX into agonist flexor muscles. When these modalities have failed, or structural problems limit elbow range of motion, operative intervention is planned.

Generally, the indications for operative intervention include fixed elbow flexion contractures greater than 40° in patients with volitional control of the elbow and hand, and more than 100° in patients without volitional control (for hygiene).[5]

In patients with CP, surgery may be considered after the child has developed functional use of the upper extremity (usually after 6 years of age). Evaluation should include multiple visits and performance evaluation; serial videotaping is helpful. Reconstruction in older patients may carry significant risk, as these patients have often developed compensatory mechanisms that can be lost after surgical intervention.

In patients with stroke, surgical intervention should be postponed until the patient is neurologically stable; this takes at least 1 year. Patients with TBI should be treated similarly; however, spontaneous neurologic recovery can occur for up to 18 months. Additionally, as noted previously, patients with TBI tend to develop heterotopic ossification around the elbow joint.

To restore active elbow extension, tendon transfers, either a posterior deltoid-to-triceps brachii tendon transfer or a biceps brachii-to-triceps brachii tendon transfer, may be considered.[6–10] The same prerequisites to perform any tendon transfer apply here, including healthy donor muscles, with a Medical Research Council (MRC) grade of 4 or 5, and a function synergistic to the one being reconstructed.[7,9,10] The transferred tendon also must have an adequate soft tissue bed without significant scarring along the anticipated new route.[9] Finally, passive range of motion must be near complete before tendon transfer surgery.[7,9] For restoration of elbow extension in a spastic elbow, surgery is usually delayed until the flexion contracture is less than 20°.[7,8]

Additionally, when considering a biceps brachii-to-triceps brachii tendon transfer for restoration of elbow extension, the patient must exhibit intact brachialis and supinator muscle function[6,8,9] so as not to impair postoperative ability to flex the elbow and supinate the forearm.[6]

SURGICAL TECHNIQUES/PROCEDURES
Preoperative Planning

Initial workup includes imaging with plain radiographs, although advanced imaging with computed tomography and/or MRI may be required. Preoperative imaging is especially important to assess for heterotopic ossification, especially in those patients who have sustained TBI or elbow trauma.

Measurement of joint range of motion, both active and passive, must be assessed using a goniometer. Muscle tone must also be assessed. These 2 factors must be considered together, as severe spastic muscle tone will limit assessment of any underlying joint contracture. In some cases, the degree of contracture remains unknown until the spasticity is treated. Some patients have volitional control of their spastic muscles, allowing for functional use of the spastic extremity after release.

To predict the required surgical intervention, Carlson and colleagues[5] classified patients into 2 categories: dynamic and static. Patients with "dynamic" deformity of the elbow included those with a fixed deformity less than 45° and these patients usually did not require intervention about the elbow joint capsule. Patients with a fixed elbow contracture greater than 45° were classified as "static," and these required more extensive surgical intervention, including anterior elbow capsule release.

In patients who are deemed candidates for tendon transfer (to restore elbow extension), maximal benefit will be achieved if the patient's elbow contracture is less than 20° to 30°, and the supinator and brachialis muscles are functioning. Evaluation of supinator and brachialis function can be determined with careful physical examination; dynamic electromyography and nerve blocks can be used to confirm individual muscle function in equivocal cases.[3]

PREPARATION AND PATIENT POSITIONING: CORRECTION OF ELBOW FLEXION CONTRACTURE
Positioning

The patient is placed in the supine position. A hand extension table is generally used. A pneumatic tourniquet is placed as high as possible toward the axilla. A sterile tourniquet may be used, especially for small children.

Procedure

1. A transverse incision is planned just proximal to the elbow flexion crease (**Fig. 2**).[3,5,11]
2. Dissection is carried through the subcutaneous tissues with spreading and retraction of the subcutaneous veins. If more proximal or distal exposure is needed, the incision can be extended in a lazy-S or Z-plasty fashion.
3. Subcutaneous dissection should proceed from medial to lateral, exposing the antecubital fossa.
4. Identify the lacertus fibrosus and biceps brachii tendon (**Fig. 3**A).
5. Identify and protect the median nerve and brachial artery medial to biceps tendon.
6. Identify and protect the lateral antebrachial cutaneous nerve lateral to the biceps muscle; it emerges between biceps and brachialis muscles.
7. Release or resect the lacertus fibrosis.
8. Expose the biceps tendon (**Fig. 3**B). Retractors are placed on each side of the tendon and it is exposed from its distal insertion (radial tuberosity) proximally to the musculotendinous junction.
9. Decision point (biceps tendon-muscle unit): fractional lengthening for mild contractures versus Z-lengthening for more severe contractures versus (controversial) transection for absent function/extreme contractures.
   - Fractional lengthening of biceps tendon (for mild contractures): On opposite sides of the

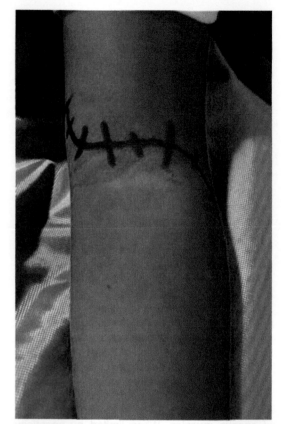

Fig. 2. Incision design to approach antecubital fossa. Start with transverse incision and extend proximally and distally if needed.

tendon, 2 transverse incisions are made 1 to 2 cm apart, halfway through the tendinous portion of the musculotendinous junction (taking care to leave muscle fibers intact). The elbow is then passively extended, allowing for separation of the tenotomy sites but keeping the muscle in continuity.
   - Z-lengthening of biceps tendon (for severe contractures): A step cut is performed over as much length of the tendon as possible (allowing for more tendon substance for a strong repair) (**Fig. 3**C).
   - Transection of biceps tendon (for extreme contractures in the nonfunctional limb): While controversial, the biceps tendon can be completely transected for extreme contractures if no restoration of function is expected.
10. The brachialis muscle will come into view with lengthening/release of the biceps muscle (**Fig. 3**D).
11. Decision point (brachialis muscle): partial release versus complete release (**Fig. 3**E).
    - Partial release of brachialis muscle: This can be performed using 1 or 2 incisions, with transverse incisions made over the

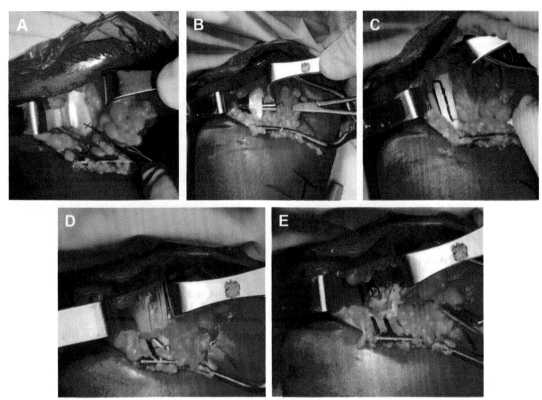

Fig. 3. Release of elbow flexion contracture. (*A*) The "x" marks lacertus fibrosus. (*B*) Exposed biceps tendon. (*C*) Biceps tendon planned Z-lengthening incision. (*D*) Exposed brachialis fascia. (*E*) Fractional lengthening of brachialis fascia.

aponeurosis on the superficial aspect of the muscle, leaving the muscle intact. If 2 incisions are planned, the proximal one should be performed first; if the distal is performed first, the brachialis fascia/aponeurosis retracts under the biceps muscle belly, making the second incision difficult.

- Complete release of brachialis muscle: In patients with severe contractures without volitional control, the brachialis can be completely transected.

12. Assess brachioradialis muscle. If contracted, first identify and protect the radial nerve; it emerges between the brachioradialis and brachialis muscles.
13. Decision point (brachioradialis muscle): partial release versus complete release.
    - Partial release of brachioradialis muscle: Detach origin of the brachioradialis with a combination of blunt dissection and electrocautery, allowing brachioradialis to slide distally.
    - Complete release of brachioradialis muscle: Performed directly through muscle belly of brachioradialis. Take care to identify and protect the radial nerve.

14. Assess anterior elbow joint. Consider anterior capsulectomy.
15. If Z-lengthening of the biceps tendon was performed, it should be repaired using either side-to-side or Pulvertaft weave and 3-0 or 2-0 nonabsorbable sutures, with the elbow flexed to 30°.
16. Assess the skin and consider Z-plasty or local flap transposition for skin closure.
17. Release the tourniquet and ensure hemostasis.
18. After skin closure, which may require local flaps or skin grafting (see later in this article), apply a long-arm splint that keeps the elbow at 30° of flexion.

Preparation and positioning: Posterior deltoid-to-triceps brachii tendon transfer for elbow extension restoration:

1. A lateral incision is planned over the deltoid.
2. The posterior third to half of the deltoid muscle is elevated from its humeral insertion.
3. The axillary nerve is identified and protected.
4. Because the deltoid has a short tendon at its insertion, this can be elevated with a bony segment from the humerus. Alternatively, it can be augmented with a tibialis anterior

free tendon graft, Dacron tape, or fascia lata graft.

5. The central third of the triceps tendon is elevated from its insertion on the olecranon process. This is elevated from distal to 1 to 2 cm from the musculotendinous junction of the triceps.

6. The triceps tendon is then woven through the deltoid tendon and sutured with nonabsorbable sutures.

7. Tension is set to have no more than 45° of passive elbow flexion.

8. Triceps tendon that remains attached to the olecranon medial and lateral to the elevated portion are sutured together.[6]

Preparation and positioning: Biceps brachii-to-triceps brachii tendon transfer for restoration of elbow extension:

1. A 3-cm incision is planned anteriorly over the antecubital fossa and a 7-cm longitudinal incision is planned over the medial aspect of the distal arm, at the level of the medial intermuscular septum.

2. The anterior and medial incisions can be connected.

3. The musculocutaneous nerve lateral to the biceps tendon is identified and protected.[7]

4. The lacertus fibrosis is incised.[6,7] Care is taken to protect the underlying median nerve and brachial artery.

5. The biceps tendon is followed distally in the forearm to its insertion into the radial tuberosity.[7]

6. The biceps tendon is released 1 cm proximal to its insertion on the radial tuberosity and a nonabsorbable braided suture is placed within the tendon.[6,7]

7. In the medial incision, the medial intermuscular septum is released and the ulnar nerve is identified.

8. The biceps tendon is passed into the arm incision and further dissected free from the surrounding tissues to facilitate its excursion.[7] This is continued until the most distal motor branches of the musculocutaneous nerve entering the muscle are identified.[6]

9. The biceps tendon is passed around the medial side of the humerus, superficial to the ulnar nerve.[7,8]

10. A third 7-cm incision is made on the posterior aspect of the distal third of the arm and is curved laterally around the olecranon and the subcutaneous border of the ulna.[6]

11. The triceps tendon is identified and split over the tip of the olecranon process.[7]

12. A unicortical hole is drilled from the tip of the olecranon and gradually enlarged to accept the biceps tendon.[7,8]

13. The biceps tendon is passed from the medial incision to the posterior incision.[7]

14. The biceps tendon is then passed through the medial portion of the triceps tendon into the split made in the triceps tendon.[7]

15. Two small drill holes are placed through the opposite posterior cortex via the unicortical hole.[8]

16. With the elbow maintained in full extension, a suture passer is placed in each one of these holes via the posterior cortex to retrieve the sutures within the biceps tendon, passing the tendon into the unicortical hole. The sutures are then tied over the bone.

17. Fixation is further secured by adding nonabsorbable sutures between the biceps and triceps tendons.[7]

COMPLICATIONS AND MANAGEMENT
Injury to Neurovascular Structures

- A number of critical neurovascular structures may be encountered during the course of dissection and muscle release. Oftentimes, these are a limiting factor in achieving release of the elbow contracture.
- If injured intraoperatively, named nerves and major vessels should be repaired.
- Ensure that tension on the brachial artery does not lead to distal ischemia of the forearm and hand.
- In some rare occasions, the lateral antebrachial cutaneous nerve may be cut to achieve desired contracture release. If cut, it should be cut as proximally as possible to ensure the end retracts beneath muscle, preventing a symptomatic neuroma.[1]
- Postoperative neurovascular checks should be performed, and splint adjustments should be made as needed.

Skin and Soft Tissue Coverage of Antecubital Fossa

- If primary closure of the skin is not possible, a complete release of the biceps muscle from its origin as well as the brachialis fascia beneath the biceps can be performed. The muscle can be released distally, and the muscle flap placed over the neurovascular structures of the antecubital fossa. A split-thickness skin graft is then placed over the muscle.[1]

Loss of Elbow Flexion Strength

- Although patients who undergo fractional lengthening of the biceps experience minimal loss of volitional elbow strength, those who undergo Z-lengthening or transection can expect to lose elbow flexion strength.
- *Avoid* full extension of the elbow in patients with volitional control, as they may experience difficulty with elbow flexion when full release is performed. This can be an even greater problem for the patient than the initial flexion contracture.[11]
- Consider limiting biceps lengthening to less than 2 cm.[12]

Loss of Active Supination

- Lengthening, effectively weakening, of the biceps muscle will result in a reduction in supination strength.
- Preoperative assessment of supinator muscle function through physical examination and dynamic electromyography can help prevent this complication.
- Techniques, such as pronator rerouting and flexor carpi ulnaris transfer, may improve a co-existing pronation contracture.

Postoperative Hematoma

- Hematoma formation after this procedure is typically secondary to muscle bleeding from myotomy or injury to large subcutaneous veins.
- To prevent postoperative hematoma, use needle-point electrocautery to perform myotomy. Also, consider placement of a drain, especially when myotomy has been performed.

Complications Related Specifically to Tendon Transfers for Elbow Extension Restoration

- Tendon rupture with sudden loss of function during the rehabilitation period should prompt a return to the operating room for exploration.[9]
- Stretching of the tendon transfer during the rehabilitation period should prompt modification of the rehabilitation protocol and the use of protective orthoses.[9]
- Lateral routing of the biceps tendon during the biceps brachii-to-triceps brachii tendon transfer has been plagued by radial nerve injuries; therefore, the medial routing technique is preferred.[8]

POSTOPERATIVE CARE
Spastic Elbow Biceps Lengthening

- At 14 to 21 days postoperatively, the splint and dressings are removed and the incisions are assessed.

- If only fractional lengthening of the biceps was performed, the patient can be started in therapy immediately with protected range-of-motion exercises, encouraging active range of motion.
- If Z-lengthening of the biceps was performed, the splint is maintained at 30° of flexion for an additional 4 weeks, followed by night splints for an additional 3 weeks.
- Long-term therapy and night bracing are used to prevent recurrence.

Tendon Transfer for Restoration of Elbow Extension

- The elbow is maintained in a long-arm cast in full extension for 4 weeks followed by nighttime extension splinting in a custom-made splint.
- During the day, the patient wears a dial-hinge brace that acts as a flexion block at 15°.
- Each week, the brace is adjusted to allow 15 more degrees of flexion.
- This brace is worn until elbow flexion reaches 90° without any extension lag.
- An extension splint, worn at night, is maintained until the 12th postoperative week.
- Strengthening exercises are initiated 3 months after the surgery.[7]

OUTCOMES

With respect to improvement of the flexion contracture after complete release (including anterior capsulotomy), results from Mital[13] demonstrate that fixed elbow contractures may be improved from approximately 48° to 10°, and up to 95° of active flexion can be preserved. Carlson and colleagues[5] report similar results, demonstrating improvement in active extension range from 77° to 39° and improvement of passive extension from 59° to 22°. Impressively, Carlson's group[5] also demonstrated preserved postoperative active flexion to 123°. Generally, fractional lengthening of the biceps results in 10° to 30° of improvement with no appreciable loss of flexion power, whereas Z-lengthening for the biceps results in 45° to 60° of improvement with a more obvious loss of flexion power.[11]

It is difficult to measure the functional improvement patients may obtain after operations that improve elbow extension. According to Carlson and colleagues,[5] many hemiplegic patients report the newfound ability to participate in activities they could not do before surgery, including bicycle riding, kayaking, or holding a plate in their lap. In patients with tetraplegia, Wangdell and Friden[6] reported improvements in all activities of daily living, particularly propelling a wheelchair and reaching for overhead objects.

Mulcahey and colleagues[8] conducted a prospective randomized study in patients with C6 or C7 spinal cord injuries in which each arm was assigned to either a posterior deltoid-to-triceps brachii tendon transfer or a biceps brachii-to-triceps brachii transfer. Both patient groups demonstrated a statistically significant increase in elbow extension strength from baseline to their 24-month follow-up visit. There was no statistically significant difference in the postoperative elbow extension strength between groups. However, 7 of the 8 biceps brachii-to-triceps brachii tendon transfer patients achieved MRC 3 or greater strength, whereas only 1 in 8 patients having undergone posterior deltoid-to-triceps brachii achieved MRC 3 strength.[8]

A meta-analysis of 14 studies and more than 500 cases showed a mean MRC score increase from 0 to 3.3 after reconstruction of elbow extension.[9] As documented by Barus and Kozin,[3] the results for mild spasticity tend to be better than that for severe spasticity. They also note that functional benefits related to elbow spasticity surgery are dependent on the degree of hand spasticity and function.

SUMMARY

Elbow spasticity typically results from an injury to the brain or spinal cord. The resultant, typically flexed, posture of the elbow becomes a functional problem, a hygiene problem, and a cosmetic deformity. Treatment is initially conservative, including therapy and medication. When those modalities fail, surgical intervention is performed. In mild and moderate cases of elbow spasticity, surgical intervention is aimed at improving function and appearance. In severe cases of elbow spasticity, operative intervention mainly seeks to improve access to the antecubital fossa for hygiene. The typical techniques focus on lengthening or sectioning those structures that contribute to the deformity, namely the flexors of the elbow, and if necessary, the joint capsule. Heterotopic ossification is occasionally seen, especially in patients who have suffered TBI, and this must also be addressed when treating flexion contractures of the elbow.

REFERENCES

1. Lomita C, Ezaki M, Oishi S. Upper extremity surgery in children with cerebral palsy. J Am Acad Orthop Surg 2010;18(3):160–8.
2. Manske PR, Langewisch KR, Strecker WB, et al. Anterior elbow release of spastic elbow flexion deformity in children with cerebral palsy. J Pediatr Orthop 2001;21(6):772–7.
3. Barus D, Kozin SH. The evaluation and treatment of elbow dysfunction secondary to spasticity and paralysis. J Hand Ther 2006;19(2):192–205.
4. Morrey BF. Post-traumatic contracture of the elbow. Operative treatment, including distraction arthroplasty. J Bone Joint Surg Am 1990;72(4):601–18.
5. Carlson MG, Hearns KA, Inkellis E, et al. Early results of surgical intervention for elbow deformity in cerebral palsy based on degree of contracture. J Hand Surg 2012;37(8):1665–71.
6. Wangdell J, Friden J. Activity gains after reconstructions of elbow extension in patients with tetraplegia. J Hand Surg Am 2012;37(5):1003–10.
7. Kozin SH, D'Addesi L, Chafetz RS, et al. Biceps-to-triceps transfer for elbow extension in persons with tetraplegia. J Hand Surg 2010;35(6):968–75.
8. Mulcahey MJ, Betz RR, Smith BT, et al. A prospective evaluation of upper extremity tendon transfers in children with cervical spinal cord injury. J Pediatr Orthop 1999;19(3):319–28.
9. Fridén J, Gohritz A. Tetraplegia management update. J Hand Surg 2015;40(12):2489–500.
10. Dunn JA, Sinnott KA, Rothwell AG, et al. Tendon transfer surgery for people with tetraplegia: an overview. Arch Phys Med Rehabil 2016;97(6 Suppl):S75–80.
11. Sebastin S, Chung K. Release of a spastic elbow flexion contracture. In: Chung K, editor. Operative techniques: hand and wrist surgery. 2nd edition. Philadelphia: Elsevier Saunders; 2012. p. 264–70.
12. Lightdale-Miric N, de Roode C. Cerebral palsy. In: Abzug JM, Kozin SH, Zlotolow DA, editors. The pediatric upper extremity. New York: Springer; 2015. p. 769–802.
13. Mital MA. Lengthening of the elbow flexors in cerebral palsy. J Bone Joint Surg Am 1979;61(4):515–22.

Surgical Management of Spasticity of the Shoulder

Dan A. Zlotolow, MD[a,b,*]

KEYWORDS

- Shoulder • Spasticity • Hemiplegia • Quadriplegia • Cerebral palsy • Traumatic brain injury
- Stroke

KEY POINTS

- There are multiple etiologies for developing spasticity of the shoulder.
- All etiologies involve deregulation of the lower motor neurons.
- Athetoid movements are difficult to manage.
- All or some muscles of the shoulder can be involved.
- Treatment depends on the needs of the patient and the muscles involved.

INTRODUCTION

Although much has been written about cerebral palsy (CP) and spasticity of the upper limb, relatively little has been devoted to the shoulder.[1–4] Even the textbook, *The Pediatric Upper Extremity*, contains a chapter that only covers surgical options distal to and including the elbow.[5] Perhaps this is because most surgery for spasticity is performed by either general pediatric orthopedists or adult hand surgeons, both of whom are generally less comfortable treating the shoulder. More likely, however, is that the shoulder is less problematic in this patient population than other joints and merits less attention. The more common position of shoulder adduction and internal rotation is rarely the limiting factor for patient function; this more commonly depends on terminal limb (hand) control (**Fig. 1**). Hygiene may be an issue if the adduction contracture is severe, particularly if accompanied by an internal rotation contracture. Donning and doffing clothing also may be an issue. Even more rarely, we have seen patients with difficulty fitting into chairs or getting through doorways because of bilateral external rotation and abduction contractures. Although shoulder spasticity is relatively uncommon, it may present significant functional problems for those affected.

PREOPERATIVE ASSESSMENT

Regardless of etiology, injuries to the brain are difficult to manage peripherally with the tools available to a hand surgeon. Although we can rearrange the muscles that remain under the control of the central nervous system and release, replace, or remove those muscles that are not, we are not able to directly impact the underlying problem of control. After splinting and therapy have failed to provide sufficient improvement, surgery may be appropriate in some cases.

Patients tend to fall into 2 broad categories: those with some volitional motion and those without (**Fig. 2**). For patients with no volitional motion, the goals are not to improve function (that is not possible), but rather to facilitate care. Patients with volitional motion can be further subdivided into those limited by spasticity and those limited by lack of coordination (athetoid movements);

Disclosure Statement: Ownership or Royalty Agreement: Osteomed, Arthrex, McGinley Orthopaedics, Elsevier, Springer.
[a] Department of Orthopaedics, The Hospital for Special Surgery, 535 East 70th Street, New York City, NY 10021, USA; [b] Shriners Hospital for Children Philadelphia, 3551 North Broad Street, Philadelphia, PA 19140, USA
* 3551 North Broad Street, Philadelphia, PA 19140.
E-mail address: DZLOTOLOW@YAHOO.COM

Hand Clin 34 (2018) 511–516
https://doi.org/10.1016/j.hcl.2018.06.008

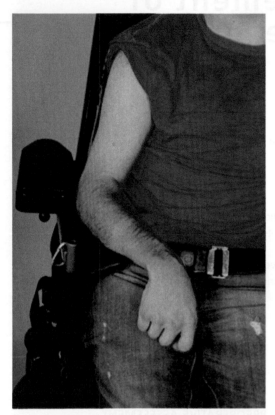

Fig. 1. Typical posture of the shoulder in patients with spastic shoulder girdle muscles. (Used with permission of Shriners Hospitals for Children–Philadelphia, Philadelphia, PA. All rights reserved.)

athetoid movements are a relative contraindication for surgery.

The cause of spasticity needs to be considered before any surgical intervention. Function in patients with progressive brain lesions, such as tumors and multiple sclerosis, will deteriorate over time, making any gains from surgical intervention less enduring. Relatively static lesions, such as

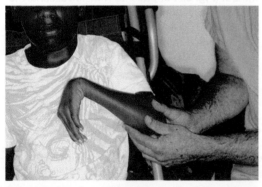

Fig. 2. Testing the volitional strength of the deltoid. (Used with permission of Shriners Hospitals for Children–Philadelphia, Philadelphia, PA. All rights reserved.)

CP, may also have peaks of spasticity that will impact timing of surgical intervention. We tend to delay definitive surgery for CP until after the peak of spasticity, typically approximately 12 years of age. Lesions that are in evolution, such as in the acute period following a stroke or traumatic brain injury, may require a wait-and-see approach until spasticity stabilizes. The goals in the acute period are instead to minimize joint contractures with therapy, splinting, and chemodenervation. Afterward, antispasmodic agents should be titrated until spasticity is minimized without compromising global function.

Once the level of spasticity has relatively stabilized, a thorough assessment of the patient's functional goals and neurologic, muscular, and joint assets and liabilities is performed; goals may need to be curtailed or expanded based on what is realistically possible. Managing expectations of patients and family members becomes a primary concern during the surgical planning phase.

Preoperative assessment tools, such as electrodiagnostic studies, motion analysis, and spasticity-specific instruments, such as the Shriners Hospital for Children Upper Extremity Evaluation (SHUEE),[6] can be very helpful. In particular, the SHUEE can be used to assess the efficacy of the surgical intervention by comparing preoperative and postoperative scores. Electromyography (EMG) is helpful for ascertaining volitional control and baseline spasticity of individual muscles. Motion analysis can demonstrate joint contractures and movement patterns.

We also consider botulinum toxin A (Botox) to be a preoperative assessment tool. Injection of an affected muscle with Botox offers a preview of what a release or permanent denervation may yield. If the improvements in function or posture are clinically significant after chemodenervation, the results provide greater confidence that a permanent solution may also yield similar benefits.

SURGICAL PLANNING

Surgical plans are built from the inside out; the first concern is to release restrictive joint contractures. More than almost any other joint in the body, the shoulder relies on capsular and muscular constraints for stability. When peri-glenoid muscles lose their excursion, the resultant loss of motion leads to capsular contracture. If the patient's active range of motion matches his or her passive motion, then no tendon or nerve transfer will augment motion. However, if there is a motion lag, muscles can then be transferred or differentially innervated or denervated, as needed, to augment active motion. Last, the skin may need to be rearranged to allow or improve joint motion. Surgery always proceeds in a proximal to distal direction.

In the case of patients with athetoid movements, the goals of surgery are to augment joint mobility and restore lost function. Attempts to manage or improve on the athetoid movements have had little success. One exception is the emerging technique of nerve transfer to treat spasticity. Muscles that display good volitional control can be sacrificed, if expendable, and their motor nerves transferred to vital muscles that display athetoid movements.

Nerve transfers can restore lost innervation or replace hyperactive signals from uninhibited anterior horn cells with absent or decreased cortical modulation. The shoulder is an ideal joint for nerve transfers because of its proximity to donor nerves. Nerve donors can include the spinal accessory nerve, intercostal nerves, long thoracic nerve, medial pectoral nerve, radial nerve branches to triceps, and contralateral C7. For patients with hemiplegia and no involvement of the contralateral side, the contralateral C7 nerve transfer offers significant promise, and preliminary studies have shown good results.[7,8] Hypothetical concerns about sacrificing function on the unaffected side have not, as of yet, been confirmed. However, only young children are capable of the cortical retraining required for the contralateral C7 transfer to be functional without mirror movements. In adults, the goals of nerve transfers may instead focus on spasticity, pain, and contracture minimization rather than for motor patterning, control, dexterity, or strength gains.

Unlike nerve transfers for lower motor nerve injuries, in which the focus is on providing motor input to supply to the weak or flaccid muscle, the goals of nerve transfers for the spastic upper extremity are primarily to relieve spasticity. Nerve transfer recipients, therefore, tend to be the stronger spastic muscles, rather than the weaker, nonspastic muscles. Nerve transfers in this population have not been performed long enough for the evolution of consensus guidelines for treatment, but the principle of prioritizing the spastic muscles will likely persist.

Most spastic conditions result in adduction and internal rotation contractures of the shoulder, but any combination of contractures can occur. Some contractures may put the shoulder in an optimal position for function and should not be addressed unless there is sufficient voluntary function to warrant release. In high-functioning patients, the key is to restore balance to the shoulder. This can be accomplished with a combination of tendon transfer, nerve transfers, and tendon releases.

MUSCLE RELEASE/DENERVATION

The most commonly performed release in our practice is a pectoralis major lengthening to address internal rotation and adduction contractures.[9,10] The pectoralis tendon can be approached through a short transverse incision near the insertion of the tendon onto the humerus. If a large correction is required, we use a Z-plasty skin and tendon incision with the middle segment parallel to the muscle fibers. The tendinous portion of the muscle is inferior to the muscle insertion, and can be divided completely without creating a cosmetic deformity at the anterior axillary fold. However, if the contracture is severe and the pectoralis is not functional, the entire muscle may be released. Another option is to perform a medial pectoral neurectomy. The nerve pierces the pectoralis minor and can be found on the undersurface of the pectoralis major. The medial pectoral nerve innervates the more caudal, costal portion of the pectoralis major that is primarily responsible for the contracture. The upper pectoralis is innervated by the lateral pectoral nerve and contributes more to forward flexion of the shoulder.

The teres major and latissimus dorsi muscles are innervated by the lower subscapular (C6/7) and the thoracodorsal (C7) nerves, respectively. They can be major contributors to internal rotation and adduction contractures along with the pectoralis major. Because the teres major and latissimus dorsi insertions are just posterior to the pectoralis major, these tendons also can be accessed through an anterior axillary incision.

The subscapularis muscle can also contribute to internal rotation contractures, but typically does not cause an adduction deformity because its insertion is on the humeral head. Release of the muscle can be accomplished by releasing the upper rolled border (tendinous) portion, while maintaining the lower muscular portion incontinuity. Like the pectoralis major, the subscapularis is segmentally innervated by the C5-7 nerve roots via the upper and lower subscapular nerves. The lower subscapular nerve can be accessed through a posterior or anterior axillary incision. The upper subscapular nerve occasionally travels with the suprascapular nerve, but more commonly branches off the posterior cord near the upper border of the subscapularis.

If the shoulder is still tight after release of all the internal rotators, an anterior and inferior capsular release is indicated. This can be performed most safely through an open approach in which the pectoralis major and subscapularis tendon have been divided in a Z step-cut for later repair, giving wide exposure of the anterior and inferior capsule. The axillary nerve can be seen lying directly superficial to the axillary pouch of the capsule. Alternative techniques include an arthroscopic release, or an inferior open release through an inferior axillary incision (**Fig. 3**). The inferior capsular release, however, does not divide the rolled border of the subscapularis.

The suprascapular nerve-innervated supraspinatus and infraspinatus muscles and the axillary-innervated teres minor muscle are rarely an issue, as these muscles are relatively weak compared with the muscles causing adduction and internal rotation. To prevent instability, release is best performed as a muscle slide. A longitudinal incision along the medial portion of the scapula can provide access to all 3 muscles. The interval between the teres minor and the infraspinatus is sometimes difficult to find. The interval between the teres minor and major is best found distally where the muscle insertions diverge.

The deltoid is often the primary culprit of abduction contractures. Each head has its own tendon, so fractional lengthening or Z-lengthening can be tailored to the specific head or heads primarily contributing to the contracture. Care should be taken to stay below the equator of the muscle to minimize risk to the axillary nerve.

TENDON TRANSFER

Tendon transfers are rarely performed about the shoulder. Our requirement for a tendon transfer donor is voluntary control over a muscle of at least 4/5 strength (ie, active movement against gravity and moderate resistance). Muscles that fire out-of-phase can still be used, and may be ideal if reoriented for in-phase motions. For example, the latissimus dorsi and/or teres major tendons may be transferred for external rotation and abduction if they contract when the patient attempts those particular functions.[11] The underlying principle is the conversion of a harmful antagonist into a helpful agonist by changing the muscle insertion. The latissimus dorsi and the teres major tendons can be transferred individually or as a conjoined tendon. Transfer to the supraspinatus tendon footprint yields humeral head depression and an abduction moment. Transfer to the infraspinatus footprint yields external rotation. Because both functions are commonly desired, the tendons are transferred to the junction between the infraspinatus and supraspinatus footprints.

Transfer of either the upper or lower trapezius are additional alternatives to recreate shoulder abduction or external rotation, respectively.[12] We have found the upper trapezius transfer to be contraindicated in skeletally mature patients because the attachment of the muscle to bone moves distally as the humerus grows predominantly from the proximal physis. This results in superior subluxation of the humeral head on the glenoid.

NERVE TRANSFER

Nerve transfers have only recently been applied for upper extremity spasticity. In theory, any controllable, expendable, and adequately sized (in terms of axonal count) nerve can be transferred to any other nerve in which function is lacking or spasticity is problematic. One big advantage of nerve transfers in patients with spasticity is that the muscles retain their contractile ability, unlike patients with lower motor neuron or axonal injuries. There is, therefore, no urgency to embark on surgery, as there is no risk for irreversible denervation. One disadvantage, however, may be that a spastic muscle develops fibrosis over time and may have limited excursion.[13–16] It is unclear whether removing the spastic signal and replacing it with an unaffected nerve pathway will reverse muscle fibrosis and over what time period this might occur.

For hemiplegic patients, the contralateral C7 (CC7) transfer has been shown to improve function without compromising function from the donor

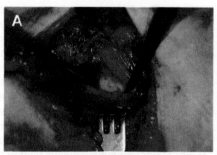 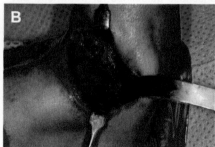

Fig. 3. (*A*) Anterior and inferior capsular release via a posterior axillary approach. (*B*) A latissimus dorsi and teres major tendon transfer can be performed through the same approach. (Used with permission of Shriners Hospitals for Children–Philadelphia, Philadelphia, PA. All rights reserved.)

Table 1
Nerve transfers

Donor	Recipients
Spinal accessory	Suprascapular nerve
Radial (triceps)	Axillary
Ulnar	Axillary
Median	Axillary
Long thoracic	Axillary, suprascapular nerve, upper or lower subscapular nerve
Thoracodorsal	Axillary, suprascapular nerve, upper or lower subscapular nerve
Medial pectoral	Axillary, suprascapular nerve, upper or lower subscapular nerve
Intercostals	Axillary, suprascapular nerve, upper or lower subscapular nerve
Contralateral C7	C7, lower trunk

side.[7,8] So far, the CC7 has been transferred only to the lower and middle trunks, not the upper trunk. The transfer takes advantage of the inherent ability of the contralesional cerebral hemisphere to participate in the recovery of the injured limb by contributing neural signals via native connections.[17] Approximately 20% of the axons of the brachial plexus can be found in C7, and because C7 contributes primarily to the axonal redundancy of the upper limb with few specific functions, the risk of a clinically measurable loss on the donor side is minimal. The technique in a brachial plexus without prior injury is fairly straightforward, as compared with a CC7 transfer in the setting of a brachial plexus root avulsion. However, it does require a thorough understanding of and experience in brachial plexus surgery to mitigate the significant risks.

If there is EMG evidence of normal innervation of the muscles acting on the shoulder, other nerve transfer donors are available, including the spinal accessory, radial, ulnar, median, long thoracic, thoracodorsal, medial pectoral, and intercostals (**Table 1**).

SUMMARY

Managing spasticity of the shoulder, as with any other joint, requires a global understanding of the patient's unique abilities, limitations, and goals. Improving shoulder function has been notoriously difficult in this population. As a result, realistic goals of surgery typically include improvements in joint contracture, passive shoulder

manipulation, and hygiene. Unlike in the forearm, wrist, and hand, tendon transfers for shoulder-related spasticity are rarely performed, as functional donors are uncommonly available. Nerve transfers are emerging as a potential option, with the promise of replacing spasticity by reconnecting viable upper motor neurons with their target muscle.

REFERENCES

1. Van Heest AE, House JH, Cariello C. Upper extremity surgical treatment of cerebral palsy. J Hand Surg Am 1999;24(2):323–30.
2. Carroll RE. The surgical treatment of cerebral palsy. I. The upper extremity. Surg Clin North Am 1950;31(2):385–90.
3. Seruya M, Johnson J. Surgical treatment of pediatric upper limb spasticity: the shoulder. Semin Plast Surg 2016;30(1):45–50.
4. Makki D, Duodu J, Nixon M. Prevalence and pattern of upper limb involvement in cerebral palsy. J Child Orthop 2014;8:215–9.
5. Lightdale-Miric N, de Roode CP. Cerebral palsy. In: Kozin SH, Abzug J, Zlotolow DA, editors. The pediatric upper extremity. New York: Springer; 2014. p. 769–802.
6. Davids JR, Peace LC, Wagner LV, et al. Validation of the Shriners Hospital for Children Upper Extremity Evaluation (SHUEE) for children with hemiplegic cerebral palsy. J Bone Joint Surg Am 2006;88(2):326–33.
7. Xu WD, Hua XY, Zheng MX, et al. Contralateral C7 nerve root transfer in treatment of cerebral palsy in a child: case report. Microsurgery 2011;31:404–8.
8. Zheng M-X, Hua X-Y, Feng J-T, et al. Trial of contralateral seventh cervical nerve transfer for spastic arm paralysis. N Engl J Med 2018;378(1):22–34.
9. Domzalski M, Inan M, Littleton AG, et al. Pectoralis major release to improve shoulder abduction in children with cerebral palsy. J Pediatr Orthop 2007;27(4):457–61.
10. Namdari S, Alosh H, Baldwin K, et al. Outcomes of tendon fractional lengthenings to improve shoulder function in patients with spastic hemiparesis. J Shoulder Elbow Surg 2012;21(5):691–8.
11. Greenhill DA, Smith WR, Ramsey FV, et al. Double versus single tendon transfers to improve shoulder function in brachial plexus birth palsy. J Pediatr Orthop 2017. [Epub ahead of print].
12. Elhassan B, Bishop A, Shin A, et al. Shoulder tendon transfer options for adult patients with brachial plexus injury. J Hand Surg Am 2010;35(7):1211–9.
13. Booth CM, Cortina-Borja MJ, Theologis TN. Collagen accumulation in muscles of children with cerebral palsy and correlation with severity of spasticity. Dev Med Child Neurol 2001;43:314–20.

14. Burke D, Wissel J, Donnan GA. Pathophysiology of spasticity in stroke. Neurology 2013;80(3 Suppl 2): S20–6.

15. Peterson MD, Gordon PM, Hurvitz EA, et al. Secondary muscle pathology and metabolic dysregulation in adults with cerebral palsy. Am J Physiol Endocrinol Metab 2012;303(9):E1085–93.

16. Raghavan P, Lu Y, Mirchandani M, et al. Human recombinant hyaluronidase injections for upper limb muscle stiffness in individuals with cerebral injury: a case series. EBioMedicine 2016;9(C):306–13.

17. Buetefisch CM. Role of the contra-lesional hemisphere in post-stroke recovery of upper extremity motor function. Front Neurol 2015;6:214.

Management of Joint Contractures in the Spastic Upper Extremity

Kristi S. Wood, MD, MSc, FRCSC[a], Aaron Daluiski, MD[a,b],*

KEYWORDS

• Cerebral palsy • Joint contracture • Spastic contracture • Flexion contracture

KEY POINTS

• Limited joint range of motion in a patient with upper extremity spasticity not due to bony constraint can result from muscle spasticity or contractures of the muscle or joint.
• Splinting or serial casting can be a useful initial treatment.
• Chronic spasticity can lead to secondary changes in the muscle resulting in muscle contracture, which can subsequently lead to joint contracture.
• Identifying the cause of the deformity is critical for successful treatment.
• Botulinum toxin A (Botox) is a useful adjunct to differentiate between spasticity and contracture and to guide treatment; when Botox no longer provides relief of a spastic deformity, surgical intervention may be warranted.

INTRODUCTION

Joint contractures are common in patients with upper extremity spasticity and, as such, any treatment of spasticity should include means to prevent contractures. This lack of joint mobility is due to both primary spasticity and secondary contractures resulting from longstanding spasticity. Contractures can result in poor limb function, difficulties with activities of daily living, such as hygiene and dressing, and psychological distress due to appearance. The overarching goals of treatment for these patients include improving function, which allows for greater independence, hygiene, and appearance.

CAUSE OF JOINT CONTRACTURES

Joint contractures are defined by decreased range of motion (ROM) of the affected joint. Although this term is nonspecific, patients with upper extremity spasticity-related joint contractures typically result from 3 interrelated physiologic mechanisms:

1. Primary spasticity
2. Muscular fibrosis/contraction
3. Intrinsic joint contracture

These mechanisms typically occur sequentially and are summarized in **Fig. 1**.

Spasticity

As referenced in O'Dwyer[1], Lance concisely defined spasticity as a "motor disorder characterized by a velocity-dependent increase in tonic stretch reflexes ("muscle tone") with exaggerated tendon jerks, resulting from hyperexcitability of the stretch reflex, as one component of the upper motor neuron syndrome".[1] Spasticity of particular

Disclosure: The authors have no commercial or financial conflicts of interest to disclose.
[a] Department of Pediatric Orthopaedic Surgery, Hospital for Special Surgery, 535 East 70th Street, 5th Floor, New York, NY 10021, USA; [b] Department of Hand and Upper Extremity, Hospital for Special Surgery, 523 East 72nd Street, 4th Floor, New York, NY 10021, USA
* Corresponding author. Department of Hand and Upper Extremity, Hospital for Special Surgery, 523 East 72nd Street, 4th Floor, New York, NY 10021.
E-mail address: DaluiskiA@HSS.EDU

Hand Clin 34 (2018) 517–528
https://doi.org/10.1016/j.hcl.2018.06.011

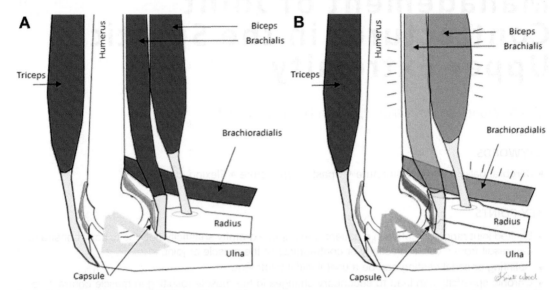

Fig. 1. (*A*) A normal elbow and (*B*) an elbow with spastic contractures. Contracture can be due to spastic and/or fibrotic flexors (biceps, brachialis, brachioradialis), tight capsule, tight ligaments, and/or dislocated radial head.

muscle groups or imbalance of muscular forces around a joint leads to limited ROM of a joint. It is important to appreciate the role of spasticity as the initiating factor in muscle and joint contracture development.

Muscle Contracture

A muscle contracture refers to a shortening of muscle length due to a decrease in the number of sarcomeres in series along the myofibrils, accompanied by an increase in the resistance to passive stretch.[1–5] Immobilization with the muscle in a shortened position produces decreased muscle fiber length, along with shortening of muscle connective tissue and an increase in muscle stiffness.[1] In patients with disruption of central command execution (ie, those at risk for spasticity), numerous peripheral effects occur because of immobilization of a joint in a fixed position or maintaining a muscle in a shortened position. In addition to actual spastic shortening, secondary causes for muscle shortening or contraction include muscle atrophy, sarcomere loss, accumulation of intramuscular connective tissue, increased muscular fat content, degenerative changes at the myotendinous junction, and an increase in mechanical spindle stimulation by stretch.[6] One study found that the muscle shortening occurs at the fascicle level in patients after spinal cord injury.[7] Taken together, these suggest that chronic spasticity will lead to changes in the muscle resulting in less contractility and elasticity due to increased

muscle stiffness; this ultimately can lead to contracture. Maintaining muscle length and joint mobility is therefore important in preventing the onset of contractures.[8]

Once an upper extremity joint contracture occurs, successful treatment requires an understanding of the primary cause. Elucidating whether the cause of the limited ROM is due to spasticity alone or the secondary effects of muscle contracture can be challenging. Botulinum toxin type A (Botox) can be a useful diagnostic tool in making this distinction.

Shear wave elastography is an ultrasound tool that provides direct quantitative in vivo measurement of tissue material properties.[9–11] Multiple ultrasound push beams are used to induce the shear waves, and subsequently, to measure the shear wave speed in muscle. The shear wave speed is related to material properties, such that shear waves travel faster through stiffer tissues. As such, higher velocities indicate stiffer tissues[9] and can be associated with increased spasticity.[12]

Studies on the use of shear wave sonoelastography evaluation of muscle have shown potential for assessing structural changes in muscles, which may in turn prove useful in prognostication, evaluation, and treatment of spasticity.[11,13–16] When combined with the Modified Ashworth Scale, spasticity can be better quantified.[14] In addition, it may become a readily available tool that can assess the effect of Botox on a spastic muscle[17] or potentially predict poor candidates through assessing the extent of chronic changes within muscle structure.[18]

Joint Contracture

Joint contracture is typically due to a combination of soft tissue contracture of the ligaments around a joint and the joint capsule itself. The mechanism of joint contracture in spastic paresis is similar to that of immobilized limbs. Animal studies on immobilized limbs have demonstrated "proliferation of fibrofatty connective tissue within the joint space, adhesions between synovial folds, adherence of fibrofatty connective tissue to cartilage surfaces, atrophy of cartilage, ulcerations at points of cartilage-cartilage contact, disorganizations of cellular and fibrillary ligament alignment and regional osteoporosis of the involved extremity."[6] Gracies[6] and Trudel and colleagues[19] also describe increasing evidence that immobilized joints adapt to their new position by modifying the length of some compartments of the synovial intima. It has been shown that adhesions of synovial villi rather than a proliferation of pannus are the main intra-articular changes leading to contracture after immobility.[6,20]

JOINT SUBLUXATIONS AND DISLOCATIONS

Limited joint ROM in patients with spasticity can also result from a subluxated or dislocated joint. Radiologic imaging of a joint with limited motion is therefore a critical component of evaluating and managing spasticity associated with joint contractures. Literature on upper extremity dislocations secondary to spasticity is sparse, with only case reports regarding the shoulder and elbow.

Shoulder

Although rare, glenohumeral subluxation can occur due to spasticity and can be a source of pain.[21] Although this is more commonly seen in patients after stroke and traumatic brain injury (TBI), there are case reports in patients with cerebral palsy (CP).[22,23] Spasticity and increased muscle tone can occur within a few weeks after stroke and TBI and usually affect the shoulder adductors and internal rotators. Spasticity can be, and subluxation is often, self-limited, although in some patients these findings persist.[24]

Even with dynamic electromyography (EMG), identifying affected muscles can be difficult. Botox may play a diagnostic role by identifying which muscles are involved and thus most amenable to surgery. Botox may be therapeutically useful in patients with more severe spasticity immediately following a brain injury in order to prevent the development of fixed contractures with associated glenohumeral subluxation.

A biceps suspension procedure is one technique used for inferior glenohumeral subluxation with functional impairment. In one report, more than half of the 11 patients that underwent this procedure also had extra-articular tenotomies to treat coexisting muscular contractures.[24] They reported significant improvements in abduction and external rotation as well as in extension and forward elevation, suggesting that additional soft tissue releases may be beneficial. It is also important to evaluate for dislocation or degenerative disease of the shoulder if motion is limited, because treatment approaches may differ from management of spasticity.

Elbow

Nontraumatic radial head dislocation occurring in the setting of spasticity is primarily seen in patients with CP, as opposed to other causes of spasticity. Although infrequently reported, the association of radial head dislocation with flexion contracture of the elbow and contracture of the forearm pronators is known to exist.[25] Pletcher and colleagues[26] described 9 elbows with radial head dislocations in patients with CP, with 8 being bilateral and posterior and 1 being unilateral and anterior. Of the 368 elbows surveyed, the incidence was 2.4% overall and 27% in those with elbow flexion and forearm pronation contractures. Yasuda and colleagues[27] reported an incidence of 3% in 100 patients with CP. A radiographic retrospective review of 96 patients with CP identified a 2% incidence of radial head dislocation.[28] Another report of 10 radial head dislocations in 8 patients compared treatment with radial head excision to open reduction of the radial head with reconstruction of the annular ligament. All excision patients remained pain free, and all reconstruction patients redislocated within 16 weeks. As a result, they recommended excision of the radial head in patients with established symptomatic dislocation.[29] However, Garg and colleagues[30] presented a patient managed with release of aponeurosis of the flexor-pronator origin and the bicipital aponeurosis, followed by reconstruction of the annular ligament with triceps aponeurosis and proximal radioulnar joint pinning. This patient had maintenance of reduction at 5-year follow-up. Although the existing data are inconclusive regarding optimal management of this rare entity, the authors' experience suggests that these patients do not have symptoms related to their radial head subluxation and therefore do not benefit from surgical reconstruction.

Although the reported incidence is between 2% and 3%, the true incidence of radial head dislocation as sequelae of chronic pronation-flexion spasticity and muscle imbalance is unknown. The unknown nature is multifactorial and relates to the presence of painless dislocations, dislocations with minimal limitations of function, severe contractures of the elbow limiting examination, and other spine and lower extremity deformities taking precedence.[29,30]

COMMON JOINT CONTRACTURES

The more commonly found contractures of the upper extremity are shoulder adduction and internal rotation (more than abduction and external rotation), elbow flexion, forearm pronation, wrist flexion, thumb-in-palm (adduction) deformity, and finger flexion contractures.[21,31–33] Around the shoulder, the pectoralis major, latissimus dorsi, teres major, and long head of triceps are most commonly involved.[31] Elbow flexion contracture results from spasticity of the biceps brachii, brachialis, and brachioradialis.[33] Pronation deformity occurs primarily because of spasticity of the pronator teres (PT), and although secondary contracture of the interosseous membrane has been described, the authors have never encountered this in their patient population.

Wrist and finger flexion is caused by spastic or contracted wrist flexors coupled with weak wrist extensors. The flexed position can weaken grip by decreasing the tenodesis effect that occurs with wrist extension. Thumb-in-palm deformity is complex and can be due to spasticity or contracture of adductor pollicis, flexor pollicis brevis, first dorsal interosseous, flexor pollicis longus, abductor pollicis longus, extensor pollicis brevis, and extensor pollicis longus. Metacarpophalangeal (MCP) joint and proximal interphalangeal (PIP) joint contractures tend to occur in conjunction. The most common finding resulting from spastic intrinsic muscles is MCP joint flexion and PIP joint extension, which may ultimately result in a swan-neck deformity. Typically, the deformity is more of a cosmetic concern, however can become functionally limiting if severe. MCP joint flexion can worsen after correction of a wrist flexion deformity because of the effective loss of extensor digitorum communis strength.[33]

PATIENT EVALUATION

A limb with fixed joints may be due to any of the causes previously discussed: severe spasticity or contracture of muscles, tendons, or joint capsule and ligaments. Evaluation should proceed with each of these possibilities in mind. The patient should be observed for asymmetry in form or movement. Muscles should be palpated for tone and assessed for muscle strength. ROM, both passive and active, may provide clues to motor control. Triceps brachii, biceps brachii, and brachioradialis reflexes should be tested with a reflex hammer as a means to assess for the presence of spasticity. Spasticity can also be graded by resistance to passive movement, using the Ashworth scale.[31]

TREATMENT OPTIONS
Nonoperative: General

Physical therapy, including passive ROM, splint use, and teaching of adaptive strategies, is a key component to nonoperative management of spasticity and secondary contractures. Therapy is aimed not only at preserving or improving joint mobility but also at stimulating the region of the sensorimotor cortex homunculus dedicated to the hand.[34] Bimanual activity encourages the use of the affected extremity. Constraint-induced therapy (CIT) is used in hemiplegic patients and involves intensive functional training of the more affected upper extremity during which the less affected side is restrained. A recent randomized controlled trial reported better spatial and temporal efficiency, in the form of smoother movement, more efficient grasping, and better movement preplanning and execution for functional improvement up to 6 months after treatment compared with traditional rehabilitation using unimanual or bimanual therapy.[35] However, in general, intensive activity-based, goal-directed interventions, such as both bimanual therapy and CIT, are more effective than standard therapy,[36] and a recent systematic review comparing bimanual therapy and CIT could not conclude superiority of either method.[37]

Splinting can be initiated as a primary treatment method to both prevent and treat joint contractures. Various options exist including static progressive, dynamic, and static resting splints. Splinting is contraindicated in severe spasticity, however, because "rebound" spasticity can lead to skin breakdown.[33] The choice of splint is dependent on the patient, their level of spasticity, and degree of contracture. An in-depth review of splinting options and indications is beyond the scope of this article.

Botox chemically blocks the release of acetylcholine at the presynaptic neuromuscular junction, resulting in temporary weakness of the injected muscle.[33,38] It can be useful not only as a therapeutic intervention for spasticity but also as a diagnostic aid in determining muscle involvement in spastic joint deformities. Based on muscle response, this may provide insight into potential beneficial interventions.[39] For example, preoperative administration of Botox might reveal that a tendon lengthening would be ineffective in the setting of a joint capsule contracture or if muscle contracture is due to fibrosis, rather than spasticity alone. Botox injection can also be used to temporarily decrease spasticity to allow more intense therapy to resolve tightness. The use of Botox may be helpful, for example, in children during times of rapid growth when spasticity can increase, resulting in increased stiffness.

Operative Management: General

As the contracture may result from either soft tissue (muscle/tendon) or joint capsule contracture, both must be considered when addressing the fixed deformity. Results of previous clinical examinations and treatments may help guide surgical decisions and predict postoperative outcomes. Care must be taken to avoid neurovascular injury due to stretch from a shortened position after other structures are released. After appropriate musculotendinous releases have been performed, if the joint still remains contracted, a joint capsular release can be considered.

Joint-Specific Management

Shoulder
Nonoperative Physical therapy should be aimed at improving joint ROM. Resistance bands may be a useful tool to stretch the shoulder in abduction and external rotation.

Operative
Subscapularis Z-lengthening or release
This procedure has been reported to increase shoulder ROM, but is rarely needed in the authors' practice.

Indications include failed nonoperative treatment of shoulder internal rotation contracture or recurrent axillary hygiene issues.[33,40,41]

Indications
- Failed nonoperative treatment of shoulder internal rotation contracture
- Recurrent axillary hygiene issues

Technique
- Deltopectoral or axillary incision
- Pectoralis major tendon identified along the posterior surface of the muscle
- Fractional lengthening at the pectoralis major musculotendinous junction (MTJ)
- Deepen deltopectoral interval to expose subscapularis
- Identify the subscapularis tendon insertion on the lesser tuberosity

- Divide or Z-lengthen the subscapularis tendon
  - Z-lengthening preserves some tendon function, preventing excessive external rotation and helping to prevent anterior shoulder dislocation
- Subscapularis lengthening can also be done using a muscle slide through a longitudinal incision along the lateral border of the scapula
- Subscapularis is elevated extraperiosteally from the anterior scapula beginning inferiorly and progressing superiorly

Postoperative management
- Shoulder abduction sling for 4 to 6 weeks
- Therapy for ROM to begin at 4 to 6 weeks, or earlier if no tendon repair is performed

Humerus rotational osteotomy
A rotational osteotomy is used to reposition the limb.[33] Indications include an extremely contracted shoulder not amenable to soft tissue release.

Technique
- Medial, lateral, or deltopectoral approach
- Expose humeral diaphysis
- Choose a 6- or 8-hole plate; plate thickness depends on humerus size (3.5 mm often adequate)
- Fix to humerus proximal to planned osteotomy site
- Elevate periosteum only at osteotomy site
- A Kirschner wire (K wire) is placed in the distal fragment to mark the desired rotation, to be in line with a hole of the plate once rotated. A second K wire can be used in a plate hole to more easily measure the planned degree of rotation
- Alternatively, 2 K wires can be placed separate from the plate and the angle between them measured to calculate their ultimate position after rotational correction to ensure the desired rotation is obtained
- Remove plate and perform osteotomy with oscillating saw; irrigate to reduce thermal injury
- Rotate the humerus to the desired amount of correction, so the distal K wire and screw holes align, or so the angle between the 2 K wires measures the calculated amount
- Affix the plate to the proximal fragment
- Reduce the osteotomy and place screws in the distal fragment, using standard compression techniques

Postoperative management
- Bulky dressing (hand to shoulder)
- Sling to prevent stress across osteotomy site
- Remove dressings and provide custom humeral brace 3 weeks after surgery

- Brace is worn for 4 to 6 weeks until radiographic and clinical union

Elbow

As indicated previously, it is critical to identify the cause of the deformity, in order to target the exact structures to be released or lengthened.

Elbow flexor tendon lengthenings for dynamic or fixed spastic contractures

For contracture originating from muscle, individual lengthening or release of the biceps, brachialis, and/or brachioradialis can be performed.[33,41–49] The authors prefer fractional lengthening for most cases; however, in severe contractures, a Z-lengthening of biceps may be required.

Indications include spastic flexion contracture of the elbow.

Contraindications include skin (relative) and joint contractures and weakness in active elbow flexion, because this can be worsened after lengthening and compromise hand-to-mouth function.

Technique

- Lazy-S incision in antecubital fossa (**Fig. 2**)
- Mobilize or ligate antecubital veins
- Identify and protect
  - Lateral antebrachial cutaneous nerve, extending between biceps and brachialis
  - Median nerve and brachial artery deep to lacertus fibrosus
  - Radial nerve exiting between brachioradialis and brachialis

- Release the lacertus fibrosis, extending medially off of the biceps tendon
- Treat contracted muscles
  - Brachioradialis: isolate from extensor carpi radialis brevis (ECRB) and radial nerve and myotomize directly from humerus using cautery
  - Brachialis: fractional lengthening of the tendon at myotendinous junction
  - Biceps: fractional lengthening or Z-lengthening depending on severity of flexion and supination preoperatively
- The neurovascular bundle may limit attempts at full passive extension; this finding may eliminate the benefit of any simultaneous capsular release. If the neurovascular structures are not under tension, release the capsule
- If the biceps tendon is Z-lengthened, repair tendon via tendon weave or end-to-end repair
- Skin closure with absorbable sutures

Postoperative management

- Long arm cast with elbow in the maximum allowable extension, for 3 to 4 weeks, longer if more severe contracture
- Custom splint and initiate therapy at 3 weeks
- Serial casting can be used if further gains in elbow position are required after all releases

Forearm

Forearm contractures are typically positioned in pronation. Surgical options for forearm

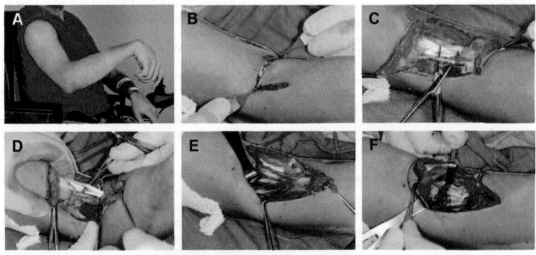

Fig. 2. Elbow contracture release. (*A*) Preoperative elbow flexion contracture; passive extension lacking at least 90°. (*B*) "Z"-plasty incision in antecubital fossa. (*C*) Identify and protect the lateral antebrachial cutaneous nerve. (*D, E*) After incising the lacertus fibrosus on the medial edge of biceps tendon, the biceps tendon is Z-lengthened. Repair is performed at the completion of the release before closure. (*F*) Brachialis is identified and the neurovascular bundle is retracted gently medially. A fractional lengthening of brachialis is performed. Brachioradialis has been isolated and myotomized with cautery off of the humerus (not shown). Care must be taken to protect the radial nerve and ECRB. (Used with permission of Shriners Hospitals for Children–Philadelphia. All rights reserved.)

contracture include a simple release, tendon transfer (PT rerouting), osteotomy of the radius and/or ulna, or the one-bone forearm procedure. Although a flexor-pronator origin muscle slide can release a pronation contracture as well as an elbow flexion contracture, it is more commonly used for wrist flexion contracture.

Pronator teres rerouting
This procedure is done to convert the PT into a forearm supinator.[33,50–54]

Indications include active control of pronation and lack of active supination, with full passive supination.

Contraindications include patients lacking active control of pronation, which will cause the tendon to tether rather than actively supinate.

Technique
- Longitudinal incision over the radial aspect of the forearm
- Develop the interval between the brachioradialis and the wrist extensors
- Protect the radial sensory nerve found deep to brachioradialis
- Identify the PT proximal insertion just proximal to the radial sensory nerve
- Release PT insertion with periosteal sleeve and mobilize the tendon proximally
- Incise a window in the interosseous membrane
- Pass the PT tendon through the window from volar to dorsal and around the radius, attaching to its original insertion site with transosseous sutures or suture anchors with the forearm supinated

Postoperative management
- Immobilization with forearm in neutral or partial supination for 4 weeks
- Removable splint for an additional 4 weeks in the same position
- Initiate therapy at 4 weeks postoperatively

Wrist and Digits

Nonoperative
Static wrist splints can be used to prevent progression of a contracture. The authors do not use static progressive splinting at the wrist.

Operative
To provide the most appropriate surgical management of the wrist and digits, it is critical to evaluate the extent of joint contracture, in addition to tone and muscle spasticity of the flexors and extensors.[33] Utilization of median and/or ulnar nerve block may help uncover joint involvement.[55]

In severe fixed wrist capsular contractures, a proximal row carpectomy (PRC) may be helpful to allow extension of the wrist to neutral before a tendon transfer can be performed. However, PRC yields only a small gain in passive wrist extension. Wrist arthrodesis may be used in severe cases. Although this may decrease function due to the loss of the tenodesis effect at the wrist, a solid fusion typically results and remains durable. **Fig. 3** describes the steps in a PRC/arthrodesis. In the authors' practice, bony procedures are reserved for skeletally mature patients.

Flexor-pronator slide
Indications include wrist flexion contracture and forearm pronation contracture in a highly functioning patient.[33,56,57] Contraindications include differential involvement of the finger and wrist flexors, because this procedure does not allow for release of individual muscles.

Technique

- Extensile incision along medial forearm from above the elbow to the ulnar styloid at the wrist
- Identify ulnar nerve and trace through cubital tunnel, ensuring complete release proximally from fascia and arcade of Struthers to allow for anterior transposition
- While protecting the brachial vessels and median and ulnar nerves, the flexor-pronator mass is incised directly off ulna, down to the medial collateral ligament, which is preserved
- Release flexor-pronator muscle mass sequentially to the wrist
- Continue in an ulnar to radial direction
- Protect anterior interosseous nerve and artery during dissection superficial to these structures until radius is encountered
- Release any taut muscle that originates from the radius proximally, until wrist and fingers can be extended completely
- Standard layered closure

Postoperative management

- Long-arm cast applied with wrists and digits in extension, forearm in midsupination
- Cast for 4 weeks: elbow at 45° flexion, forearm supinated, wrist and digits extended
- Removable splint for 4 more weeks, allowing ROM and therapy
- After 8 weeks, splinting at night only for 1 month

Flexor Tendon Tightness

Thumb and digital joint contractures are typically managed with soft tissue (skin and muscle)

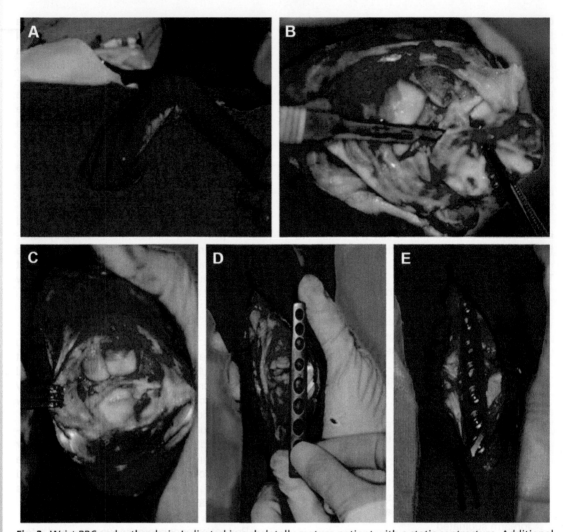

Fig. 3. Wrist PRC and arthrodesis. Indicated in a skeletally mature patient with a static contracture. Additional wrist flexor tenotomy may be required. (*A*) Resting wrist flexion contracture. (*B, C*) After dorsal incision and elevation/retraction of the extensor compartments, excision of proximal carpal row. Cartilage surfaces are denuded. (*D, E*) Plate fixation of the wrist from the radius to the third metacarpal in neutral flexion, with compression through the plate. Cancellous bone from excised carpals of the proximal row can be used as bone graft. (Used with permission of Shriners Hospitals for Children–Philadelphia. All rights reserved.)

releases. If the contracture remains despite soft tissue release, the joint capsule should also be released.

Thumb adductor release
Indications include adducted thumb metacarpal with no volitional control of the adductor pollicis.[33,58,59]

Technique
- Use a double-opposing Z-plasty of the first web space
- Identify the 2 heads of adductor pollicis and release from the thumb metacarpal
- Identify the origin of the first dorsal interosseous dorsal to the adductor and release
- Consider a capsulodesis or arthrodesis of the MCP joint if unstable
- Use 0.045-in K wires to stabilize the carpometacarpal joint in maximal extension and the MCP joint in 10° of flexion
- Immobilize with a thumb spica cast for 4 weeks
- Remove K wires at 4 weeks and apply a thumb spica splint for an additional 4 weeks
- Initiate ROM therapy at 4 weeks postoperatively

Fractional tendon lengthening

Indications include a functional hand where the digits can be fully straightened with the wrist flexed, but not with the wrist held passively at neutral.[33,60]

Contraindications include inability to fully extend the digits with the wrist flexed. This finding would require Z-lengthening or superficialis to profundus (STP) transfer in order to achieve an adequate release.

Technique
- Palpate MTJ of digital flexor tendons on mid-aspect of volar forearm
- Through a 4-cm longitudinal incision centered over this area, make 2 transverse tenotomies at least 1 cm apart in the MTJ of each tendon to be lengthened
- The distal tenotomy should be at least 2 cm proximal to the distal aspect of the MTJ
- Keep the muscular portion intact (only divide the tendinous portion)
- Hold the wrist in neutral and gently passively extend the digits just short of the desired length. Note: overcorrection will result in excessive weakening of flexor tendons
- Immobilize arm with the wrist in neutral for 4 weeks
- Unrestricted finger motion is allowed. Instruct patient on digital extension exercises
- Removable wrist splint after 4 weeks to allow ROM and therapy. Discontinue at 8 weeks.

Interosseous muscle slide

Indications include MCP joint flexion inhibiting hand function or causing interdigital hygiene problems.[33,61,62]

Relative contraindications include concerns regarding cosmesis in the absence of functional deficits.

Technique
- Transverse incision on dorsum of hand at mid-metacarpal level, or 2 longitudinal incisions in the interspaces between the index/long and ring/little fingers
- Interosseous muscles identified with retraction of extensor tendons
- Subperiosteal dissection to release both the dorsal and the volar interosseous muscles
- MCP joints brought into full extension with PIP joints flexed
- If MCP joint extension is tight, use a K wire to hold the joint in extension for 4 weeks
- Immobilize in full extension for 4 weeks and then switch to a removable splint for an additional 4 weeks

Intrinsic lateral band release

Indications include intrinsic muscle contracture for which a dynamic EMG shows no volitional activity.[33,63]

Technique
- Midline longitudinal incision over dorsum of MCP joint and proximal phalanx of each finger
- Dissection on ulnar and radial sides of extensor mechanism
- Identify palmar edge of lateral bands and then transect both the lateral band and the oblique fibers of the extensor hood
- Be careful to preserve the transverse fibers of the sagittal extensor hood
- Consider concomitant neurectomy of the motor branch of the ulnar nerve in the Guyon canal to prevent recurrent deformity

Swan-neck deformity

Central slip tenotomy is a reliable treatment of dynamic swan-neck deformity in CP without an MCP joint flexion deformity.[64]

Indications include greater than 20° of hyperextension at the PIP joint.

Contraindications include inability to flex PIP joint when the digit is held with the deformity corrected.

Technique
- Central slip released through transverse incision proximal to PIP joint, while preserving the adjacent lateral bands
- PIP joint pinned in 10° of flexion for 4 weeks
- Active extension to 10° short of full extension, blocked with oval-8 splint

Metacarpophalangeal joint arthrodesis

Indications include significant MCP joint flexion deformity and fixed contracture that does not improve with ulnar nerve block.[33,65]

Contraindications include nonfunctioning long digital flexors; otherwise MCP joint fusion will eliminate any functional digit flexion.

Technique
- Longitudinal incision over each MCP joint to be fused
- Incise extensor hood and capsule longitudinally
- Release collateral ligaments from metacarpal head
- Remove articular surfaces of metacarpal head and base of proximal phalanx with oscillating saw
- Perform osteotomies to ensure appropriate cascade, from 25° for the index to 40° to the small finger, increasing by 5° with each digit

- Ensure no radial or ulnar angulation
- Fixation can be held with a 2.0-mm contoured plate, a headless compression screw, or K wires
- Close capsule and extensor hood with interrupted nonabsorbable sutures
- Immobilize hand for 4 weeks in forearm-based extension splint with wrist in neutral and digits extended followed by a custom palm-based splint across MCP joints with PIP joints free until bony union

Intrinsic-minus deformity

This deformity manifests as a claw hand, with hyperextension of the MCP joints and flexion of the PIP and DIP joints.[66] Although an exhaustive description of all surgical options will not be covered in this section, there are a few points relevant to management of this deformity. The MCP joint capsule may require surgical release, followed by pinning of the MCP joints in a reduced position for 4 weeks. The digital flexion deformity may also require lengthening of the extrinsic digital flexors or an STP transfer. In cases whereby the hyperextension deformity is not correctable with a soft tissue release alone, a closing wedge flexion osteotomy of the distal metacarpal corrects the deformity and lessens the chance of compromising the viability of skin overlying the dorsal MCP joint. The osteotomy is fixed with a small dorsal plate or wires.

SUMMARY

Contractures of the spastic upper extremity may be due to spasticity alone, muscle contracture, or joint contracture. Determination of the underlying cause is critical to ensuring successful treatment. Initial management consists of physical therapy and splinting. Botox can be a useful adjunct, not only in relieving spasticity but also by helping determine the underlying cause of the contracture. Surgical management consists of release or lengthening of the causative muscle/tendon unit with subsequent joint capsular release, as required. Postoperative splinting maintains the newly gained ROM and protects any associated tendon lengthening or transfer.

REFERENCES

1. O'Dwyer NJ, Ada L, Neilson PD. Spasticity and muscle contracture following stroke. Brain 1996;119(Pt 5):1737–49.
2. Lance J. Symposium synopsis. In: Feldman RG, Young RR, Koella WP, editors. Spasticity: disordered motor control. Miami (FL): Symposia Specialists; 1980. p. 485–94.
3. Tardieu C, Huet de la Tour E, Bret MD, et al. Muscle hypoextensibility in children with cerebral palsy: I. Clinical and experimental observations. Arch Phys Med Rehabil 1982;63(3):97–102.
4. Bax MC, Brown JK. Contractures and their therapy. Dev Med Child Neurol 1985;27(4):423–4.
5. O'Dwyer NJ, Neilson PD, Nash J. Mechanisms of muscle growth related to muscle contracture in cerebral palsy. Dev Med Child Neurol 1989;31(4): 543–7.
6. Gracies JM. Pathophysiology of spastic paresis. I: paresis and soft tissue changes. Muscle Nerve 2005;31(5):535–51.
7. Kwah LK, Herbert RD, Harvey LA, et al. Passive mechanical properties of gastrocnemius muscles of people with ankle contracture after stroke. Arch Phys Med Rehabil 2012;93(7):1185–90.
8. Cloodt E, Rosenblad A, Rodby-Bousquet E. Demographic and modifiable factors associated with knee contracture in children with cerebral palsy. Dev Med Child Neurol 2018;60(4):391–6.
9. Lee SS, Gaebler-Spira D, Zhang LQ, et al. Use of shear wave ultrasound elastography to quantify muscle properties in cerebral palsy. Clin Biomech (Bristol, Avon) 2016;31:20–8.
10. Bercoff J, Tanter M, Fink M. Supersonic shear imaging: a new technique for soft tissue elasticity mapping. IEEE Trans Ultrason Ferroelectr Freq Control 2004;51(4):396–409.
11. Jakubowski KL, Terman A, Santana RVC, et al. Passive material properties of stroke-impaired plantarflexor and dorsiflexor muscles. Clin Biomech (Bristol, Avon) 2017;49:48–55.
12. Wu CH, Ho YC, Hsiao MY, et al. Evaluation of poststroke spastic muscle stiffness using shear wave ultrasound elastography. Ultrasound Med Biol 2017; 43(6):1105–11.
13. Mathevon L, Michel F, Aubry S, et al. Two-dimensional and shear wave elastography ultrasound: a reliable method to analyse spastic muscles? Muscle Nerve 2018;57(2):222–8.
14. Ceyhan-Bilgici M, Bekci T, Ulus Y, et al. Quantitative assessment of muscle stiffness with acoustic radiation force impulse elastography after botulinum toxin A injection in children with cerebral palsy. J Med Ultrason (2001) 2018;45(1):137–41.
15. Jiang L, Wei X, Wang Q, et al. Study based on sonoelastography technology for spastic gastrocnemius in rat with spinal cord injure. Zhonghua Yi Xue Za Zhi 2016;96(5):364–9 [in Chinese].
16. Eby SF, Zhao H, Song P, et al. Quantifying spasticity in individual muscles using shear wave elastography. Radiol Case Rep 2017;12(2):348–52.
17. Brandenburg JE, Eby SF, Song P, et al. Quantifying effect of onabotulinum toxin A on passive muscle stiffness in children with cerebral palsy using ultrasound shear wave elastography. Am J Phys Med

Rehabil 2018. https://doi.org/10.1097/PHM.0000000000000907.

18. Liu KH, Bhatia K, Chu W, et al. Shear wave elastography–a new quantitative assessment of post-irradiation neck fibrosis. Ultraschall Med 2015;36(4):348–54.

19. Trudel G, Jabi M, Uhthoff HK. Localized and adaptive synoviocyte proliferation characteristics in rat knee joint contractures secondary to immobility. Arch Phys Med Rehabil 2003;84(9):1350–6.

20. Trudel G, Seki M, Uhthoff HK. Synovial adhesions are more important than pannus proliferation in the pathogenesis of knee joint contracture after immobilization: an experimental investigation in the rat. J Rheumatol 2000;27(2):351–7.

21. Manara JR, Taylor J, Nixon M. Management of shoulder pain after a cerebrovascular accident or traumatic brain injury. J Shoulder Elbow Surg 2015;24(5):823–9.

22. Namdari S, Keenan MA. Treatment of glenohumeral arthrosis and inferior shoulder subluxation in an adult with cerebral palsy: a case report. J Bone Joint Surg Am 2011;93(23):e1401–5.

23. de-Boer KS, Rozing PM, Arendzen JH. Treatment of recurrent posterior dislocation of the shoulder in cerebral palsy by injection with botulinum toxin A into the M. subscapularis. Clin Rehabil 2004;18(7):764–6.

24. Namdari S, Keenan MA. Outcomes of the biceps suspension procedure for painful inferior glenohumeral subluxation in hemiplegic patients. J Bone Joint Surg Am 2010;92(15):2589–97.

25. Subbarao JV, Kumar VN. Spontaneous dislocation of the radial head in cerebral palsy. Orthop Rev 1987;16(7):457–61.

26. Pletcher DF, Hoffer MM, Koffman DM. Non-traumatic dislocation of the radial head in cerebral palsy. J Bone Joint Surg Am 1976;58(1):104–5.

27. Yasuda H, Sakai K, Higashi T, et al. Physical and radiographic assessment of wrist joint for cerebral palsied adult. Central Jpn J Orthop Surg Traumatol 1988;33:1354–5. (in Japanese).

28. Nishioka E, Yoshida K, Yamanaka K, et al. Radiographic studies of the wrist and elbow in cerebral palsy. J Orthop Sci 2000;5(3):268–74.

29. Abu-Sneineh AK, Gabos PG, Miller F. Radial head dislocation in children with cerebral palsy. J Pediatr Orthop 2003;23(2):155–8.

30. Garg R, Fung BK, Chow SP, et al. Surgical management of radial head dislocation in quadriplegic cerebral palsy – a 5 year follow-up. J Hand Surg Eur Vol 2007;32(6):725–6.

31. Namdari S, Baldwin K, Horneff JG, et al. Orthopedic evaluation and surgical treatment of the spastic shoulder. Orthop Clin North Am 2013;44(4):605–14.

32. Tafti MA, Cramer SC, Gupta R. Orthopaedic management of the upper extremity of stroke patients. J Am Acad Orthop Surg 2008;16(8):462–70.

33. Kozin S, Lightdale-Miric N. Spasticity: cerebral palsy and traumatic brain injury. In: Wolfe SW, Hotchkiss RN, Kozin SH, et al, editors. Green's operative hand surgery, Vol. 2, 7th edition. Philadelphia: Elsevier; 2017. p. 1080–121.

34. Friel KM, Kuo HC, Fuller J, et al. Skilled bimanual training drives motor cortex plasticity in children with unilateral cerebral palsy. Neurorehabil Neural Repair 2016;30(9):834–44.

35. Chen HC, Chen CL, Kang LJ, et al. Improvement of upper extremity motor control and function after home-based constraint induced therapy in children with unilateral cerebral palsy: immediate and long-term effects. Arch Phys Med Rehabil 2014;95(8):1423–32.

36. Sakzewski L, Ziviani J, Boyd RN. Efficacy of upper limb therapies for unilateral cerebral palsy: a meta-analysis. Pediatrics 2014;133(1):e175–204.

37. Tervahauta MH, Girolami GL, Øberg GK. Efficacy of constraint-induced movement therapy compared with bimanual intensive training in children with unilateral cerebral palsy: a systematic review. Clin Rehabil 2017;31(11):1445–56.

38. Autti-Rämö I, Larsen A, Peltonen J, et al. Botulinum toxin injection as an adjunct when planning hand surgery in children with spastic hemiplegia. Neuropediatrics 2000;31(1):4–8.

39. Koman LA, Paterson Smith B, Balkrishnan R. Spasticity associated with cerebral palsy in children: guidelines for the use of botulinum A toxin. Paediatr Drugs 2003;5(1):11–23.

40. Landi A, Cavazza S, Caserta G, et al. The upper limb in cerebral palsy: surgical management of shoulder and elbow deformities. Hand Clin 2003;19(4):631–48, vii.

41. Koman LA, Gelberman RH, Toby EB, et al. Cerebral palsy. Management of the upper extremity. Clin Orthop Relat Res 1990;(253):62–74.

42. Anakwenze OA, Namdari S, Hsu JE, et al. Myotendinous lengthening of the elbow flexor muscles to improve active motion in patients with elbow spasticity following brain injury. J Shoulder Elbow Surg 2013;22(3):318–22.

43. Carlson MG, Hearns KA, Inkellis E, et al. Early results of surgical intervention for elbow deformity in cerebral palsy based on degree of contracture. J Hand Surg Am 2012;37(8):1665–71.

44. Dy CJ, Pean CA, Hearns KA, et al. Long-term results following surgical treatment of elbow deformity in patients with cerebral palsy. J Hand Surg Am 2013;38(12):2432–6.

45. Goldner J. Upper extremity reconstructive surgery in cerebral palsy or similar conditions. Instr Course Lect 1961;18:169–77.

46. Manske PR. Cerebral palsy of the upper extremity. Hand Clin 1990;6(4):697–709.

47. Manske PR, Langewisch KR, Strecker WB, et al. Anterior elbow release of spastic elbow flexion deformity in children with cerebral palsy. J Pediatr Orthop 2001;21(6):772–7.

48. Mital MA. Lengthening of the elbow flexors in cerebral palsy. J Bone Joint Surg Am 1979;61(4):515–22.

49. Skoff H, Woodbury DF. Management of the upper extremity in cerebral palsy. J Bone Joint Surg Am 1985;67(3):500–3.

50. Bunata RE. Pronator teres rerouting in children with cerebral palsy. J Hand Surg Am 2006;31(3):474–82.

51. de-Roode CP, James MA, Van Heest AE. Tendon transfers and releases for the forearm, wrist, and hand in spastic hemiplegic cerebral palsy. Tech Hand Up Extrem Surg 2010;14(2):129–34.

52. Gschwind CR. Surgical management of forearm pronation. Hand Clin 2003;19(4):649–55.

53. Sakellarides HT, Mital MA, Lenzi WD. Treatment of pronation contractures of the forearm in cerebral palsy by changing the insertion of the pronator radii teres. J Bone Joint Surg Am 1981;63(4):645–52.

54. Strecker WB, Emanuel JP, Dailey L, et al. Comparison of pronator tenotomy and pronator rerouting in children with spastic cerebral palsy. J Hand Surg Am 1988;13(4):540–3.

55. Manske P, Strecker W. Cerebral palsy, brain injury, stroke - spastic disorders of the upper extremity. In: Peimer C, editor. Surgery of the hand and upper extremity, Vol. 2. New York: McGraw-Hill; 1996. p. 1517–38.

56. El-Said NS. Selective release of the flexor origin with transfer of flexor carpi ulnaris in cerebral palsy. J Bone Joint Surg Br 2001;83(2):259–62.

57. Thevenin-Lemoine C, Denormandie P, Schnitzler A, et al. Flexor origin slide for contracture of spastic finger flexor muscles: a retrospective study. J Bone Joint Surg Am 2013;95(5):446–53.

58. Hoffer MM, Perry J, Garcia M, et al. Adduction contracture of the thumb in cerebral palsy. A preoperative electromyographic study. J Bone Joint Surg Am 1983;65(6):755–9.

59. Keats S. Surgical treatment of the hand in cerebral palsy: correction of thumb-in-palm and other deformities. Report of nineteen cases. J Bone Joint Surg Am 1965;47:274–84.

60. Le-Viet D. Flexor tendon lengthening by tenotomy at the musculotendinous junction. Ann Plast Surg 1986;17(3):239–46.

61. Matsuo T, Matsuo A, Hajime T, et al. Release of flexors and intrinsic muscles for finger spasticity in cerebral palsy. Clin Orthop Relat Res 2001;(384):162–8.

62. Smith R. Intrinsic muscles of the fingers: function, dysfunction and surgical reconstruction. Instr Course Lect 1975;24:200–20.

63. Keenan M, Kozin S, Berlet AC. Contracture releases in the non-functional arm. In: Keenan M, Kozin S, Berlet A, editors. Manual of orthopaedic surgery for spasticity. New York: Raven Press; 1993.

64. Carlson MG, Gallagher K, Spirtos M. Surgical treatment of swan-neck deformity in hemiplegic cerebral palsy. J Hand Surg Am 2007;32(9):1418–22.

65. Ledgard JP, Tonkin MA. Simultaneous four finger metacarpophalangeal joint fusions - indications and results. Hand Surg 2014;19(1):69–76.

66. Sapienza A, Green S. Correction of the claw hand. Hand Clin 2012;28(1):53–66.

Technical Pearls of Tendon Transfers for Upper Extremity Spasticity

Samir K. Trehan, MD[a], Kevin J. Little, MD[a,b],*

KEYWORDS

- Tendon transfers • Cerebral palsy • Tetraplegia • Wrist deformity • Wrist spasticity
- Finger spasticity

KEY POINTS

- Successful tendon transfer surgery depends on a thorough preoperative clinical evaluation, understanding of tendon transfer biomechanics, appropriate donor and recipient selection, technical execution, and postoperative rehabilitation.
- Tendon transfer pillars include matching donor and recipient work capacity, excursion, and synergy; maintaining a straight line of pull; ensuring single donor function; and minimizing tendon donor morbidity.
- Flexor carpi ulnaris to extensor carpi radialis brevis, extensor carpi ulnaris to extensor carpi radialis brevis, and flexor digitorum profundus to superficialis transfers are some of the most common tendon transfers used for patients with upper extremity spasticity.

INTRODUCTION

Patients with upper extremity spasticity due to cerebral palsy, tetraplegia, traumatic brain injury, or stroke frequently display an imbalance of muscular forces acting across their joints. The treating surgeon must carefully evaluate their function and have a thorough knowledge of the fundamentals of treatment before initiating care. Surgical treatment may be indicated depending on functional goals and the magnitude of deformity and joint range of motion. Surgical options include tendon transfer, tendon lengthening, tenotomy, tenodesis, and arthrodesis. The goal of tendon transfer surgery in this setting is the restoration of muscle balance and active muscle control. Success after tendon transfer surgery depends on a thorough preoperative clinical evaluation, an understanding of tendon transfer biomechanics, appropriate donor and recipient muscle selection, technical execution, and postoperative rehabilitation.

PREOPERATIVE PATIENT EVALUATION

Tendon transfer surgical planning requires a thorough preoperative clinical evaluation. Before examining the involved extremity, overall functional status, social infrastructure, and psychological status should be assessed. Additionally the patients' and caregivers' goals for intervention should be assessed so that appropriate treatment strategies that best fit these goals can be devised. In patients with tetraplegia, the priorities for reconstruction are (from first to last): wrist extension, pinch, grasp, release, and intrinsic reconstruction.[1] Extremity examination should be detailed and methodical,

Disclosure Statement: The authors have no relevant financial disclosures.
[a] Pediatric Hand and Upper Extremity Center, Cincinnati Children's Hospital Medical Center, 3333 Burnet Avenue, ML 2017, Cincinnati, OH 45229, USA; [b] University of Cincinnati School of Medicine, 3230 Eden Avenue, Cincinnati, OH 45267, USA
* Corresponding author. Pediatric Hand and Upper Extremity Center, Cincinnati Children's Hospital Medical Center, 3333 Burnet Avenue, ML 2017, Cincinnati, OH 45229.
E-mail address: Kevin.Little@cchmc.org

Hand Clin 34 (2018) 529–536
https://doi.org/10.1016/j.hcl.2018.06.009
0749-0712/18/© 2018 Elsevier Inc. All rights reserved.

including observation of the skin and resting posture, joint stability and range of motion, muscle strength and activity, and neurovascular examination. Surgical indications are beyond the scope of this article; however, before considering tendon transfer surgery, several aspects of the physical examination are emphasized:

1. Joints affected by the planned procedure should be supple and without contracture. Joint stability must also be assessed because joint mobility outside of the anticipated range of motion can alter the line of pull of the tendon transfer and lead to suboptimal tensioning or joint contracture.
2. The function and activity of potential donor and recipient muscles (in addition to synergist or antagonist muscles) must be understood. Clinical examination can be supplemented with other data sources, such as dynamic electromyography, motion analysis, and video review of patients performing standardized tasks.[2–4] A thorough understanding of muscular balance is required to ensure appropriate donor and recipient muscle selection and prevent iatrogenic harm.
3. Potential donor muscle strength should be at least 4+/5 because of the anticipated loss of at least 1 grade of strength postoperatively.[5,6]
4. Tendon transfer surgery timing is generally delayed until at least age 6 years in patients with cerebral palsy and at least 1 year after injury in spinal cord injury patients.

Contraindications to tendon transfer surgery in patients with upper extremity spasticity disorders include fixed joint contractures, spasticity in the planned donor muscle beyond voluntary control (dyskinesia), and lack of social infrastructure and/or psychological ability to comply with postoperative rehabilitation.[1] It is also important to note that tendon transfers can be performed in combination with other techniques such as arthrodesis and/or tenodesis.

Patient evaluation by the surgeon or therapist may include 1 of several scales to assess baseline functional status and/or improvement. The House classification ranges from grade 0 (does not use) to 8 (spontaneous, complete use). Grades 1 to 3 are characterized by a passive assist hand, grades 4 to 6 by an active assist hand, and grades 7 to 8 by spontaneous use.[7] The Manual Ability Classification System (MACS) evaluates the patient's ability to handle objects required for activities of daily living.[8] The scale ranges from 1 (handles objects easily and successfully) to 5 (does not handle objects and has severely limited ability to perform even simple actions). In general, the MACS and House classifications are inverse scales, such that a MACS 1 corresponds to a House spontaneous use (7/8) hand and a MACS 5 corresponding to an unused (House 0) hand.[9] The Assisting Hand Assessment (AHA) evaluates bimanual hand function in patients with conditions affecting a unilateral upper extremity (eg, cerebral palsy or brachial plexus birth injury) via 15 minutes of simulated bimanual tasks.[10] Using the AHA at age 18 months, children's hand functions can be divided into high or low. The evidence suggests that children with high hand function at 18 months functionally plateau around age 3 years. Despite this, they end up at a higher functional level than patients with low hand function, who typically plateau around age 7 years.[11] Finally, the Zancolli classification evaluates the interrelationship between finger and wrist flexor spasticity and contracture by assessing at what angle of wrist flexion full passive finger extension can be achieved.[9,12] Patients with minimal flexor spasticity can achieve full passive finger extension in positions of wrist extension or neutral (Zancolli 1), whereas patients with severe spasticity can only achieve full passive finger extension in full wrist flexion (Zancolli 3). The Zancolli classification helps guide treatment strategies for tendon lengthening, tendon releases, and/or flexor digitorum superficialis (FDS) to profundus transfer to improve hand function and/or resting posture.

TENDON TRANSFER SELECTION

Appropriate tendon transfer selection is based on the following principles (**Box 1**):

1. The work capacity of the donor and recipient muscles should be matched.[13,14] Muscle fiber volume is proportional to work capacity and the muscle cross-sectional area is proportional

---

Box 1
Six pillars of tendon transfer surgery

1. Match work capacity of donor and recipient muscles
2. Match excursion of donor and recipient muscles
3. Transferred tendon linear vector of pull
4. One donor, 1 function
5. Acceptable morbidity of donor muscle sacrifice
6. Consider synergistic donor and recipient muscles to ease rehabilitation

to maximum tension.[14] The work capacity of muscles in the forearm is listed in **Table 1**.[15]

2. The excursion of the donor and recipient muscles should be matched.[13,14] The average muscle fiber length is proportional to excursion. The Boyes 3-5-7 rule provides a helpful mnemonic regarding excursion of wrist and finger flexors or extensors.[16] The wrist flexors and extensors have 33 mm of excursion, the finger extensors and extensor pollicis longus have 50 mm of excursion, and the finger flexors have 70 mm of excursion. The brachioradialis has been reported to have up to 61 mm of excursion on complete mobilization.[17] Importantly, in the setting of tendon transfer surgery, excursion may increase owing to donor muscle intraoperative mobilization and/or spanning additional joints.[15,16] For example, tendon transfers crossing the wrist can gain an additional 20 to 30 mm of excursion via the tenodesis effect.[16]

3. The tendon transfer should result in a linear vector of pull to maximize efficiency and minimize potential deforming forces.

Table 1 Forearm muscle work capacity	
Muscle	**Work Capacity (MKg)**
Flexor Digitorum Superficialis	4.8
Flexor Digitorum Profundus	4.5
Flexor Carpi Ulnaris	2.0
Brachioradialis	1.9
Extensor Digitorum Communis	1.7
Pronator Teres	1.2
Flexor Pollicis Longus	1.2
Extensor Carpi Radialis Longus	1.1
Extensor Carpi Ulnaris	1.1
Extensor Carpi Radialis Brevis	0.9
Flexor Carpi Radialis	0.8
Extensor Indicis Proprius	0.5
Palmaris Longus	0.1
Extensor Pollicis Brevis	0.1
Extensor Pollicis Longus	0.1
Abductor Pollicis Longus	0.1

Data from Ingari JV, Green DP. Radial nerve palsy. In: Wolfe SW, Hotchkiss RN, Pederson WC, et al, editors. Green's operative hand surgery. 6th edition. Philadelphia: Churchill Livingstone; 2011. p. 1075–92.

4. One donor muscle should perform only 1 function.[15] The transfer of a single donor tendon to 2 recipients that perform opposing functions across a given joint will result in decreased transfer force, amplitude, and efficiency.

5. Donor muscle sacrifice should have minimal morbidity. Specifically, the function of other muscles that can compensate for lost donor muscle function, as well as prevent potential postoperative muscular imbalance, must be confirmed.

6. Finally, rehabilitation following tendon transfer surgery is facilitated by selecting donor and recipient muscles with synergistic effects. For example, transferring a wrist flexor muscle to a finger extensor muscle provides synergistic function because these motions are naturally coupled via tenodesis.

SURGICAL EXPOSURE

Incision planning and exposure are important steps during tendon transfer surgery. A curvilinear incision will maximize transferred tendon coverage by subcutaneous tissue and minimize direct apposition with the incision (ie, scar) line. As part of the surgical exposure, the donor muscle must be adequately mobilized to maximize excursion and create a linear vector of pull on transfer.[15,16] Finally, the transferred musculotendinous unit should travel in a path of sufficient width such that there is no impediment to gliding. In cases in which the donor and recipient muscles are approached through different incisions, a subcutaneous tunnel can be created with a hemostat or Allis clamp in atraumatic fashion.

TENSIONING, TRANSFER, AND SUTURE TECHNIQUES

Tendon transfer tensioning is a critical operative step that requires assessment of multiple variables, such as antagonist muscle tone and strength, joint stability or instability, and patient age. Maximum force is generated from muscle contraction at its resting length due to the optimal overlap of myosin and actin.[18] Thus, muscle length during tendon transfer tensioning should correspond to the resting length of the muscle.[16,19] Tendon transfer tensioning should be performed before suture fixation and then must be rechecked after securing the first suture.

Numerous tendon transfer coaptation techniques have been described. The Pulvertaft weave was initially described in 1956 and remains a very commonly used technique.[20] The Pulvertaft weave involves interlacing the donor tendon through orthogonal slits in the recipient tendon, which are sequentially secured with stitches.[20] The number of interlacing weaves, type of stitch, and type of suture vary depending on surgeon preference, tendon size, and tendon excursion. The potential downsides of this technique relate to required recipient tendon length, surgical time, and construct bulk once completed. Other described tendon transfer techniques have been reported, such as the side-to-side, end weave, lasso, loop-tendon, wrap-around, double-loop, and spiral techniques.[21–26] Brown and colleagues[27] reported that the side-to-side repair using a cross-stitch technique was stronger and stiffer than the Pulvertaft weave using horizontal mattress sutures, with comparable bulk and tendon length, in a study of cadaveric finger flexor tendons. Bidic and colleagues[23] reported that the lasso technique had equivalent strength, required 7 mm less tendon length, had more bulk, and was twice as fast to perform than the Pulvertaft weave, in a study of porcine flexor tendons. Fuchs and colleagues[24] reported that the wrap-around technique had equivalent strength and less bulk than the Pulvertaft weave, in a study of porcine extensor tendons. Jeon and colleagues[25] reported that the loop-tendon method had greater strength than the end-weave method, in a study of rabbit tendons. Kulikov and colleagues[26] reported that the spiral technique had equivalent strength to the Pulvertaft weave, in a study of porcine extensor tendons.

Regardless of transfer technique, other technical variables include suture material, type of stitch, number of stitches, and the number of weaves or passes (the latter is only applicable to certain techniques; eg, the Pulvertaft weave). Wagner and colleagues[28] reported that vertical mattress sutures were inferior to the pulley, running locked, and figure-of-8 suture techniques for side-to-side tenorrhaphy, in a porcine flexor tendon model. Gabuzda and colleagues[21] reported increasing strength of the end-weave repair with an increasing number of weaves (up to 5, the maximum number tested), in a cadaveric flexor tendon model. In addition, they reported increased strength of the cross-stitch versus horizontal mattress for suturing the repair. Finally, Tanaka and colleagues[29] reported that the repair strength increased with the number of weaves (up to 3, the maximum number tested) in a cadaveric flexor tendon model. They also reported that the corner stitch had equal strength to the cross-stitch with the potential advantage of less impairment of tendon vascularity due to superficial suture placement.

The senior author's preferred technique is a modification of the Pulvertaft weave (**Fig. 1**).

Briefly, the recipient tendon is manipulated with an Allis clamp via rotation to fine-tune transfer tension. A Pulvertaft weave is then performed with 3 passes using a tendon passer secured by horizontal mattress 3-0 braided nonabsorbable sutures. Tendon transfer tension is rechecked on passing the first suture, ideally holding the function of the tendon transfer against gravity resistance. The second and third passes of the weave are then performed and secured with horizontal mattress sutures. Finally, the excess recipient tendon is passed proximal to the Pulvertaft weave back through the donor tendon using the tendon passer and then sutured. This final step provides an opportunity to fine-tune tendon transfer tension as needed and possibly increase construct strength with an additional weave (at the expense of additional time and increased bulk).

PEARLS FOR COMMON TENDON TRANSFERS
Flexor Carpi Ulnaris to Extensor Carpi Radialis Brevis Transfer

Described by Green and Banks[30] in 1962, the flexor carpi ulnaris (FCU) is transferred to the extensor carpi radialis brevis (ECRB) to treat a dynamic wrist flexion deformity. Preoperatively, it is critical to evaluate flexibility of the wrist flexion deformity, potential spasticity of the FCU, and finger position or flexibility with the wrist in a corrected (ie, neutral) posture. This tendon transfer is indicated in the setting of weak wrist extension (ie, unable to get to neutral), as well as functioning flexor carpi radialis and FCU. Van Heest and colleagues[31] reported a mean improvement of 2.5 or more levels according to the House functional classification in 28 subjects who underwent the FCU to ECRB transfer.[7]

In the operating room, a volar forearm incision is marked from the pisiform, along the course of the FCU, to the midforearm. Under tourniquet control, the skin is incised and dissection is carried down to the FCU. The ulnar neurovascular bundle is isolated deep to the FCU throughout the entire incision and retracted radially. The FCU is then elevated from the pisiform to maximize tendon length. The FCU is mobilized proximally from the ulna to optimize excursion and create a linear vector of pull. Proximal mobilization of the FCU can be safely performed because the dominant vascular pedicle to the FCU is located 5.9 cm from the olecranon.[32] Notably, a less invasive approach to FCU harvest has been described with a tendon stripper, a distal transverse incision at the insertion onto the pisiform, and a proximal transverse incision at the musculotendinous junction.[33,34] Tunneling of the FCU to the dorsal incision where the ECRB is

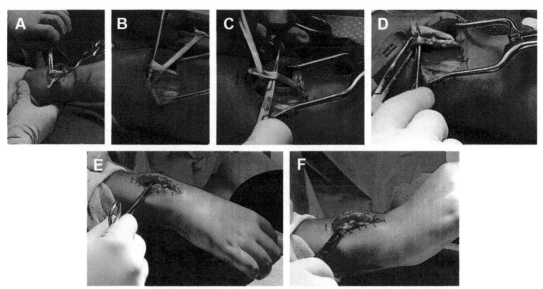

Fig. 1. Modification of Pulvertaft weave demonstrated in cerebral palsy patient undergoing flexor carpi ulnaris (FCU) to extensor carpi radialis brevis (ECRB) tendon transfer. (*A*) An Allis clamp is placed underneath the ECRB tendon. The FCU tendon is visualized on ulnar aspect of wound. (*B*) Using a tendon passer, the FCU tendon is passed through the ECRB tendon in a dorsal-volar direction. Transfer tension is fine-tuned by rotating the Allis clamp, which has been placed around the proximal aspect of the ECRB tendon. The transfer is then secured with horizontal mattress 3-0 braided nonabsorbable suture. (*C*) The FCU tendon is passed a second tine through the ECRB tendon in an orthogonal (ie, radial-ulnar) direction. (*D*) After the second and third passes of the Pulvertaft weave have been sutured, the excess FCU tendon is passed proximally using a tendon passer. At this stage, manipulation of the ECRB tendon with an Allis clamp (placed proximal to the tendon passer) allows fine-tuning of transfer tension. (*E*) Final tendon transfer tension is confirmed by observing the wrist, assuming approximately 20° of flexion with gravity when lifted from the operating room table. (*F*) Gentle traction on the ECRB with an Allis clamp demonstrates an effective wrist extension moment and secure suture fixation.

exposed can be modified depending on the forearm rotational posture.[35] A supination moment can be achieved by passing the FCU tendon around the ulna or a pronation moment can be achieved by passing the FCU radially. Alternatively, the FCU can be passed through the interosseous membrane for a linear line of pull without rotational moment. After the FCU tendon has been passed into the dorsal incision, attention is turned toward tensioning and securing the transfer.

Green initially described tensioning the transfer in forearm supination and 45° of wrist extension.[30] However, even with less aggressive tensioning parameters, late hyperextension deformity has been reported.[36] de Roode and colleagues[37] recommended tensioning the transfer in forearm pronation and the wrist in neutral to 10° of extension. Carlson and colleagues[33] recommended tensioning the transfer with the wrist in neutral and then ensuring appropriate tension by observing the wrist falling into approximately 20° of flexion with gravity when the hand and pronated forearm are gently lifted from the operating room table. We prefer to tension the transfer in neutral forearm rotation and the wrist in 20° of wrist extension. The tendon transfer is then

completed using the modified Pulvertaft weave previously described. Notably, less aggressive tensioning may be indicated in younger patients and/or patients with quadriplegic involvement given the increased rate of a late hyperextension deformity.[36]

Wounds are closed with absorbable sutures and the patient is placed into a well-padded below-elbow cast with the wrist in 10° of wrist extension for 4 weeks. At the first postoperative visit, the patient is placed in a thermoplastic splint with the wrist in 10° of extension. The splint is worn full-time for the following 4 weeks, except for hygiene and therapy consisting of active range of motion. Therapy progresses to nighttime splinting, passive range of motion, and strengthening at 3 months.

Extensor Carpi Ulnaris to Extensor Carpi Radialis Brevis Transfer

The extensor carpi ulnaris (ECU) to ECRB transfer is another option to treat a dynamic wrist flexion deformity.[34] This transfer may be favored compared with the FCU to ECRB transfer in the setting of FCU spasticity, flexor carpi radialis weakness, and/or ulnar deviation deformity in extension (due to weak radial wrist extensors).[33] Van Heest and colleagues[31] reported a mean improvement of 2.5 or more levels according to the House functional classification in 42 subjects who underwent to ECU to ECRB transfer.

In the operating room, a longitudinal incision over the dorsal aspect of the wrist is marked. Under tourniquet control, the skin is incised and dissection is carried over the ECU to its insertion on the fifth metacarpal base. The ECU is then elevated from its insertion distally to maximize tendon length. The ECU is mobilized proximally to optimize excursion and create a linear vector of pull. If present and spastic, the FCU should be addressed via either Z-lengthening or fractional lengthening through a small volar incision along the distal tendon or at the musculotendinous junction, respectively. The ECU is then transferred to the ECRB proximal to the extensor retinaculum using the modified Pulvertaft weave and tensioning parameters described for the FCU to ECRB transfer. Smooth tendon gliding without impingement at the extensor retinaculum is verified. Finally, wound closure, postoperative immobilization, and rehabilitation are identical to the FCU to ECRB transfer.

Flexor Digitorum Superficialis to Flexor Digitorum Profundus Transfer

Described by Braun and colleagues[38] in 1974, the FDS to flexor digitorum profundus (FDP) transfer (ie, superficialis to profundus transfer) is reserved for patients with severe finger flexion contractures that cannot be corrected even with the wrist in maximal flexion. This tendon transfer can provide lasting improvements in hand position and hygiene; however, functional gains are not expected because grip strength is substantially decreased postoperatively.[39]

In the operating room, a longitudinal volar incision is marked in the distal forearm. Under tourniquet control, the skin is incised, the FDS tendons are dissected distally to the wrist crease, and the FDP tendons are dissected proximally to the musculotendinous junction. The FDS tendons are then sutured together distally in side-to-side fashion with (2-0 braided nonabsorbable sutures) and FDP tendons are sutured together proximally; this is done to maintain equal tension and a normal finger cascade. The FDS tendons are then transected distally and FDP tendons are transected proximally. The tendon transfer is tensioned by placing the wrist in neutral, the metacarpophalangeal joints at 45° of flexion, and the proximal interphalangeal joints at 45° of flexion.[40] The tendons are then repaired in side-to-side fashion with (2-

0 braided nonabsorbable sutures). After placing the first stitch, tendon transfer tension is rechecked by simulating tenodesis effect; that is, full finger extension with wrist flexion and finger flexion (touching palm) with wrist extension.[34]

Alternatively, the tendons can be transferred individually from the FDS muscles into the FDP tendons. This is technically more challenging because the normal finger cascade must be reproduced for each finger; however, it can allow for independent movement of each digit if preoperative assessment reveals that the patient has control of the FDS muscles. If this alternative is pursued, the tendons are either sutured side-to-side or woven together (if length allows), starting with the index finger and progressing in an ulnar direction to ensure correct finger cascade.

The wounds are closed with absorbable sutures and the patient is placed into a well-padded below-elbow cast with the wrist in neutral and fingers in an intrinsic-plus position for 4 weeks. At the first postoperative visit, the patient is provided a thermoplastic splint that can be removed for hygiene and range of motion exercises.

SUMMARY

Tendon transfers are an important surgical option when treating patients with muscular imbalance due to cerebral palsy, traumatic brain injury, tetraplegia, or stroke. A successful surgical outcome requires a thorough preoperative clinical evaluation, an understanding of tendon transfer biomechanics, appropriate donor and recipient muscle selection, an exacting technical execution, and a thoughtful postoperative rehabilitation program. Using the pearls provided in this article, the surgeon may optimize results after tendon transfers for upper extremity spasticity.

REFERENCES

1. Van Heest AE. Tetraplegia. In: Wolfe SW, Hotchkiss RN, Pederson WC, et al, editors. Green's operative hand surgery. 6th edition. Philadelphia: Elsevier Inc; 2011. p. 1209–34, 2011.
2. Carlson MG, Spincola LJ, Lewin J, et al. Impact of video review on surgical procedure determination for patients with cerebral palsy. J Hand Surg Am 2009;34(7):1225–31.
3. Van Heest AE. Functional assessment aided by motion laboratory studies. Hand Clin 2003;19(4): 565–71.
4. Mowery CA, Gelberman RH, Rhoades CE. Upper extremity tendon transfers in cerebral palsy: electromyographic and functional analysis. J Pediatr Orthop 1985;5(1):69–72.

5. Omer GE Jr. Tendon transfers in combined nerve lesions. Orthop Clin North Am 1974;5(2):377–87.

6. Omer GE Jr. Reconstructive procedures for extremities with peripheral nerve defects. Clin Orthop Relat Res 1982;(163):80–91.

7. House JH, Gwathmey FW, Fidler MO. A dynamic approach to the thumb-in palm deformity in cerebral palsy. J Bone Joint Surg Am 1981;63(2):216–25.

8. Eliasson AC, Krumlinde-Sundholm L, Rosblad B, et al. The Manual Ability Classification System (MACS) for children with cerebral palsy: scale development and evidence of validity and reliability. Dev Med Child Neurol 2006;48(7):549–54.

9. Arner M, Eliasson AC, Nicklasson S, et al. Hand function in cerebral palsy. Report of 367 children in a population-based longitudinal health care program. J Hand Surg Am 2008;33(8):1337–47.

10. Krumlinde-Sundholm L, Lindkvist B, Plantin J, et al. Development of the Assisting Hand Assessment for adults following stroke: a Rasch-built bimanual performance measure. Disabil Rehabil 2017;1–9. [Epub ahead of print].

11. Holmefur M, Krumlinde-Sundholm L, Bergstrom J, et al. Longitudinal development of hand function in children with unilateral cerebral palsy. Dev Med Child Neurol 2010;52(4):352–7.

12. Zancolli EA, Zancolli ER Jr. Surgical management of the hemiplegic spastic hand in cerebral palsy. Surg Clin North Am 1981;61(2):395–406.

13. Brand PW, Beach RB, Thompson DE. Relative tension and potential excursion of muscles in the forearm and hand. J Hand Surg Am 1981;6(3):209–19.

14. Brand PW. Biomechanics of tendon transfer. Orthop Clin North Am 1974;5(2):205–30.

15. Ingari JV, Green DP. Radial nerve palsy. In: Wolfe SW, Hotchkiss RN, Pederson WC, et al, editors. Green's operative hand surgery. 6th edition. Philadelphia: Elsevier Inc; 2011. p. 1075–92, 2011.

16. Wilbur D, Hammert WC. Principles of tendon transfer. Hand Clin 2016;32(3):283–9.

17. Kozin SH, Bednar M. In vivo determination of available brachioradialis excursion during tetraplegia reconstruction. J Hand Surg Am 2001; 26(3):510–4.

18. Livermore A, Tueting JL. Biomechanics of tendon transfers. Hand Clin 2016;32(3):291–302.

19. Peljovich A, Ratner JA, Marino J. Update of the physiology and biomechanics of tendon transfer surgery. J Hand Surg Am 2010;35(8):1365–9 [quiz: 1370].

20. Pulvertaft RG. Tendon grafts for flexor tendon injuries in the fingers and thumb; a study of technique and results. J Bone Joint Surg Br 1956;38-B(1):175–94.

21. Gabuzda GM, Lovallo JL, Nowak MD. Tensile strength of the end-weave flexor tendon repair. An in vitro biomechanical study. J Hand Surg Br 1994; 19(3):397–400.

22. Kim SH, Chung MS, Baek GH, et al. A loop-tendon suture for tendon transfer or graft surgery. J Hand Surg Am 2007;32(3):367–72.

23. Bidic SM, Varshney A, Ruff MD, et al. Biomechanical comparison of lasso, Pulvertaft weave, and side-by-side tendon repairs. Plast Reconstr Surg 2009; 124(2):567–71.

24. Fuchs SP, Walbeehm ET, Hovius SE. Biomechanical evaluation of the Pulvertaft versus the 'wrap around' tendon suture technique. J Hand Surg Eur Vol 2011; 36(6):461–6.

25. Jeon SH, Chung MS, Baek GH, et al. Comparison of loop-tendon versus end-weave methods for tendon transfer or grafting in rabbits. J Hand Surg Am 2009;34(6):1074–9.

26. Kulikov YI, Dodd S, Gheduzzi S, et al. An in vitro biomechanical study comparing the spiral linking technique against the Pulvertaft weave for tendon repair. J Hand Surg Eur Vol 2007;32(4):377–81.

27. Brown SH, Hentzen ER, Kwan A, et al. Mechanical strength of the side-to-side versus Pulvertaft weave tendon repair. J Hand Surg Am 2010; 35(4):540–5.

28. Wagner E, Ortiz C, Wagner P, et al. Biomechanical evaluation of various suture configurations in side-to-side tenorrhaphy. J Bone Joint Surg Am 2014; 96(3):232–6.

29. Tanaka T, Zhao C, Ettema AM, et al. Tensile strength of a new suture for fixation of tendon grafts when using a weave technique. J Hand Surg Am 2006;31(6): 982–6.

30. Green WT, Banks HH. Flexor carpi ulnaris transplant and its use in cerebral palsy. J Bone Joint Surg Am 1962;44-A:1343–430.

31. Van Heest AE, House JH, Cariello C. Upper extremity surgical treatment of cerebral palsy. J Hand Surg Am 1999;24(2):323–30.

32. Payne DE, Kaufman AM, Wysocki RW, et al. Vascular perfusion of a flexor carpi ulnaris muscle turnover pedicle flap for posterior elbow soft tissue reconstruction: a cadaveric study. J Hand Surg Am 2011;36(2):246–51.

33. Carlson MG, Athwal GS, Bueno RA. Treatment of the wrist and hand in cerebral palsy. J Hand Surg Am 2006;31(3):483–90.

34. Carlson MG. Cerebral palsy. In: Wolfe SW, Hotchkiss RN, Pederson WC, et al, editors. Green's operative hand surgery. 6th edition. Philadelphia: Elsevier Inc; 2011. p. 1139–72, 2011.

35. Van Heest AE, Murthy NS, Sathy MR, et al. The supination effect of tendon transfer of the flexor carpi ulnaris to the extensor carpi radialis brevis or longus: a cadaveric study. J Hand Surg Am 1999;24(5): 1091–6.

36. Patterson JM, Wang AA, Hutchinson DT. Late deformities following the transfer of the flexor carpi ulnaris to the extensor carpi radialis brevis in children

with cerebral palsy. J Hand Surg Am 2010;35(11): 1774–8.

37. de Roode CP, James MA, Van Heest AE. Tendon transfers and releases for the forearm, wrist, and hand in spastic hemiplegic cerebral palsy. Tech Hand Up Extrem Surg 2010;14(2):129–34.

38. Braun RM, Vise GT, Roper B. Preliminary experience with superficialis-to-profundus tendon transfer in the hemiplegic upper extremity. J Bone Joint Surg Am 1974;56(3):466–72.

39. Keenan MA, Korchek JI, Botte MJ, et al. Results of transfer of the flexor digitorum superficialis tendons to the flexor digitorum profundus tendons in adults with acquired spasticity of the hand. J Bone Joint Surg Am 1987;69(8):1127–32.

40. Manske PR, Strecker WB. Cerebral palsy, brain injury, stroke: spastic disorders of the upper extremity. In: Peimer CA, editor. Surgery of the hand and upper extremity. 2nd edition. New York: McGraw-Hill; 1996. p. 1517–38.

Selective Neurectomy for the Spastic Upper Extremity

Caroline Leclercq, MD

KEYWORDS

- Spasticity • Motor nerves • Neurectomy • Hyperselective neurectomy

KEY POINTS

- Hyperselective neurectomy is effective in reducing the severity of upper limb spasticity.
- The procedure requires a thorough knowledge of the anatomy of upper extremity motor nerves and their branches to each individual muscle.
- Neurectomy should involve at least two-thirds of each motor ramus entering the target muscles.
- Magnifying loupes and microsurgical instruments are recommended for this procedure.

INTRODUCTION

Spasticity occurs as a consequence of many conditions, including cerebral palsy (CP), stroke, and traumatic brain injury. The initial treatment for spasticity is nonsurgical, including a wide range of physical and occupational therapy techniques. Pharmacologic agents may be used as an adjunct, whether orally, intrathecal, or locally administered. In select cases, surgery may be indicated following proper conservative treatment.

The goals of surgical treatment can vary greatly, depending on the extent of functional impairment. Whenever possible, surgery aims to improve function. In some cases, however, it will be limited to improving hygiene and comfort, reducing pain, or correcting a severe deformity. The goal of functional surgery is to correct the deformities by rebalancing existing forces.[1] Multiple surgical techniques are used to address different components of the upper extremity deformity, such as spasticity, muscle contracture, joint contracture, and paralysis; this goal-specific surgical plan underscores the need for a preliminary thorough physical examination. Surgical options aimed at spasticity reduction include root procedures (eg, selective radicotomy

and dorsal root entry zone lesioning) as well as peripheral procedures (eg, partial neurectomy).

Partial neurectomy was described by Stoffel[2] in 1913, and expanded by Brunelli and Brunelli[3] in 1983. The conceptual basis of this technique is to decrease the spastic component of the deformity, while retaining some active control of the involved muscles. Satisfactory outcomes of this technique have been reported,[4–14] but the results are difficult to interpret because of a lack of standardized use of postoperative outcomes instruments. Further, there is a general perception that recurrence is frequent. In light of our recent anatomic studies,[15–17] new guidelines for a "hyperselective" neurectomy (HSN) have been described and we have conducted a prospective study to reevaluate the results of this treatment. In this article, we discuss the essential components of a preoperative examination, indications for HSN, technical details, and outcomes of treatment.

PREOPERATIVE EXAMINATION

Selective neurectomy is effective only for the spastic component of the deformity. Therefore, it must be distinguished from other potential

Disclosure: The author does not have any commercial or financial conflicts of interest or funding sources to disclose.
Institut de la Main, Clinique Bizet, 21 rue Georges Bizet, Paris 75116, France
E-mail address: caroline.leclercq@free.fr

Hand Clin 34 (2018) 537–545
https://doi.org/10.1016/j.hcl.2018.06.010

deforming factors, namely muscle contracture, joint deformities, and paralysis. The clinical picture may vary greatly from one individual to another, depending on the amount and location of the initial brain insult. Further, clinical manifestations within the same patient may vary, depending on ambient temperature, emotional state, and stress, for example, Clinical examination is a critical part of the assessment. It is best performed as a multidisciplinary team, including the physiatrist, neurologist, physical and occupational therapist, and surgeon. This should ideally be done in a warm, quiet, and friendly environment to limit spasticity. For the same reason, it is unwise to decide on surgery after a single session, and assessment should be repeated before any decision-making. Physical examination findings are recorded on standardized charts, and video recording of each patient is performed before and after every step of treatment. A thorough examination of the upper limb is essential to rule out any other associated neurologic disorders and/or potential contraindications to surgery.

Evaluation of Spasticity

Spasticity is usually easy to diagnose based on clinical characteristics, but can be difficult to quantify.[4] The Ashworth scale was developed to assess the efficacy of antispasticity treatment in patients with multiple sclerosis. It is descriptive and, despite subsequent modification, remains subject to personal interpretation, with suboptimal interobserver reliability.[18] There is evidence that the Tardieu scale[19] is currently the most reliable tool for evaluating spasticity.[20–24]

Muscle Contracture

Unlike spasticity, muscle contracture is permanent and cannot be overcome. However, the distinction between contracture and spasticity may be difficult to establish clinically. Despite this challenge, it is critical to discern contracture from spasticity to formulate the best treatment plan. In such cases, nerve blocks or botulinum toxin (Botox) are very helpful; spasticity yields completely, whereas contracture persists.[25,26]

Joint Deformity

Passive motion of the involved joints may be difficult to assess because of muscle contractures. In this setting, motor blocks are not very helpful because they cannot alleviate muscle contracture. Sometimes it is not until surgical release of the muscle contracture that the actual range of passive motion can be evaluated. Joint contracture is rare in patients with CP, who present more

frequently with joint instability, especially at the thumb metacarpophalangeal (MCP) joint (eg, hyperextension), and at the finger proximal interphalangeal (PIP) joints (eg, swan-neck deformity).

Motor Impairment

Motor examination of the upper limb may be difficult, especially when severe contractures are present. Rather than individual muscles, it is easier to evaluate muscle groups contributing to a particular function. The palsy usually predominates in the distal part of the upper limb and involves the extensor and supinator muscles, whereas the spastic flexor, adductor, and pronator muscles usually retain some voluntary control. Assessment of the weak extensor and supinator muscles may be difficult when the antagonist flexors and pronators are severely spastic. Botox serves as a diagnostic aid in this regard; when injected in the spastic antagonist muscles, it allows one to more accurately evaluate the function of the seemingly paralyzed muscles. In many cases, these muscles may end up demonstrating satisfactory voluntary control.

We have not found electromyographic studies to be helpful in quantifying the motor function of either the pseudo-paralytic or the spastic muscles. Although promising, 3-dimensional movement analysis is complex in the upper limb, and not routinely used.[27,28] Involuntary movements, whether spontaneous (eg, chorea, athetosis) or during use (eg, dystonia) are recorded; they may be contraindications to surgery.

Sensory Impairment

Sensory examination is essentially impossible before the ages of 4 or 5. Light touch and 2-point discrimination are generally intact in children with CP, whereas complex sensations (eg, fine sensibility, proprioception, stereognosis) are more readily affected. In patients with stroke, all types of sensations may be severely impaired. Pain may be present, but is difficult to evaluate and discern causation. It may be linked to severe contractures, a deformed joint, or, rarely, Kienböck's disease secondary to a severe wrist flexion deformity.[29]

Functional Assessment

The International Classification of Functioning, Disability and Health (ICF) provides a standard language and framework for assessing function and disability.[30] The ICF is unique in its ability to distinguish capacity and performance. Capacity is the ability to execute a task at the highest possible level of functioning. Performance is the spontaneous use of the hand during activities or play. In short, the ICF differentiates what patients can do versus what they actually do, in an effort to better understand their ability.[31] Other validated tools for assessing capacity include some multitask tests (Melbourne Assessment of Unilateral Upper Limb Function, Shriners Hospital Upper Extremity Evaluation, Jebsen Taylor) and unitask tests (Box and Block, Nine Hole Peg). Performance can be accessed through questionnaires (AbilhandKids, Children's Hand-Use Experience Questionnaire) and tests (Assisting Hand Assessment, Video Observations Aarts and Aarts).

General Preoperative Assessment

The aim of the general examination is to determine the possibility for functional improvement after surgery, taking into account other neurologic impairments, the patient's age, intellectual status, motivation, and family environment. In general, surgery is not indicated for abnormal movements or dystonia. Contraindications may also include anticipated lack of compliance, emotional disorders, or unrealistic expectations. Cognitive problems are not a contraindication, per se, but must be carefully evaluated before surgery.

THE ROLE OF BOTOX

In addition to systemic medications, which are used for treating generalized spasticity, some agents are effective for local muscle spasticity.[32] Rather than lidocaine, alcohol, or phenol,[15] Botox has become the mainstay for muscle-specific treatment of spasticity. Botox is injected directly into the muscle of interest and results in a reduction of spasticity lasting up to several months. It is now routinely used in the spastic upper limb with measurable and reproducible effects.[33,34]

Botox may be repeated as required, sometimes yielding a permanent improvement if the antagonist muscles increase in strength, thus balancing the spasticity more effectively. In such cases, Botox plays an educational role in simulating the effect of surgery.[35,36] Botox is also useful as a preoperative test, in order to decide which muscles require a permanent surgical reduction of spasticity. This is particularly informative when multiple muscles contribute to the same function. If spasticity recurs after injection, a more definitive surgical procedure can be considered.

SURGICAL TREATMENT: THE ROLE OF SELECTIVE NEURECTOMY
Neurotomy

Neurotomy (complete sectioning of a nerve trunk) may be indicated in nonfunctional upper limbs

with severe spasticity to facilitate hygiene, nursing, and to improve cosmesis. The primary application is neurotomy of the motor branch of the ulnar nerve at the wrist. This procedure creates a flaccid palsy of the involved muscles, but is ineffective for established muscle contractures.

Selective or Partial Neurectomy

Selective or partial neurectomy (division of only select fascicles of a major motor nerve) had been suggested as early as 1913 in an attempt to retain some function.[2] This technique has gained popularity after Brunelli and Brunelli[3] published a clinical series in 1983 and coined the term "hyponeurotization." The procedure is performed at the entry point of the nerve into the muscle, where it usually divides into several small fascicles. Under magnification, part of the fascicles are resected. Brunelli and Brunelli[3] initially advocated dividing 50% of the fascicles, but after experiencing recurrence of spasticity, they recommended resection of a greater number of fibers. They also recommended planning a second partial neurectomy 6 months later, in cases of recurrence. The author has adapted this technique and feel that the term "hyperselective" neurectomy (HSN) better describes the procedure.[37]

Anatomic Study

We performed several anatomic studies to establish a cartography of the motor branches of the musculocutaneous, median, ulnar, and radial nerves. In 16 cadaver dissections, the musculocutaneous nerve gave off 1 to 5 trunks for the biceps, which reached the muscle from 18% to 64% of the arm length. The musculocutaneous nerve then gave off 1 to 3 branches for the brachialis, which reached the muscle from 35% to 75% of the arm length[15] (**Fig. 1**). Therefore, during HSN, we recommend dissecting the musculocutaneous nerve from 18% to 75% of the arm length to visualize the appropriate branch patterns.

In 20 cadaver dissections, motor branches of the median nerve in the forearm had the most complex and variable distribution.[16] The median nerve gave off 1 or 2 trunks for the pronator teres, starting at 3% of the forearm length, 1 trunk only for the flexor carpi radialis (FCR), usually as a common trunk with other branches from 21% to 41% of the forearm length. For both the flexor digitorum superficialis muscles (FDS), and the flexor digitorum profundi (FDP), part of the terminal branches were located under the muscle bellies, requiring detaching these muscles for access to the nerve-muscle junction. The flexor pollicis longus (FPL) was most frequently innervated by 1 branch from the anterior interosseous nerve, which reached

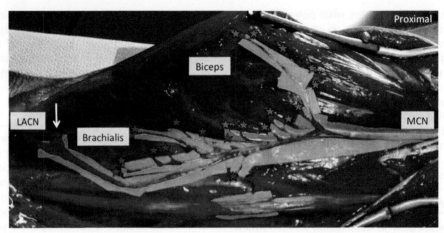

Fig. 1. Cadaver dissection of the musculocutaneous nerve and its motor branches to the biceps and brachialis muscles. LACN (*arrow*), lateral antebrachial cutaneous nerve; MCN, musculocutaneous nerve. *Yellow stars* indicate the points where the 11 terminal rami of the motor branches enter the biceps muscle, and *orange stars* the points where the 9 terminal rami of the motor branches enter the brachialis muscle.

the muscle between 44% and 63% of the forearm length. As such, for HSN directed at the wrist flexors, we recommend dissection of the median nerve from the elbow flexion crease up to 41% of the forearm length, in combination with intraoperative nerve stimulation for identification of the rami dedicated to the FCR; the FPL branch can be identified at between 44% and 63% of the forearm length. We do not recommend this technique for the finger flexors because of the aggressive muscle dissection required for fascicular identification.

Our group also evaluated the ulnar nerve branching pattern in 20 upper limbs.[17] The ulnar nerve gave off 1 to 4 trunks for the flexor carpi ulnaris, which reached the muscle between 0% and 50% of the forearm length. Most of these branches originated from the posterior aspect of the ulnar nerve. The FDP received, in most cases, a single branch from the ulnar nerve, originating, on average, 50 mm from the medial epicondyle, and no forearm muscle motor branches were found after the ulnar artery joined the nerve. Therefore, the ulnar nerve should be dissected from the medial epicondyle until 50% of the forearm length.

A combined approach to the median and ulnar nerves during HSN of the wrist flexors may be performed through a single L-shape incision starting above the elbow crease and curving toward the anterior aspect of the forearm (**Fig. 2**). Similar studies by our group have been performed for the radial nerve and the terminal motor branch of the ulnar nerve in the palm (20 cadaver dissections each, unpublished data [Merlini L & Leclercq C, 2018; Bini N & Leclercq C, 2016]). These studies indicate that HSN is feasible for these particular peripheral nerves, as well. With regard to the brachioradialis,

there are several motor branches, the most distal one potentially emerging as a common branch with the extensor carpi radialis longus (5% of cases). For the adductor pollicis and first dorsal interosseous motor nerves, a skin incision in the flexor crease allows satisfactory identification and partial division of all terminal branches of the ulnar nerve.

Indications and Contraindications

HSN is indicated when one wishes to reduce spasticity permanently. It has no effect on muscle or joint contractures; muscle contractures should be addressed by muscle or tendon lengthening, and joint contractures by arthrolysis, bone shortening, or arthrodesis. Paralysis of the antagonist muscles must be addressed, when possible, by reconstructive procedures (eg, tendon transfers). However, weak antagonists may spontaneously

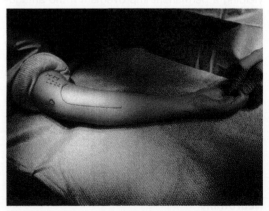

Fig. 2. Skin incision for HSN of the wrist flexors; combined approach of the median and the ulnar nerve motor branches.

improve after HSN has reduced the tone of the spastic agonist muscles.

General contraindications for surgery in patients with spasticity of the upper limb also apply to this technique: dystonia or abnormal movements, lack of compliance, unrealistic expectations. Cognitive problems are not necessarily a contraindication to this technique, as long as the patient can cope with a surgical procedure and the postoperative regimen.

Surgical Technique

Depending on the patient and the involved nerve, HSN can be performed under axillary block or general anesthesia. Because of the need for intraoperative nerve stimulation, paralysis is contraindicated. The skin incision follows the guidelines mentioned previously. Once the nerve trunk has been exposed, the motor branches are meticulously dissected. There are usually several rami for each involved muscle, and all of them must be identified to achieve a satisfactory result. Each ramus is dissected up to the neuromuscular junction (**Fig. 3**). Then, using microsurgical instruments and magnification, the required number of fascicles are resected from each ramus: most commonly our group divides at least two-thirds of the involved nerve branch, depending on the amount of spasticity and the desired result. Some investigators coagulate the proximal stump to prevent nerve regrowth.[5]

Postoperative care consists of a soft, nonadherent dressing until the wound is healed. Gentle exercises of the involved muscles are subsequently initiated. A temporary paresis of the target muscles is common during the first few weeks. Not infrequently, this technique is performed concomitantly with other rebalancing procedures (eg, tendon lengthening, tendon transfers), and the postoperative regimen will vary according to the requirements of these other procedures.

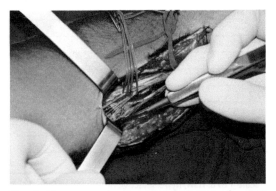

Fig. 3. Neuromuscular junction between the FCR branches from the median nerve and the muscle.

RESULTS

We have performed HSN for more than 100 patients. In 2012, we initiated an ongoing prospective study to assess the long-term results of this procedure. We have since enrolled 47 patients (22 adults and 25 children) who underwent 52 HSN procedures. Patient age ranged from 7 to 74 years old (average 33 years old). In our study, the cause of spasticity was CP in 23, stroke in 19, traumatic brain injury in 2, and brain tumor in 4 patients. Patient selection was based on serial clinical examination and the results of preoperative Botox injections. All patients had previous medical treatment for spasticity, including medications, physical and occupational therapy, orthoses, and Botox injections (average 2.3 injections per patient).

Preoperative and postoperative assessment was based on spontaneous limb position, active and passive motion, and muscle strength as measured by the Medical Research Counsel scale. Spasticity was assessed using both the modified Ashworth and the Tardieu scales. Functional results were evaluated with the House score and an activities of daily living questionnaire. Patient satisfaction was rated according to the Visual Analogue Satisfaction scale. The results were evaluated at 6 months, and at the longest follow-up.

HSN involved 133 muscles (**Table 1**), amounting to 2.8 neurectomies per surgery. Other procedures were performed simultaneously in 27 cases, including 31 muscle lengthening, 3 tendon

Table 1 Detail of the 133 target muscles treated by hyperselective neurectomy in 47 patients	
Muscle Involved	**Number Treated**
Supraspinatus	3
Infraspinatus	3
Teres minor	2
Subscapularis	1
Biceps	27
Brachialis	19
Brachioradialis	6
Flexor carpi radialis	18
Flexor carpi ulnaris	14
Palmaris longus	13
Pronator teres	12
Extensor carpi radialis	1
Flexor pollicis longus	1
Thumb adductor	1
First dorsal interosseous	1

transfers, and 1 midcarpal arthrodesis. There were 2 postoperative complications: 1 hematoma in a patient on warfarin, and a technical failure related to difficulties identifying the infraspinatus motor branch.

In our ongoing study, 36 patients have a follow-up longer than 6 months: 20 adults (25 HSN) with an average follow-up of 15.2 months (range 6–63 months), and 16 children (16 HSN) with an average follow-up of 19 months (range 6–40 months). The outcome has been analyzed separately for each involved joint and for adults compared with children. The results of the 2 most significant groups, adult elbow flexors (AE) (15 patients), and 11 children wrist flexors (CW) (11 patients) are listed in **Tables 2** and **3**. The data show a dramatic improvement in the spontaneous posture (AE 60%, CW 92%), an increase in antagonist strength (AE 0.9 points, CW 2.1 points) without a decrease in flexion strength. Despite these gains, there was a limited improvement in average active range of motion (AE 22°, CW 14°). We also found a significant decrease in spasticity at 6 months in both groups, but a slight recurrence at last follow-up in adults, particularly as measured by the Tardieu scale. Patient satisfaction at final follow-up was high in both groups (average 8.8).

DISCUSSION

Favorable results have been reported after partial neurectomies in the upper limb.[5–13] However, there is little consensus regarding indications, technique, and postoperative outcomes. In an effort to address these challenges, we systematically reviewed the literature regarding different techniques for partial neurectomy in the upper limbs of patients with spasticity.[14] We identified 14 articles that met inclusion criteria, amounting to 425 cases of partial neurectomy.

First, the terminology was confusing in 5 articles, in which the term partial neurectomy (or neurotomy) described resection of the entire motor branch with conservation of the sensory branch (1 musculocutaneous nerve, 4 terminal motor branches of the ulnar nerve in the hand). The techniques also varied: some investigators, following the original description of Brunelli and Brunelli,[3] follow the motor branches until they enter the muscle, and perform a partial neurectomy at this level.[9,11] Others, to simplify the procedure, perform a partial neurectomy at the level of the main nerve trunk, without approaching the target muscle(s). In these studies, the motor fascicles are identified proximally using a stimulator and partially resected.[4,9,12,13] Although faster with limited requisite exposure, this technical variation is less precise with possible insufficient reduction of spasticity secondary to inadequate nerve branch division as well as potential injury to sensory fibers.[4] Some investigators coagulate the proximal stump or ligate the nerve with a metal clip[5] in an attempt to block nerve regrowth. Others, however, leave the proximal stump undisturbed, fearing damage to the remaining fibers.

Critical assessment regarding the studies using the original technique of Brunelli and Brunelli[3] indicate that incisions were often quite small, compared with the branching pattern of the motor nerves, and thus some motor branches may have been missed.[14] Using data from our cadaveric studies,[15–17] skin incisions should be longer than that generally reported in the literature. With

Table 2
Results of HSN of the elbow flexors in 15 adult patients at 4-month and 16-month follow-up

HSN = 15	Preoperative	4-mo Postoperative	16-mo Postoperative
Spontaneous posture	105° flexion	35° flexion	42° flexion
Active extension	83°	29°	34°
Active flexion	136°	110°	109°
Strength extension (MRC)	3.4	2.4	4.3
Strength flexion (MRC)	3.3	2.8	3.9
Ashworth	2.5	0.2	0.7
Tardieu V1-V3	51	4	25
Tardieu T	2.1	0.5	1
House	0.7	2.4	1.5
VAS			9.9

Abbreviations: Ashworth, modified Ashworth (scale 0–4); House, scale 1 to 8; HSN, hyperselective neurectomy; MRC, Medical Research Council (scale 0–5); Tardieu, Tardieu scale: V1 (angle of passive motion) minus V3 (angle of stretch reflex), T: 1 to 3; VAS, Visual Analogue Satisfaction (scale 0–10).

Table 3
Results of HSN of the wrist flexors in 11 children at 5-month and 20-month follow-up

HSN = 11	Preoperative	5-mo Postoperative	20-mo Postoperative
Resting posture	70° flexion	37° flexion	5° flexion
Active extension	17°	25°	30°
Active flexion	80°	68°	81°
Strength extension (MRC)	1.9	3.8	4.0
Strength flexors (MRC)	4.1	4.4	4.9
Ashworth	2.2	0.1	0
Tardieu V1-V3	37	5	0
Tardieu T	2.6	0.7	0
House	3	5	7
Box & Block	19.7	29.5	31
VAS			Children 8.1/Parents 7.2

Abbreviations: Ashworth, modified Ashworth (scale 0–4); House, scale 1 to 8; HSN, hyperselective neurectomy; MRC, Medical Research Council (scale 0–5); Tardieu, Tardieu scale: V1 (angle of passive motion) minus V3 (angle of stretch reflex), T: 1 to 3; VAS, Visual Analogue Satisfaction (scale 0–10).

regard to the FDS and FDP motor branches, our data suggest that HSN is not feasible without harming the muscles, in contradiction with the experience of Brunelli and Brunelli.[3] Therefore, we do not recommend HSN for the finger flexor muscles, and instead favor tendon-lengthening procedures.

In our previous review of the literature,[14] the amount of fibers resected varied from 33% to 80%. Some investigators decide on the amount of neurectomy depending on the Ashworth score,[38] whereas others rely on the response to perioperative stimulation after resection of 50% of the fibers.[11] Brunelli and Brunelli[3] initially advocated dividing 50% of the fascicles, but after identifying multiple patients with recurrence, they subsequently recommended resection of a larger amount of fibers. Recurrence was explained not by nerve regrowth from the transected stumps, but by what he termed the "adoption" phenomenon; this describes the adoption of orphan muscle fibers by the remaining nerve branches, equivalent to the "sprouting" phenomenon described elsewhere.[39,40] They also recommended a planned second neurectomy 6 months later in cases of recurrence; this was performed in 90% of cases.[3] Despite these recommendations, stable results after a single procedure have been reported by several investigators.[5,11] For example, Maarrawi and colleagues[38] report 5% recurrence at 1 year. Our results at 19-month follow-up seem to indicate a slight recurrence in adults, but none in children. Functional outcomes are difficult to analyze, given the wide variety of baseline function and surgical techniques. In our review of 14 studies, 9 of the

studies involved mainly nonfunctional hands (65%–100% of cases), and the neurectomy was often performed in cases of failure of all other treatments.

After extensive cadaver studies, we have developed guidelines for HSN of the major motor nerves of the upper limb. A prospective study of 36 HSNs has shown a significant reduction of spasticity as measured by validated outcomes assessment tools, without any loss of strength. Except for 1 technical failure, the goal of surgery, whether functional, nursing, or cosmesis, has been attained in all cases.

SUMMARY

Surgery is only one element of the rehabilitative care of patients with upper extremity spasticity. Initial management focuses on splinting, occupational therapy, and pharmacologic treatment, as needed. A careful clinical examination and local chemodenervation are required to select the proper candidates for partial neurectomy. Although many variations of selective neurectomy exist, the results of our technique of HSN in spasticity of the upper limb have been promising, showing effective reduction of spasticity and improved motion, without any loss of strength. These results have remained stable over time in the medium-term, except in adults, which tend toward a slight recurrence of spasticity. We hypothesize that the significant increase in strength of the antagonist muscles, through rebalancing of forces, is responsible for the stability of the results. A longer follow-up will be necessary to evaluate the long-term outcomes of this procedure. Management of patients with upper limb spasticity can be challenging and poses the risks of recurrence, limited improvement, and weakening. HSN is a relatively new technique that expands the armamentarium of the upper extremity surgeon and attempts to address some of the historical limitations of surgical management of the spastic upper limb.

REFERENCES

1. Tonkin MA. The upper limb in cerebral palsy. Curr Orthop 1995;9:149–55.
2. Stoffel A. Treatment of spastic contractures. Am J Orthop Surg 1913;210:611.
3. Brunelli G, Brunelli F. Partial selective denervation in spastic palsies (hyponeurotization). Microsurgery 1983;4:221–4.
4. Decq P, Shin M, Carrillo-Ruiz J. Surgery in the peripheral nerves for lower limb spasticity. Operat Tech Neurosurg 2005;7:136–40.
5. Reddy S, Puligopu AK, Purohit AK. Results of selective motor fasciculotomy in spastic upper limbs due to cerebral palsy (a review of 30 children and adults). Indian J Cereb Palsy 2015;1:21–7.
6. Garland DE, Thompson R, Waters RL. Musculocutaneous neurectomy for spastic elbow flexion in nonfunctional upper extremities in adults. J Bone Joint Surg Am 1980;62:108–12.
7. Msaddi AK, Mazroue AR, Shahwan S, et al. Microsurgical selective peripheral neurotomy in the treatment of spasticity in cerebral-palsy children. Stereotact Funct Neurosurg 1997;69:251–8.
8. Decq P, Filipetti P, Feve A, et al. Peripheral selective neurotomy of the brachial plexus collateral branches for treatment of the spastic shoulder: anatomical study and clinical results in five patients. J Neurosurg 1997;86:648–53.
9. Purohit AK, Raju BS, Kumar KS, et al. Selective musculocutaneous fasciculotomy for spastic elbow in cerebral palsy: a preliminary study. Acta Neurochir (Wien) 1998;140:473–8.
10. Sindou MP, Simon F, Mertens P, et al. Selective peripheral neurotomy (SPN) for spasticity in childhood. Childs Nerv Syst 2007;23:957–70.
11. Buffenoir K, Rigoard P, Ferrand-Sorbets S, et al. Étude rétrospective du résultat à long terme des neurotomies sélectives périphériques dans le traitement du membre supérieur spastique. [[Retrospective study of the long-term results of selective peripheral neurotomy for the treatment of spastic upper limb]]. Neurochirurgie 2009;55:S150–60 [in French].
12. Puligopu AK, Purohit AK. Outcome of selective motor fasciculotomy in the treatment of upper limb spasticity. J Pediatr Neurosci 2011;6:S118–25.
13. Sitthinamsuwan B, Chanvanitkulchai K, Phonwijit L, et al. Surgical outcomes of microsurgical selective peripheral neurotomy for intractable limb spasticity. Stereotact Funct Neurosurg 2013;91:248–57.
14. Gras M, Leclercq C. Spasticity and hyperselective neurectomy in the upper limb. Hand Surg Rehab 2017;36:391–401.
15. Cambon-Binder A, Leclercq C. Anatomical study of the musculocutaneous nerve branching pattern: application for selective neurectomy in the treatment of elbow flexors spasticity. Surg Radiol Anat 2015;37:341–8.
16. Parot C, Leclercq C. Anatomical study of the motor branches of the median nerve to the forearm and guidelines for selective neurectomy. Surg Radiol Anat 2016;38:597–604.
17. Paulos R, Leclercq C. Motor branches of the ulnar nerve to the forearm: an anatomical study and guidelines for selective neurectomy. Surg Radiol Anat 2015;37:1043–8.
18. Bohannon RW, Smith MB. Interrater reliability of a modified Ashworth scale of muscle spasticity. Phys Ther 1987;67:206–7.
19. Tardieu G, Shentoub S, Delarue R. Research on a technic for measurement of spasticity. Rev Neurol (Paris) 1954;91:143–4.
20. Boyd RN, Barwood SA, Ballieu C, et al. Validity of a clinical measure of spasticity in children with cerebral palsy in a double blinded randomised controlled clinical trial. Dev Med Child Neurol 1998;40:7.
21. Mackey AH, Walt SE, Lobb G, et al. Intraobserver reliability of the modified Tardieu scale in the upper limb of children with hemiplegia. Dev Med Child Neurol 2004;46:267–72.
22. Yam WK, Leung MS. Interrater reliability of Modified Ashworth Scale and Modified Tardieu Scale in children with spastic cerebral palsy. J Child Neurol 2006;21:1031–5.
23. Patrick E, Ada L. The Tardieu Scale differentiates contracture from spasticity whereas the Ashworth Scale is confounded by it. Clin Rehabil 2006;20:173–82.
24. Gracies JM, Burke K, Clegg NJ, et al. Reliability of the Tardieu Scale for assessing spasticity in children with cerebral palsy. Arch Phys Med Rehabil 2010;91:421–8.
25. Braun RM, Hoffer MM, Mooney V, et al. Phenol nerve block in the treatment of acquired spastic hemiplegia in the upper limb. J Bone Joint Surg Am 1973;55:580–5.
26. Roper B. Evaluation of spasticity. Hand 1975;7:11–4.
27. Fitoussi F, Diop A, Maurel N, et al. Kinematic analysis of the upper limb: a useful tool in children with cerebral palsy. J Pediatr Orthop B 2006;15:247–56.

28. Scallon G, Van Heest A. Kinematic motion analysis in upper extremity cerebral palsy. Phys Med Rehabil Int 2016;3(5):1097.

29. Leclercq C, Xarchas C. Kienböck's disease in cerebral palsy. J Hand Surg Br 1998;23:746–8.

30. World Health Organization (WHO). International classification of functioning, disability and health. Geneva (Switzerland): World Health Organization; 2001.

31. Klingels K, Jaspers E, Van de Winckel A, et al. A systematic review of arm activity measures for children with hemiplegic cerebral palsy. Clin Rehabil 2010;24:887–900.

32. Chung CY, Chen CL, Wong AM. Pharmacotherapy of spasticity in children with cerebral palsy. J Formos Med Assoc 2011;110:215–22.

33. Koman A, Paterson Smith B, Williams R, et al. Upper extremity spasticity in children with cerebral palsy: a randomized, double-blind, placebo-controlled study of the short-term outcomes of treatment with Botulinum A toxin. J Hand Surg 2013;38A:435–46.

34. Ozcakir S, Sivrioglu K. Botulinum toxin in poststroke spasticity. Clin Med Res 2007;5:132–8.

35. Buffenoir K, Decq P, Lefaucheur JP. Interest of peripheral anesthetic blocks as a diagnosis and prognosis tool in patient with spastic equines foot: a clinical and electrophysiological study of the effect of block of nerve branches to the triceps surae muscle. Clin Neuropsychol 2005;116:1596–600.

36. Hodgkinson I, Sindou M. Decision-making for treatment of disabling spasticity in children. Oper Tech Neurosurg 2005;7:120–3.

37. Leclercq C, Gras M. Hyperselective neurectomy in the treatment of the spastic upper limb. Phys Med Rehabil Int 2016;3(1):1075.

38. Maarrawi J, Mertens P, Luaute J, et al. Long-term functional results of selective peripheral neurotomy for the treatment of spastic upper limb: prospective study in 31 patients. J Neurosurg 2006;104:215–25.

39. Dengler R, Konstanzer A, Hesse S, et al. Collateral nerve sprouting and twitch forces of single motor units in conditions with partial denervation in man. Neurosci Lett 1989;97:118–22.

40. Einsiedel LJ, Luff AR. Activity and motor unit size in partially denervated rat medial gastrocnemius. J Appl Physiol (1985) 1994;76:2663–71.

Neurosurgical Management of Spastic Conditions of the Upper Extremity

Karl Balsara, MD, Andrew Jea, MD,
Jeffrey S. Raskin, MS, MD*

KEYWORDS

- Spasticity • Movement disorder • Upper extremity • Baclofen therapy • Neuromodulation

KEY POINTS

- Upper extremity spasticity is an unfortunate hypertonic consequence of many central pathologic conditions affecting the stretch reflex.
- Many surgical and nonsurgical approaches are used to treat upper extremity spasticity and its consequences.
- Despite treating the hypertonia associated with spasticity, surgical techniques for neuromodulation of muscle tone are unable to significantly improve the upper extremity functional impairment.

INTRODUCTION

Spasticity is best described as an uninhibited velocity-dependent activation of skeletal muscle reflexes resulting from upper motor neuron injury.[1,2] Surgical intervention for spasticity was first developed by the English neurophysiologist, Sir Charles Scott Sherrington. He experimentally induced a spastic condition in cats by separating the brainstem from the spinal cord and was able to abolish it by dividing their posterior rootlets.[3] This work, which was published in the 1890s and later awarded a Nobel Prize, was the foundation for practitioners who developed the dorsal rhizotomy (ie, sectioning of the dorsal nerve root or rootlets). Technological advancements over the past century have allowed surgeons to select abnormally firing dorsal roots with greater precision. Dorsal rhizotomy, when performed on the cervical roots, is effective in reducing spasticity in the upper extremities. However, the reduction in spasticity has not consistently resulted in functional improvement; for this reason, most cases were treated nonsurgically through the end of the twentieth century. Neurosurgical management of spasticity affecting the upper extremity is an evolving field. Despite modern technological gains, the goal of reliable functional improvement in the spastic patient remains elusive.

UPPER EXTREMITY SPASTICITY

Upper extremity spasticity may negatively affect quality of life and make activities of daily living difficult. The affected limb typically assumes a posture marked by internal rotation of the shoulder, a flexed elbow and wrist, and a clenched fist. Spasticity-related contractures may also interfere with residual function in the affected extremity. An effective treatment should relieve pain, address

Disclosure Statement: None of the authors have any financial disclosures.
Section of Pediatric Neurosurgery, Department of Neurosurgery, Goodman Campbell Brain and Spine, Riley Hospital for Children, Indiana University School of Medicine, 705 Riley Hospital Drive, Suite #1134, Indianapolis, IN 46202, USA
* Corresponding author.
E-mail address: jraskin@goodmancampbell.com

Hand Clin 34 (2018) 547–554
https://doi.org/10.1016/j.hcl.2018.06.012

contractures, and, when possible, restore function. Because of the extensive fine motor function of the upper extremity, a satisfactory functional improvement is difficult to achieve.

Spasticity may result from any injury to the upper motor neuron, and the causes vary. There are congenital injuries, such as cerebral palsy (CP), and acquired ones, such as stroke, multiple sclerosis, and traumatic brain or spinal cord injury (SCI). The assessment of spasticity may be complicated by the presence of dystonia, a sustained series of muscle contractions that results in a writhing or twisting motion. Spasticity and dystonia often occur together and are difficult to distinguish.[4] In patients with mixed-movement disorders, reduction of spasticity may exacerbate underlying dystonia and worsen the overall functional impairment.

For the purposes of treatment, the underlying cause of spasticity is not as significant as the location and degree of the resulting symptoms. The treatment of upper extremity spasticity is typically a combination of surgical and nonsurgical; however, it always starts with conservative modalities, such as therapy and orthotics, intramuscular administration of botulinum toxin (Botox), and oral medications, such as muscle relaxants and anxiolytics.

Surgery for neuromodulation of muscle tone is reserved for cases that fail medical management. Targets have been explored throughout the neuromuscular pathway from cortex to muscle. These techniques include dorsal rhizotomy, intrathecal baclofen therapy (ITB), motor cortex stimulation, and deep brain stimulation (DBS). Musculoskeletal procedures to normalize the biomechanics of the upper extremity, such as tendon lengthening, tendon transfers, and osteotomies, may be used in combination with neurosurgical procedures. Regardless of the surgical approach, postoperative rehabilitation remains the cornerstone for the child or adult patient with spasticity. Furthermore, physical and occupational therapy are most effective when paired with a supportive home environment.

Improvements in muscle tone following Botox injections may be significant. However, studies demonstrate that without concurrent rehabilitation there is minimal to no correlated functional improvement.[5] For example, Russo and colleagues[6] found a clear functional benefit to post-Botox occupational therapy in a randomized controlled study of children with upper extremity spasticity; the improved spasticity lasted longer than Botox injections alone. This underscores the concept that integrated approaches are more successful than either therapy or Botox alone.[7]

MEDICAL TREATMENT

Therapy and orthotics are essential to prevent the development of contractures. These modalities, which can be delivered alone or in conjunction with medication, injections, or surgical treatments, are the mainstay of maintaining and improving function and accomplishing activities of daily living. There are a multitude of approaches; a full discussion is beyond the scope of this article, but a general methodology that promotes compensation strategies and active motor learning patterns have proven superior to passive manipulation and motion pattern normalization.[8–10]

Baclofen is the most commonly used medication for spasticity; nonetheless, there are other effective medications. Tizanidine, diazepam, and dantrolene are widely prescribed for spasticity, and several others, including clonidine, gabapentin, and cannabinoids, have been used to a lesser extent. Despite widespread acceptance and anecdotal reports of success, there is limited high-level evidence to guide the use of these medications.[11]

Intramuscular administration of Botox or intraneural injection of phenol for neurolysis has been described as effective nonsurgical treatments for spasticity. Botox acts by blocking the presynaptic release of acetylcholine, thereby reducing muscle contraction. It is an injectable agent with an expected duration of action of between 3 and 8 months. The medication may be administered multiple times; however, between 3% and 10% of patients develop antibodies to the toxin, which will reduce the effective duration. Botox is indicated for focal application to prevent the development of fixed contractures, to reduce spasticity compromising function, and for patient comfort.[12]

MUSCULOSKELETAL PROCEDURES

Serial casting may be used to lengthen a muscle shortened by contractures. There is robust evidence for this technique in the lower extremity, but it is not yet well accepted in the upper extremity.[13] The goal of upper extremity surgery in cases of spasticity is typically to improve function and posture of the affected upper limb. In cases of spasticity-related joint deformities, joint release, arthrodesis, tendon lengthenings, tendon transfers, and tendon rerouting may be used. Specific functional indications exist for various aspects of motor control in the elbow, wrist, fingers, and thumb. A careful assessment is required to determine which cases may benefit from this type of intervention.[14]

NEUROSURGICAL PROCEDURES

Since the dawn of neurosurgery in the late 1800s, procedures aimed at improving neurologic function have been broadly categorized as destructive, ablative, or lesional. This categorization is also true of neurosurgical approaches to treat spasticity, where there has been a marked increase in treatment options coincident with the growing neuromodulation industry. Here, the original lesional surgeries, subsequent neurostimulation approaches, and more recently described infusion of ITB are discussed.

Dorsal Rhizotomy

In 1908, Otfrid Foerster[15] developed dorsal rhizotomy for use first in the lumbosacral spine. In 1913, he published a report of 159 total cases of dorsal rhizotomy, 23 of which involved sectioning the dorsal roots of the cervical spine for upper extremity spasticity. His technique evolved over time: initially sectioning the posterior cervical roots from C4 to T2 while sparing C6, subsequently modifying the technique to sectioning three-fifths to four-fifths of each root. His conclusion from this series, however, was not favorable, and he reported satisfactory outcomes in only a few cases. The technique then went largely unreported on until 1967, when Claude Gros[16], a French neurosurgeon, reintroduced the procedure with a measure of selectivity. In the 1970s, Kottke[17] and Heimburger both proposed rhizotomy for control of neck and arm spasticity. Both studies were limited interventions on the upper cervical nerve roots. Heimburger and colleagues[18] limited their interventions to the C1-4 roots, citing improvement in spasticity in 13/15 patients. Only 1 of these patients, however, was reported to have a meaningful functional improvement.

The lumbar dorsal rhizotomy continues to show great promise in alleviating spasticity and improving function in the lower extremities of the spastic diplegic. There are also reports that lumbar selective dorsal rhizotomy has some effect on relieving upper extremity spasticity, including 1 report noting at least 1 point gross motor function classification (GMFC) score improvement in at least 2 upper extremity muscles in 92% of patients (23/25).[19] However, the selective dorsal rhizotomy technique applied to the cervical roots was not largely successful as a therapeutic modality primarily because relieving spasticity in the upper extremities does not lead to the same kinds of functional gains that are realized in the lower extremities. Although the procedure continues to be explored in the modern era, successful functional recovery remains unpredictable and patient specific.[20]

Dorsal Root Entry Zone Lesioning

In the 1970s, dorsal root entry zone (DREZ) lesioning was introduced as a treatment of certain persistent pain syndromes. The goal of lesioning in patients with spasticity is the disruption of both the nociceptive and myostatic tonigenic fibers coming from the dorsal root, without the disruption of the medial large-caliber fibers that reach the dorsal column by selective lesioning. Candidates for this therapy are those limited by severe pain in addition to spasticity or a hypofunctioning limb without central impairment. As with the more peripherally directed dorsal rhizotomy procedure, minimal functional improvement could be expected and only as a result of unmasking previous function limited by spasticity.[21,22] Furthermore, persistent and significant hypotonia is a known adverse effect of DREZ lesioning. As a result, this technique poses significant risks in an otherwise functional patient and is seldom used.

Cerebellar/Dorsal Column Stimulation

In the 1970s and 1980s, multiple studies evaluated cerebellar and dorsal column stimulation with the procedural goal of interrupting hypertetanic spastic impulses. Despite early enthusiasm for the technique, research did not demonstrate effectiveness of either method. In the case of the cerebellar stimulation, patients did, in fact, demonstrate improvement, but study participants also improved during the placebo period of stimulation.[23,24] With regard to cervical stimulation, no improvement was detected by multiple outcomes measures.[25] Further exploration has yielded limited improvements in upper extremity function.

Motor Cortex Stimulation

Motor cortex stimulation has been shown effective in case reports and case series, especially in spastic hemiparesis. Transcranial direct current stimulation (tDCS), in which a low direct current is delivered by scalp electrodes, has been investigated as an adjunctive therapeutic modality in upper extremity spasticity resulting from stroke. A meta-analysis of 8 retrospective articles from 6 groups showed a small to moderate effect for tDCS when applied to upper limb motor function after stroke. Importantly, none of the contributing trials exceeded 13 patients.[26] A broader Cochrane review of tDCS for all stroke functions was similarly limited.[27] Further investigation is needed to better define the role and effectiveness of tDCS.

Transcranial magnetic stimulation (TMS) uses magnetic impulses to induce an electrical current at a designated focal point. Several recent studies have investigated the utility of repetitive stimulation applied in this fashion to the brain and specifically the motor cortex of patients with spasticity. This technique has been shown to be safe, with mild or no adverse effects reported in any trial, although a theoretic risk of seizure induction is described for high-frequency TMS. No study to date has focused on the efficacy or utility of this therapy in the upper extremity. Existing trials have shown that outcomes were generally diagnosis specific, with no effect in patients suffering from CP. Patients with stroke, multiple sclerosis, and incomplete SCI are reported to achieve significant improvements in spasticity, but results are temporary. Complete SCI patients are the only subgroup that demonstrated statistically significant persistent improvements. The general efficacy of this technique for spasticity has yet to be determined.[28,29]

Deep Brain Stimulation

Dystonic posturing may be localized to a specific muscle group or extremity, or it may generalize. It is classified by time of onset, distribution, temporal pattern, and associated features and may be inherited, acquired, sporadic, or idiopathic. Treatment of dystonia often improves spasticity. As with spasticity, however, there is no cure for dystonia, and treatment is directed at specific symptoms. Therapy for dystonia may be classified by responsiveness to levodopa. Whereas Botox injection is a second-line treatment for nonresponders, certain focal dystonias respond well. Cervical dystonia (ie, spasmodic torticollis) is the most well-established focal dystonia, but studies have suggested responses in blepharospasm, focal upper limb dystonia, and laryngeal dystonia.[30]

DBS may be a reasonable option in patients with mixed findings of spasticity and dystonia. DBS is thought to selectively treat dystonia, but it may also improve function. Use of DBS is largely confined to primary dystonia because this subtype is unresponsive to medications or Botox. With rare exception, patients with secondary dystonia do not respond well to DBS.[31] The globus pallidus interna is the most well-studied target for therapy, yet the subthalamic nucleus has also been investigated.[32] Studies demonstrate significant improvements in quality of life and reduction in disability, which are sustained at 3 to 5 years after the procedure. Most complications are device related, including malpositioning and infection.[33,34]

Spinal Cord Stimulation

Spinal cord stimulation (SCS) is delivered via a variety of epidural neuromodulatory devices designed to convey transdural electrical potentials into the spinal cord. This modality may be relatively sophisticated and include wireless programming technology, complex electrode geometry, and high-frequency stimulation. During the 1980s and 1990s, SCS was used to treat spasticity of the upper extremity following SCI with variable benefit, but with high cost and risk for device complications.[35,36] Given the currently available evidence, SCS is used most commonly for neuropathic pain.

Intrathecal Baclofen Therapy

Baclofen is a gamma-aminobutyric acid (GABA) derivative that works as a $GABA_B$ agonist. Activation of metabotropic $GABA_B$ receptors functionally dampens the excitatory neurotransmitters and thereby inhibits segmental monosynaptic and polysynaptic reflexes, resulting in relief of spasticity. However, in sufficient concentration, baclofen also has a depressing effect on central nervous system function, commonly resulting in side effects, such as confusion, dizziness, drowsiness, or nausea. These symptoms may limit oral dosing below a level that would otherwise be effective in controlling spasticity. If the oral dosing requirement for spasticity exceeds the maximum tolerated dose, the patient can be converted to intrathecal administration (**Fig. 1**). In this fashion, the overall systemic dose can be greatly reduced while still maintaining sufficient concentrations within the thecal space to reduce spasticity. Pharmacokinetic studies have shown that 4-fold increases in intrathecal baclofen concentration are achievable with 1/100th of the plasma concentration as compared with oral administration. Once in the intrathecal space, it acts on the superficial layers of the spinal cord to effectively reconstitute the function of the deficient GABA.

The earliest reported use of ITB for the purposes of treating spasticity was in the 1980s. Resulting from subsequent single-center studies and a multicenter clinical trial, the US Food and Drug Administration approved ITB for the treatment of spasticity of cerebral origin in 1996. A follow-up study by the investigators of the clinical trial confirmed the previously reported outcomes: statistically significant declines in spasticity as measured by Ashworth scores in both upper and lower extremities, which were enduring at 6, 12, and 24 months. Moreover, although baclofen dosages delivered by pump generally increased gradually over the first 2 years, they tended to remain stable thereafter.[37] Finally, baclofen was also

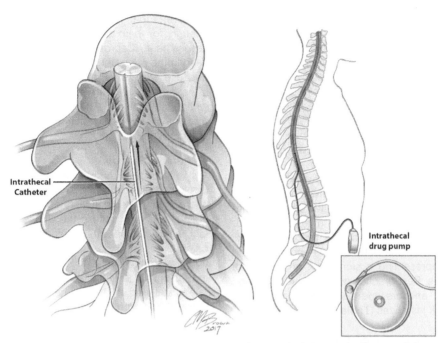

Fig. 1. Baclofen is delivered to the intrathecal space via a catheter, which is proximally passed through a Tuohy needle and tunneled to the desired level and distally connected to a refillable implanted pump. (*Courtesy of* C.M. Brown, BFA, MS, Indianapolis, IN.)

effective irrespective of the inciting cause of spasticity.[2]

ITB is typically considered for patients with severe spasticity or dystonia who, because of severity of symptoms or as a result of side effects from oral therapy, cannot tolerate oral medication in sufficient doses to resolve the spasticity. The size of the device does limit implantation in smaller patients, and, as such, the device is rarely implanted in patients younger than 6 years old. There are, however, selective reports of implantation in patients as small as 9 months of age and 18 pounds, yet most children younger than 4 respond well to oral medications.[38]

Pump implantation is generally indicated in moderate to severe spasticity with Ashworth 3 or higher scores. Pump use has been described in spastic hemiplegic patients in whom, with careful dose titration, spasticity is relieved without causing hypotonia on the unaffected side. ITB is considered second-line therapy for spastic diplegia, because these patients are usually better served with a selective dorsal rhizotomy.

This treatment modality has several advantages. It can be trialed with a single therapeutic lumbar puncture introducing 50 to 100 μg of baclofen. An intrathecal baclofen trial is indicated when a mixed-movement disorder is present, or when a patient or family desires evidence of the benefits of ITB. Similar to upper extremity rhizotomy, ITB

does not confer meaningful functional benefits. However, because the effects are titratable by dose, the effect can be adjusted according to each patient's evolving needs.[37,39,40]

The complication rate from pump placement ranges from 21% to 37%[41–43] and is most commonly attributed to infection, wound-related complications, and mechanical failure of the device or catheter. As with most implantable devices, infections may require removal of the device. Mechanical failure may potentiate life-threatening withdrawal as a result of the abrupt cessation of medication delivery. Studies have demonstrated a learning curve with device use, and complication rates tend to decline as institutional experience increases.[41,42] Therefore, best-practice guidelines recommend centers place at least 10 devices per year to maintain proficiency.[44]

Studies show wide variation in catheter-related complications, with published reports ranging from 3% to 75%. In practice, these problems can be difficult to diagnose. Their prompt recognition, however, is imperative because baclofen withdrawal can be fatal. ITB has been shown to downregulate expression of $GABA_B$ receptors in rats because the baclofen itself accounts for increased inhibitory tone.[45] Withdrawal potentiates a hyperexcitatory expression of symptoms, which include extreme spasticity, pruritis, anxiety, and disorientation. In severe cases, hyperthermia, rhabdomyolysis, and seizures have resulted in multiorgan failure, cardiac arrest, or death. Severe symptoms can be confused for shock or sepsis and delayed recognition of the underlying cause, and delay in repleting the baclofen can also be fatal. Although safety alarms can signal the device is low on medication or approaching the end of its battery life, an abrupt mechanical failure or catheter obstruction may not be readily detected. There are also sporadic reported instances of failure of the device itself.[42]

Reported infection rates for the ITB pump and catheter implantation are between 3% and 15%.[41–43] The use of perioperative systemic antibiotics correlates with reduced infection rate over 6 months.[46] The reported rate of cerebrospinal fluid (CSF) leak was between 6% and 15%, with children representing a significant proportion of those cases. Best practice guidelines recommend the use of anchors and purse-string sutures to reduce leak instances (**Table 1**).

Effect of catheter tip location

An important consideration for ITB is the ultimate location of the tip of the delivery catheter from which the drug diffuses. Early studies on intrathecal baclofen dosing include experiments as to how the drug concentration might change across the intrathecal space and whether this would impact efficacy or potential side effects. One study suggests a 43% drop across 20 cm, a measurement that corresponds roughly to the difference between localization at T12 and T2.[47–52] Given this property, the location of the catheter tip can have a substantial effect on the effectiveness of treatment and the medication dose required. If the target of therapy is relief for the upper extremities, then a midcervical placement should be the goal. If the patient is tetraplegic and requires 4-limb improvement, then an upper thoracic localization should be the goal.

Pump placement

In general, a subfascial abdominal placement is recommended to prevent erosions and reduce the possibility of the pump rotating in the pocket.

Table 1
Baclofen pump complications

Overall complications: 21%–37%		
Catheter-related complications	Infections	CSF leak
3%–75%	3%–15%	6%–15%

However, the pump must remain superficial enough for palpation and access for refills or assessment. Dacron pouches were commonly used in the past, but are no longer recommended because they were found to increase infection rates, particularly with revision surgery. As of this writing, several sizes of pumps are available with the primary limitation being the size and body habitus of the patient.[44]

Catheter placement

A skin incision is made at the L2-3 or L3-4 levels (avoiding the increased mobility at the L4-5 levels) and a Touhy needle is inserted paraspinally at an oblique angle to access the CSF space. A catheter with a radiopaque stiffener is advanced under fluoroscopic guidance. In order to address upper extremity spasticity or spastic tetraplegia, the tip should be localized between C5 and T2. The distal end of the catheter should then be secured with an anchor and tunneled to the pump location.[44] This technique has the advantages of being safe and less invasive than other alternatives. However, factors such as previous surgery or fusion, or the presence of a scoliotic deformity, may limit the ability to place the catheter in such a fashion even under fluoroscopic guidance.

SUMMARY

For the patient in whom oral medication has failed to control spasticity or the side effects of oral medication have proven intolerable, there are surgical alternatives that may successfully control spasticity. However, no therapeutic modality has been proven to yield functional improvement in the affected limb, except in cases where existing function is masked by spasticity. ITB has been widely accepted as the predominant neurosurgical treatment modality for its advantages of titratability and side-effect profile. However, this therapy at best is still only a means to control spasticity rather than improve functional outcome. The titratability of neurostimulation or medication infusion is alluring, although long-term outcome studies are continually needed to justify increased cost over lesional surgery. Because the treatment of spasticity is patient specific, the individual interventions described in this article should be applied within the framework of specific goals of care to optimize function and comfort and minimize side effects. Other neuromodulatory treatment modalities continue to be explored. Care must be taken to manage patient expectations in the surgical treatment of this challenging disorder.

REFERENCES

1. Albright AL. Neurosurgical treatment of spasticity and other pediatric movement disorders. J Child Neurol 2003;18(1_suppl):S67–78.

2. Chang E, Ghosh N, Yanni D, et al. A review of spasticity treatments: pharmacological and interventional approaches. Crit Rev Phys Rehabil Med 2013;25(1–2):11–22.

3. Sherrington CS. Decerebrate rigidity, and reflex coordination of movements. J Physiol 1898;22(4):319–32.

4. Gordon LM, Keller JL, Stashinko EE, et al. Can spasticity and dystonia be independently measured in cerebral palsy? Pediatr Neurol 2006;35(6):375–81.

5. Satila H, Kotamaki A, Koivikko M, et al. Upper limb function after botulinum toxin A treatment in cerebral palsy: two years follow-up of six cases. Pediatr Rehabil 2006;9(3):247–58.

6. Russo RN, Crotty M, Miller MD, et al. Upper-limb botulinum toxin a injection and occupational therapy in children with hemiplegic cerebral palsy identified from a population register: a single-blind, randomized, controlled trial. Pediatrics 2007;119(5):e1149–58.

7. Kaňovský P, Bareš M, Severa S, et al. Long-term efficacy and tolerability of 4-monthly versus yearly botulinum toxin type A treatment for lower-limb spasticity in children with cerebral palsy. Dev Med Child Neurol 2009;51(6):436–45.

8. Bar-Haim S, Harries N, Nammourah I, et al. Effectiveness of motor learning coaching in children with cerebral palsy: a randomized controlled trial. Clin Rehabil 2010;24(11):1009–20.

9. Morgan C, Darrah J, Gordon AM, et al. Effectiveness of motor interventions in infants with cerebral palsy: a systematic review. Dev Med Child Neurol 2016;58(9):900–9.

10. Novak I, McIntyre S, Morgan C, et al. A systematic review of interventions for children with cerebral palsy: state of the evidence. Dev Med Child Neurol 2013;55(10):885–910.

11. Pharmacological interventions for spasticity following spinal cord injury. Cochrane Database Syst Rev 2009;(4). https://doi.org/10.1002/14651858.CD001131. Available at: www.cochranelibrary.com.

12. Simpson DM, Gracies J-M, Graham HK, et al. Assessment: botulinum neurotoxin for the treatment of spasticity (an evidence-based review): report of the therapeutics and technology assessment subcommittee of the American Academy of neurology. Neurology 2008;70(19):1691–8.

13. Lannin NA, Novak I, Cusick A. A systematic review of upper extremity casting for children and adults with central nervous system motor disorders. Clin Rehabil 2007;21(11):963–76.

14. Van Heest AE, Bagley A, Molitor F, et al. Tendon transfer surgery in upper-extremity cerebral palsy is more effective than botulinum toxin injections or regular, ongoing therapy. J Bone Joint Surg Am 2015;97(7):529–36.

15. Foerster O. On the indications and results of the excision of posterior spinal nerve-roots in men. Surg Gynecol Obs 1913;16(16):463–74.

16. Gros C, nOuaknine G, Vlahovitch B, et al. La radicotomic selective posterieure dans le traitement neurochirurgical del'hypertonie pyramidale. Neurochirurgie 1967;13:505–18.

17. Kottke J. Modification of athetosis by denervation of the tonic reflexes. Develop Med Child Neurol 1970;12:236–7.

18. Heimburger RF, Slominski A, Griswold P. Cervical posterior rhizotomy for reducing spasticity in cerebral palsy. J Neurosurg 1973;39(1):30–4.

19. Gigante P, McDowell MM, Bruce SS, et al. Reduction in upper-extremity tone after lumbar selective dorsal rhizotomy in children with spastic cerebral palsy. J Neurosurg Pediatr 2013;12(6):588–94.

20. Bertelli JA, Ghizoni MF, Michels A. Brachial plexus dorsal rhizotomy in the treatment of upper-limb spasticity. J Neurosurg 2000;93(1):26–32.

21. Sindou M, Mifsud JJ, Boisson D, et al. Selective posterior rhizotomy in the dorsal root entry zone for treatment of hyperspasticity and pain in the hemiplegic upper limb. Neurosurgery 1986;18(5):587–95.

22. Sindou M, Georgoulis G, Mertens P. Neurosurgery for spasticity. Vienna (Austria): Springer Vienna; 2014. https://doi.org/10.1007/978-3-7091-1771-2.

23. Gahm NH, Russman BS, Cerciello RL, et al. Chronic cerebellar stimulation for cerebral palsy: a double-blind study. Neurology 1981;31(1):87–90. Available at: http://www.ncbi.nlm.nih.gov/pubmed/6969867.

24. Cooper IS, Riklan M, Amin I, et al. Chronic cerebellar stimulation in cerebral palsy. Neurology 1976;26(8):744–53. Available at: http://www.ncbi.nlm.nih.gov/pubmed/1084966.

25. Gottlieb GL, Myklebust BM, Stefoski D, et al. Evaluation of cervical stimulation for chronic treatment of spasticity. Neurology 1985;35(5):699–704. Available at: http://www.ncbi.nlm.nih.gov/pubmed/3887212.

26. Butler AJ, Shuster M, O'Hara E, et al. A meta-analysis of the efficacy of anodal transcranial direct current stimulation for upper limb motor recovery in stroke survivors. J Hand Ther 2013;26(2):162–71.

27. Elsner B, Kugler J, Pohl M, et al. Transcranial direct current stimulation (tDCS) for improving activities of daily living, and physical and cognitive functioning, in people after stroke [review]. Cochrane Database Syst Rev 2016;(3). https://doi.org/10.1002/14651858.CD009645.pub3. Available at: www.cochranelibrary.com.

28. Kumru H, Pascual-Leone A, Gunduz A. Outcomes in spasticity after repetitive transcranial magnetic and transcranial direct current stimulations. Neural Regen Res 2014;9(7):712.

29. Korzhova J, Sinitsyn D, Chervyakov A, et al. Transcranial and spinal cord magnetic stimulation in treatment of spasticity. A literature review and meta–analysis. Eur J Phys Rehabil Med 2018;54(1):75–84. Available at: http://www.ncbi.nlm.nih.gov/pubmed/28004906.

30. Costa J, Espírito-Santo C, Borges A, et al. Botulinum toxin type A versus anticholinergics for cervical dystonia. Cochrane Database Syst Rev 2005;(1): CD004312.

31. Eltahawy HA, Saint-Cyr J, Giladi N, et al. Primary dystonia is more responsive than secondary dystonia to pallidal interventions: outcome after pallidotomy or pallidal deep brain stimulation. Neurosurgery 2004;54(3):613–21.

32. Kupsch A, Benecke R, Müller JJ-U, et al. Pallidal deep-brain stimulation in primary generalized or segmental dystonia. N Engl J Med 2006;355(19): 1978–90.

33. Kiss ZHT, Doig-Beyaert K, Eliasziw M, et al. The Canadian multicentre study of deep brain stimulation for cervical dystonia. Brain 2007;130(11):2879–86.

34. Vidailhet M, Vercueil L, Houeto JL, et al. Bilateral, pallidal, deep-brain stimulation in primary generalised dystonia: a prospective 3 year follow-up study. Lancet Neurol 2007;6(3):223–9.

35. Siegfried J, Lazorthes Y, Broggi G. Electrical spinal cord stimulation for spastic movement disorders. Stereotact Funct Neurosurg 1981;44(1–3):77–92.

36. Barolat G, Myklebust JB, Wenninger W. Effects of spinal cord stimulation on spasticity and spasms secondary to myelopathy. Stereotact Funct Neurosurg 1988;51(1):29–44.

37. Albright AL. Intrathecal baclofen for spasticity in cerebral palsy. JAMA 1991;265(11):1418–22.

38. Albright AL, Ferson SS. Intrathecal baclofen therapy in children. Neurosurg Focus 2006;21(2):e3.

39. Albright AL, Gilmartin R, Swift D, et al. Long-term intrathecal baclofen therapy for severe spasticity of cerebral origin. J Neurosurg 2003;98:291–5.

40. Butler C, Campbell S. Evidence of the effects of intrathecal baclofen for spastic and dystonic cerebral palsy. Dev Med Child Neurol 2000;42(9): 634–45.

41. Motta F, Buonaguro V, Stignani C. The use of intrathecal baclofen pump implants in children and adolescents: safety and complications in 200 consecutive cases. J Neurosurg 2007;107(1 Suppl):32–5.

42. Taira T, Ueta T, Katayama Y, et al. Rate of complications among the recipients of intrathecal baclofen pump in Japan: a multicenter study. Neuromodulation 2013;16(3):266–72.

43. Albright AL, Awaad Y, Muhonen M, et al. Performance and complications associated with the Synchromed 10-ml infusion pump for intrathecal baclofen administration in children. J Neurosurg Pediatr 2004;101(2):64–8.

44. Albright AL, Turner M, Pattisapu JV. Best-practice surgical techniques for intrathecal baclofen therapy. J Neurosurg 2006;104(4 Suppl):233–9.

45. Kroin JS, Bianchi GD, Penn RD. Intrathecal baclofen down-regulates GABAB receptors in the rat substantia gelatinosa. J Neurosurg 1993;79(4):544–9.

46. Pan I, Kuo GM, Luerssen TG, et al. Impact of antibiotic prophylaxis for intrathecal baclofen pump surgery in pediatric patients. Neurosurg Focus 2015; 39(6):1–8.

47. Kroin JS, Ali A, York M, et al. The distribution of medication along the spinal canal after chronic intrathecal administration. Neurosurgery 1993;33(2): 226–30. Available at: http://ovidsp.ovid.com/ovidweb.cgi?T=JS&PAGE=reference&D=med3&NEWS=N&AN=7690122.

48. Robinson S, Robertson FC, Dasenbrock HH, et al. Image-guided intrathecal baclofen pump catheter implantation: a technical note and case series. J Neurosurg Spine 2017;26(5):621–7.

49. Liu JK, Walker ML. Posterior cervical approach for intrathecal baclofen pump insertion in children with previous spinal fusions. J Neurosurg Pediatr 2005; 102(1):119–22.

50. Dziurzynski K, Mcleish D, Ward M, et al. Placement of baclofen pumps through the foramen magnum and upper cervical spine. Childs Nerv Syst 2006; 22(3):270–3.

51. Ughratdar I, Muquit S, Ingale H, et al. Cervical implantation of intrathecal baclofen pump catheter in children with severe scoliosis. J Neurosurg Pediatr 2012;10(1):34–8.

52. Aljuboori Z, Archer J, Huff W, et al. Placement of Baclofen pump catheter through C1-C2 puncture: technical note. J Neurosurg Pediatr 2018;21(4): 389–94.

Management of Spinal Cord Injury-Induced Upper Extremity Spasticity

Andreas Gohritz, MD[a,b], Jan Fridén, MD, PhD[a,c],*

KEYWORDS

- Spasticity • Spinal cord injuries • Tetraplegia • Upper extremity • Reconstructive surgery
- Tendon operations • Rehabilitation

KEY POINTS

- Spasticity affects more than 80% of patients with spinal cord injury (SCI) and is significant challenge for the treating surgeon.
- Spasticity resulting from SCI typically presents with shoulder adduction/pronation, elbow, wrist, and finger flexion (closed fist), and forearm pronation.
- Tendon lengthening, release, transfer, and selective neurotomies may prevent further contracture and improve posture and function over the long term.

INTRODUCTION

The global incidence of spinal cord injury (SCI) has been estimated at 10 to 80 new cases per million annually, which translates into approximately 250,000 to 500,000 newly paralyzed people worldwide every year[1]. In about 50% of patients, SCI occurs at the cervical level, leading to a profoundly disabling tetraplegia (paralysis of all 4 extremities), mainly because of the lost arm and hand function.[2] As SCI remains incurable, upper extremity function is, aside from the brain, the most important functional resource of tetraplegic patients. In fact, patients judged upper extremity function to be the most desirable function to regain, before bowel, urinary, and sexual function, or walking ability. In a survey, 49% of tetraplegic individuals ranked rehabilitation of arm and hand function as the first priority, with no other goal surpassing 13%.[3] Another study reported that 77% of 565 tetraplegic patients expected important or very

important improvement in quality of life if their hand function improved.[4]

Upper extremity surgery involving tendon and nerve transfers, tenodeses, and joint stabilizations can reliably reconstruct key functions.[5–9] Restoration of elbow extension improves reaching capabilities and stabilizes the elbow, allowing for further reconstruction to achieve grasp, and the ability to swim and drive.[10] Reconstructed grip eliminates the need for adaptive equipment, allows one to self-groom, feed, catheterize, manipulate objects, write, and perform productive work, and markedly improves autonomy and spontaneity, thus enhancing self-esteem for tetraplegic patients.[11]

Spasticity affects about 80% of patients with SCI, especially those with cervical lesions and incomplete injuries. These include anterior cord syndrome, central cord syndrome, and Brown-Sequard syndrome,[12] which have increased in prevalence, mainly because of improved acute

Disclosure Statement: No conflict of interest whatsoever for any of the authors to disclose.
[a] Department of Hand Surgery, Swiss Paraplegic Centre, Guido A. Zäch Str. 1, Nottwil CH-6207, Switzerland;
[b] Department of Plastic, Reconstructive and Aesthetic Surgery, Hand Surgery, Universitätsspital, Spitalstraße 21, Basel CH-4031, Switzerland; [c] Institute of Clinical Sciences, Center for Advanced Reconstruction of Extremities, University of Gothenburg, Gothenburg, Sweden
* Corresponding author. Swiss Paraplegic Centre, Guido A. Zäch Str. 1, Nottwil CH-6207, Switzerland.
E-mail address: jan.friden@paraplegie.ch

management and long-term rehabilitation.[13–15] Spasticity in SCI represents a severe impairment and was, until recently, regarded as a contraindication for functional surgery.[16] Consequently, it represents a seldom-described and challenging problem.[12,17]

This article details surgical treatment options for spasticity of the upper extremity in patients with cervical SCI and tetraplegia. The authors summarize fundamentals of upper extremity spasticity and describe their experience with surgical methods to restore balance and control of the upper extremity.

CHARACTERISTICS OF SPASTICITY IN SPINAL CORD INJURY
Pathophysiological Features

Although the exact pathogenesis is still unknown, spasticity after SCI involves several features:
- Muscle hypertonicity
- Hyper-reflexia
- Clonus
- Clasp-knife responses
- Long-lasting cutaneous reflexes
- Muscle spasms (evoked by brief non-noxious skin stimuli)[18]

Evolution

Spasticity in SCI develops gradually over several months in a characteristic sequence:

- Spinal cord becomes areflexic (spinal shock)
- Tendon reflexes below the level of the lesion are lost
- Muscle paralysis apparent
- Flaccid muscle tone occurs[19]

Especially in individuals with incomplete SCI, spasticity may reduce the functional utility of residual voluntary motor control and thus severely compromise efforts at rehabilitation.

Muscle-Tendon-Joint Alterations

The pathophysiology of spasticity varies depending on the location of the lesion, but mostly develops in the antigravity muscles. Although neural mechanisms are thought to prevail, and alterations in muscle contractile properties may be less pronounced than that observed after stroke, an SCI also leads to major structural changes influencing tonicity of muscles. These changes include atrophy and fibrosis of muscle tissue because of several causes:

- Decreased myofibrillar elasticity
- Disregulation of sarcomere number

- A change of collagen type distribution and expression
- Accumulation of connective tissue
- An alteration of contractile properties, with a tendency toward tonic muscle characteristics[18,20,21]

Useful Versus Harmful Spasticity

The many manifestations of spasticity in incomplete SCI make the assessment of the SCI patient in daily practice often confusing and challenging. As a foundation, the upper extremity surgeon needs to have a simple starting point when assessing SCI patients with spasticity. Allieu proposed a practical classification of spasticity: useful or harmful spasticity.[22]

Useful spasticity can be helpful in several daily life situations (eg, finger flexor spasticity when holding an object or triceps spasticity when transferring to or from a wheelchair). It may also help to preserve muscle volume and joint-bone strength. Spasticity can be triggered by multiple stimuli or agents, such as pain (injury, wound, nerve compression), body temperature change (fever), mood change (stress, anxiety), infection (urinary tract, wound).

Harmful spasticity typically causes
- Increased muscle tone
- Involuntary movements
- Spasms (quick or sustained involuntary muscle contractions)
- Clonus (series of fast involuntary contractions)
- Pain or discomfort involving the muscles, joints, and tendons
- Joint contractures/deformities
- Hygiene problems, such as that seen with a hyperflexed elbow, adducted thumb, or clenched fist
- Transfer problems
- Abnormal posture
- Social inconveniences

Many individuals with spasticity after SCI have learned to use key trigger strategies to beneficially apply spasticity in daily life. Therefore, useful spasticity needs to be discerned before any surgical intervention is undertaken. In general, patients describe spasticity as a harmful and disturbing factor in their lives.

In a person who does not perform regular range-of-motion exercises, muscles and joints become less flexible, and almost any minor stimulation can cause severe spasticity. In this population, an acute exacerbation of spasticity also serves as a warning system when sensation is otherwise absent. For example, increased spasticity may be the signal of a urinary tract infection or an ingrown toenail.

Upper Extremity Deformity

Spasticity in the arm and hand after SCI is characterized by
- Shoulder adduction/internal rotation
- Forearm pronation
- Elbow, wrist, finger, and thumb flexion
- Thumb adduction (thumb-in-palm deformity)[23]

The closed-fist position of the spastic hand leads to difficulties in efficiently reaching, grasping, and releasing items. Treatment efforts aim to improve arm and hand usability by addressing the ability to grasp, release, and open the hand. Further goals include a long-term decrease of hypertonicity in the spastic muscles, as well as rebalancing the remaining functioning agonists and antagonists. Small objects are difficult to grasp when flexion of the finger joints is limited by spasticity. If the metacarpophalangeal (MCP) joints are affected, the opening of the hand is markedly reduced.

Spasticity in the hand varies from a decreased grip control to a completely clenched fist (**Fig. 1**). Some patients have spasticity in all flexor muscles, whereas some only have intrinsic involvement.

Intrinsic spasticity or tightness may be secondary to other conditions, such as established edema, hematoma, rheumatoid arthritis, ischemia, and central nervous system (CNS) lesions.

CONSERVATIVE TREATMENT

Nonoperative methods, such as splints, stretching, electrical stimulation, and pharmacologic management are frequently used. However, data supporting their effectiveness are limited, and the resulting benefits are inherently transient and potentially unpredictable. Splinting is used to address deformities, stabilize joints, aid transfer, reduce pain, facilitate optimization of remaining functions, and for preoperative test and postoperative protection of tendon surgery. It is less effective in long-standing (>6 months) contractures. Notably, dynamic splints may, in fact, trigger spasticity.

SURGICAL MANAGEMENT

Before surgery is undertaken, expectations of the patient, the surgeon, and the rehabilitation team have to align. Some patients with incomplete SCI can walk with or without aids; they require special attention in order to meet their specific goals of balance during gait and better hand use.

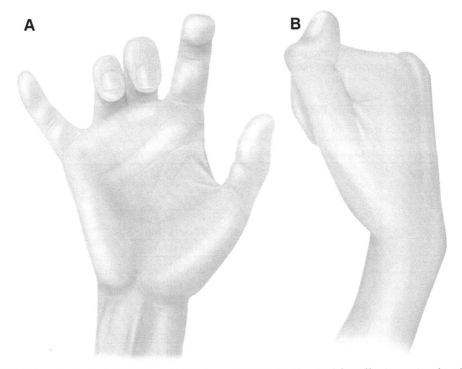

Fig. 1. (*A*) Mild spasticity limited to deep digital flexors 3 to 4. (*B*) Clenched fist affecting wrist, thumb, finger flexors, and intrinsics.

Improving shoulder range of motion and opening the hand through surgery can increase the arm swing during walking and facilitate grasping around a handle of a crutch or rollator.

Most patients with incomplete tetraplegia present with weak functions obscured by spasticity. These hidden functions should be allowed to strengthen after surgery when the influence of and deformity caused by the spastic muscles have been reduced. Also prior to surgery, antagonistic muscle training should be initiated, when suitable. A common approach is to temporarily paralyze key spastic muscles using botulinum toxin injection and thereafter electrically stimulate and voluntarily condition the remaining functioning muscles.

SELECTION AND TIMING OF PROCEDURES

Based on their experience of more than 300 operations addressing spasticity in SCI patients, the authors recommend the use of safe procedures (**Table 1**).[17] These operations can be performed in an isolated or combined fashion. Importantly, tendon transfers are excluded in this table of procedures. Reducing upper extremity spasticity will affect the balance in multiple joints, and the authors consider it contraindicated to perform a tendon transfer in this patient group before the postoperative training has reached a plateau. Not until then can the strengthened antagonist's full contribution and integration into arm and hand functionality be evaluated. However, at least 1 exception to this recommendation exists: the rare case where the extensor carpi ulnaris (ECU)

tendon has subluxated volarly at the wrist and further exaggerates the wrist flexion deformity. In these cases, the ECU should be transferred into the extensor carpi radialis brevis (ECRB) at distal forearm level concomitant with the lengthening/release procedures. Surgical treatment generally addresses spasticity by lengthening tendons and releasing muscles in an effort to relax the entire muscle tendon unit. As a result, the spastic muscles will generate less strength after surgery.

OPERATIONS FAVORED BY THE AUTHORS

The following operations are time-proven and reliably improve posture and function.

Pectoralis Major Tendon Lengthening

A common feature of shoulder dysfunction in patients with incomplete tetraplegia is related to the imbalance between weak external rotators and spastic internal rotators (**Fig. 2**). Botulinum toxin can be used successfully to reduce the internal rotation forces imparted by the pectoralis major; simultaneous electrical stimulation of rotator cuff muscles is commonly performed. Increasing the strength of rotator cuff muscles is an important adjunct to prevent glenohumeral joint dislocation. For a more permanent effect, however, the pectoralis tendon lengthening should be considered.[24]

Subscapularis Tenotomy

Subscapularis tenotomy is undertaken only when pectoralis lengthening is insufficient to allow

---

Table 1
Surgical approach to spastic joint deformities

Joint Deformity	Muscle Affected	Procedure	Technique
Spastic shoulder (adduction, pronation)	Pectoralis major Subscapularis	Tendon lengthening Tenotomy	Stair-step incision Transection
Spastic elbow (flexion)	Biceps brachii Brachialis	Tendon lengthening Muscle-fascia transection	Stair-step incision Aponeurotomy
Forearm (pronation)	Pronator teres	Muscle-tendon release	Disinsertion
Spastic wrist (flexion)	Flexor carpi radialis	Tendon lengthening	Stair-step incision
Spastic fingers (flexion)	Flexor digitorum profundus	Tendon lengthening	Stair-step incision
	Flexor digitorum superficialis	Tendon lengthening	Stair-step incision
	Interossei, lumbricals	Distal ulnar wing release	Partial aponeurectomy
Spastic thumb (flexion, Adduction)	Flexor pollicis longus Adductor pollicis	Tendon lengthening Muscle-tendon release Widening first web space	Stair-step incision Disinsertion Z-plasty

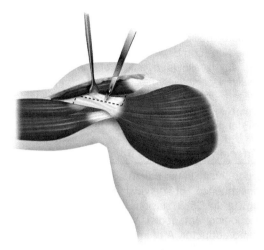

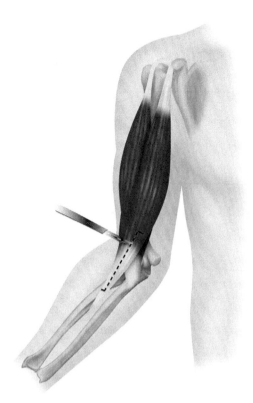

Fig. 2. Pectoralis major tendon lengthening. An angulated incision is made over the prominent and tense pectoralis major tendon. The tendon is exposed over an 8 to 10 cm distance. Using a stair-step incision (*dotted lines*), the tendon is allowed to lengthen while the arm is abducted at least 45°, and the muscle is allowed to retract. Reattach the 2 ends with sufficient overlap (ie, 2–3 cm) using the double-sided running suture back-and-forth technique. Tenotomy should be avoided, as it causes a full retraction of the muscle and a cosmetically unsightly bulk of the pectoralis muscle mass.

satisfactory passive abduction/external rotation of the shoulder. A lateral release or stair-step tendon subscapularis lengthening may be performed by an open or arthroscopic approach. The initial approach is through the deltopectoral groove, through which the cephalic vein courses. The deltoid muscle is retracted cranially/laterally, and the pectoralis muscle is retracted caudally. With maximal shoulder external rotation, the subscapularis tendon is identified and divided vertically, lateral to the musculotendinous junction. One should be aware of the axillary nerve just distal to the subscapularis and medial to the proximal humerus.[24]

Biceps Brachii Tendon Lengthening

The flexed elbow is a prominent feature and major obstacle for hand control, as well as an unfortunate stigma for many SCI patients with spasticity (**Fig. 3**). In addition, this deformity may also cause impairment of trunk posture, gait pattern in walking patients, and respiratory function, particularly in high incomplete SCI injuries affecting phrenic nerve function. In a completely nonfunctional arm, release of the flexed elbow will facilitate personal hygiene, dressing, and wheelchair transfer ability.[25]

Fig. 3. Biceps tendon lengthening. Because of the large moment arm of the biceps muscle, its distal tendon is easily palpable when spastic. A transverse incision is made in the anterior elbow and extended 6 to 8 cm in distal direction laterally and medially 6 to 8 cm in proximal direction. The adjacent median nerve and brachial vessels are protected. The lacertus fibrosus tendon is completely severed. On the biceps main tendon, a 10 cm midline incision is made through the tendon just proximal to its insertion on the radial tuberosity and proximally into the intramuscular portion of the biceps tendon. A long stair-step tendon incision secures 2 to 3 cm of overlap, even if the flexion deformity is severe. *Dotted lines* indicate incisions intended.

Brachialis Distal Aponeurotomy

The brachialis generates a substantial elbow flexion torque (**Fig. 4**). When spastic, it rapidly results in an elbow flexion contracture. In severe spastic flexion deformities of the elbow and in those without adequate triceps function, the brachialis fascia and tendon need to be surgically released.[26]

Pronator Teres Release

The authors' clinical experience suggests that the pronator teres (PT) acts a spasticity-triggering mechanism for the entire upper extremity in those with incomplete tetraplegia (**Fig. 5**). Therefore, the authors frequently perform PT release as an isolated

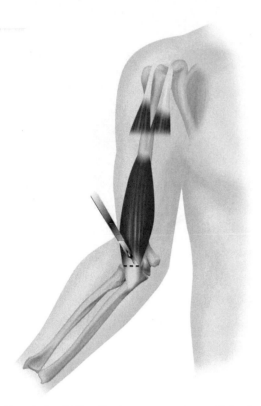

Fig. 4. Brachialis distal aponeurotomy. After the lengthening of the biceps tendon, the brachialis fascia can be exposed. The entire anterior fascia is transected together with intramuscular tendon fascicles. The elbow is then passively extended to a degree that is sufficient without putting undue tension on the median nerve and adjacent vessels. Special attention must be paid to median nerve tension, as it may be compounded if a concomitant correction of wrist flexion deformity is undertaken. *Dotted lines* indicate incisions intended.

procedure to reduce overall spasticity. Following release, the distribution and magnitude of any remaining spasticity is better evaluated and more specifically addressed in subsequent surgeries.[27]

Wrist, Finger, and Thumb Flexor Tendon Lengthening

Together with PT release, the finger, thumb, and wrist flexor lengthenings are the most frequently performed procedures to restore hand control in incomplete SCI (**Fig. 6**).[28,29]

Tendon-To-Tendon Attachment

This type of tendon-to-tendon attachment has many advantages, including strength, stiffness, and favorable gliding quality, and it is routinely used for all tendon lengthening or transfer procedures in the authors' practice (**Fig. 7**).[30]

Adductor Pollicis Release

Adductor pollicis (AdP) release is frequently performed in combination with other procedures (**Fig. 8**). It allows opening of the hand when passively or actively flexing the wrist, in order to facilitate object grasp. AdP release also enables a more functional key pinch, especially when the AdP longus (APL) function is present.[23]

Widening of First Web Space

Hypertonicity in the thumb adductor is a common consequence of cervical SCI with spasticity (**Fig. 9**). In C5-C7 lesions, there are typically no functioning antagonists to the ulnar-innervated thumb adductor. A thumb-in-palm deformity may develop rapidly unless special attention is given to thumb position during the early phase of a cervical SCI. In patients with a tight first web space, the AdP release should be combined with a widening of the first web space in order to increase working space of the thumb and avoid skin necrosis during postoperative palmar and radial abduction splinting of the thumb.

Distal Ulnar Wing Release for Correction of Intrinsic Tightness

Spastic or tight interossei are commonly found in patients with incomplete tetraplegia (**Figs. 10** and **11**). Intrinsic tightness of the proximal interphalangeal (PIP) joints may develop because of spasticity of lumbricals/interossei that are not overpowered by spastic extrinsic finger flexors. Bunnell test is commonly used to diagnose intrinsic tightness (see **Fig. 10**).[31,32] The test involves maximal passive MCP joint extension and simultaneous passive flexion of the PIP joint. Intrinsic tightness is present if the PIP joint is difficult to flex. Typically, the long finger is the most affected digit, while the small finger is least affected. Patients with affected MCP joints exhibit clenched fists with spasticity in all extrinsic flexors, and interossei/lumbricals (see **Fig. 1**B). The mild group lacking involvement of the MCP joints demonstrates focal spasticity (ie, spasticity in the interossei/lumbricals and only partial spasticity in extrinsics) (see **Fig. 1**A). The relatively simple distal ulnar wing release safely corrects intrinsic tightness (see **Fig. 11**).[33]

Hyperselective Neurectomy

Partial neurectomy is effective to reduce deformity by addressing selected spastic target muscles. Based on a thorough preoperative clinical examination, specific target muscles are identified.

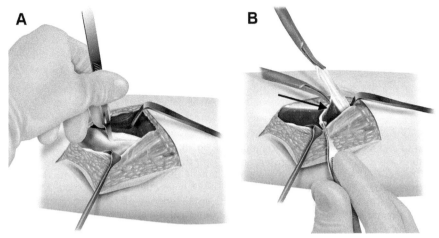

Fig. 5. Pronator teres release. (*A*) This procedure is performed through a 5 cm straight dorsoradial incision in the middle third of the forearm. Special attention should be paid to protecting the brachioradialis and the radial wrist extensors from mechanical damage that may cause adhesion, as they may be used in a subsequent tendon transfer procedure. Furthermore, it is important to bring the forearm into maximally pronated position in order to completely expose the insertion of the PT tendon, which should be thoroughly excised (3–4 cm). (*B*) Although PTu (ulnar head of PT) provides only a small (approximately 10%) portion of the total force produced by the PT, it may still restrict supination motion if left unreleased.[27] The tendinous distal cord (*arrow*) may insert separately, and it is reasonable to release or excise PTu when present.

Hyperselective neurectomy implies following every motor branch until the entry point into the target muscle and aims at improving selectivity, the amount of denervation, and the durability of spasticity reduction.[34]

POSTOPERATIVE TRAINING

The postoperative rehabilitation used for spasticity in SCI was modified from the early active protocol developed for rehabilitation after grip reconstruction and other tendon transfers in tetraplegia.[17,35,36] The cornerstones of the authors'

approach are early active mobilization of sutured tendons and surrounding tissues and maintenance of activities of daily living. Early active mobilization reduces the risks of adhesions, joint stiffness, and swelling. Active rehabilitation encourages patients to participate as much as possible within the restrictions given after surgery. Active use of the arm also facilitates activation of the muscle pump, which, when combined with intermittent elevation, prevents edema and improves circulation. Some patients hesitate to undergo surgery because of the increased dependence that follows the

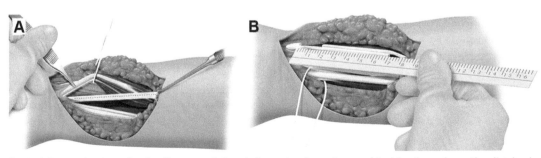

Fig. 6. (*A*) Lengthening of wrist, finger, and thumb flexor tendons. A curved incision is made on the distal volar part of the forearm; 7 to 8 cm of the tendons can be exposed. This incision should be made radial to the midline (ie, over the FCR and FPL tendons). Using this approach, the skin over the ulnarly located flexor tendons will remain intact. This is important, as multiple lengthenings and attachments FDS and FDP may be performed in this location. (*B*) Typically, a lengthening of 20 to 30 mm is required for adequate posture, which also allows for side-to-side sutures with a 4 to 5 cm overlap (see **Fig. 7**). The lengthenings should place the wrist and hand in a natural resting position. Maximal attention should be taken to restore the finger cascade. A balanced tensioning of the finger and thumb may be achieved using a simple elastic roll in the palm.

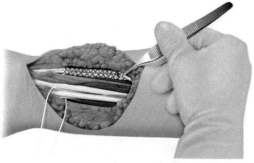

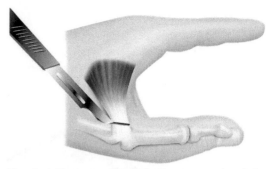

Fig. 7. Tendon-to-tendon attachment technique. Side-to-side sutures are used in tendon transfers and tendon lengthenings. The tendons are sutured side to side with cross-stitches running along on both sides, overlapping 5 cm of donor and recipient tendons. Multiple biomechanical studies have demonstrated the favorable mechanical properties (load-to-failure and stiffness) of this attachment technique. The minimal bulkiness compared with the tendon-to-tendon weave technique makes it particularly suitable in the palmar aspect of the distal forearm.

Fig. 8. Adductor pollicis release. An angulated (or z-incision, when indicated) dorsoulnar incision is made at the thumb MCP joint. The insertion of the AdP is identified and released. Make sure that the distal tendons of both the oblique and transverse heads of the adductor are thoroughly released.

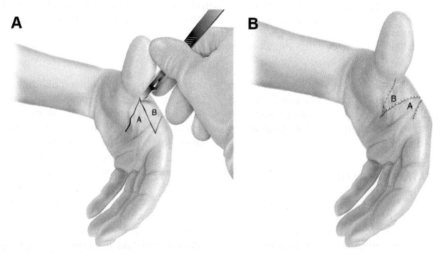

Fig. 9. (A, B) Z-plasty for widening of first web space. A single a-plasty incision is made across the midpoint of the first dorsal interosseus to the dorsoulnar aspect of the MCP joint of the thumb, along the tight skin ridge to the radial aspect of the MCP joint of the index, and then palmarly to a point allowing reach by the dorsal flap; each incision is approximately 2 cm.

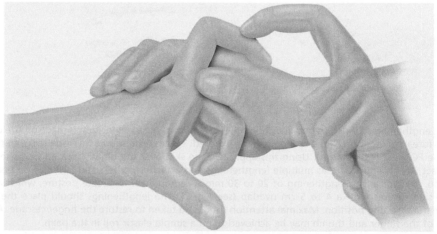

Fig. 10. Bunnell test for intrinsic tightness. Examiner extends MCP joint maximally and simultaneously flexes the PIP joint. Intrinsic tightness is present if the PIP joint is difficult/impossible to flex.

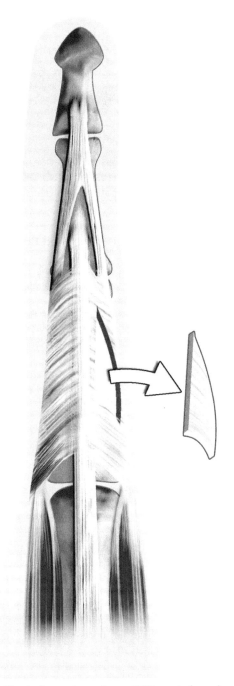

Fig. 11. Distal ulnar wing release. With an L-shaped incision on the dorsum of the proximal phalanx, the extensor tendon apparatus is exposed and a triangular segment including the lateral band and the oblique fibers of the ulnar portion of the aponeurosis is resected. Full passive PIP joint flexion should be verified when testing for intrinsic tightness.

postsurgical phase. For these patients, minimizing postoperative restrictions is an essential component of the patient's decision to pursue surgery.

Immediately after the operation, custom-made splints are fashioned, and these facilitate prolonged soft tissue stretch and prevent postoperative edema. With the exception of training sessions, the splints are worn at all times to provide additional stretch during the first 3 weeks. Elastic bands further reduce swelling and hypertrophic scar formation and secure hand position. Active training of lengthened tendons and antagonists starts within 24 hours after surgery in order to maintain active range of motion, identify functioning muscles hidden by previously overpowering muscle hypertonicity, and prevent adhesions.[37] Muscle control training focuses on accurate application of muscle force for smooth and isolated movements, learning new movements to take advantage of the improved range of motion, strengthening the antagonist muscles, and learning new activation patterns and control of the arm and hand. Activity training starting at 3 weeks aims to improve grasp and release coordination by relearning of movement patterns and intense practice in the most task- and context-specific environment; this is followed by a relaxation period. Splints are usually worn only at night, as the hand should be used as much as possible in daily life.

At 3 to 6 months postoperatively, patients undergo adjustment of strength training of the antagonists together with coordination and muscle control training, as well as analysis and education to increase active use of the hand in daily activities and to facilitate the transfer of improved function into daily use. Relearning in daily life is a long process that can continue up to 1 year after surgery. Control of training is usually independent of therapists, with only a few patients requiring occasional therapy in their home community.[35,36]

MEASURING OUTCOMES

There are currently no validated methods available to assess spasticity-reducing or deformity-correction surgery due to spasticity. The Canadian Occupational Performance Measurement (COPM) assesses patient-reported satisfaction and performance. It is, therefore, an important outcomes tool that is useful to understand the impact of surgery on activities of daily living.[38] Because the SCI population rarely suffers from cognitive deficiencies, this is an appropriate and easily administered outcomes measure.[39] A hand that can be safely controlled, is better balanced, and easier to open certainly contributes to making daily living more comfortable, as evidenced by substantial improvement of COPM scores and better grasp control after surgery (**Fig. 12**).[40]

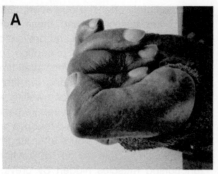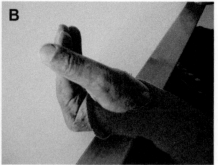

Fig. 12. (*A*) Preoperative and (*B*) postoperative hand positions in a tetraplegic patient with clenched-fist deformity who underwent tendon lengthening of his spastic FCR and FDS.

SUMMARY

Time-proven, reliable, and safe surgical procedures to reduce spasticity and correct deformity, followed by rigorous postoperative training will successfully increase mobility and independence in patients with upper extremity spasticity resulting from SCI.

ACKNOWLEDGMENTS

Multiple professionals have been instrumental for the development of the basic science, surgical procedures, and rehabilitation concepts described in this article. The authors are particularly grateful to Lina Bunketorp Käll, Sabrina Koch-Borner, Richard L Lieber, Carina Reinholdt, Joakim Strömberg, and Johanna Wangdell.

REFERENCES

1. Bickenbach J, editor. International perspectives on spinal cord injury. Geneva (Switzerland): World Health Organization; 2013.
2. Fridén J, Gohritz A. Novel concepts integrated in neuromuscular assessments for surgical restoration of arm and hand function in tetraplegia. Phys Med Rehabil Clin N Am 2012;23:33–50.
3. Anderson KD. Targeting recovery: priorities of the SCI population. J Neurotrauma 2004;21:1371–83.
4. Snoek GJ, Ijzerman MJ, Hermens HJ, et al. Survey of the needs of patients with spinal cord injury: impact and priority for improvement in hand function in tetraplegics. Spinal Cord 2004;42:526–32.
5. Moberg E. The upper limb in tetraplegia. A new approach to surgical rehabilitation. Stuttgart (Germany): Thieme; 1978.
6. Fridén J, Gohritz A. Tetraplegia management update. J Hand Surg Am 2015;40:2489–500.
7. Fridén J, Reinholdt C, Turcsanyii I, et al. A single-stage operation for reconstruction of hand flexion, extension, and intrinsic function in tetraplegia: the alphabet procedure. Tech Hand Up Extrem Surg 2011;15:230–5.
8. Reinholdt C, Fridén J. Outcomes of single-stage grip-release reconstruction in tetraplegia. J Hand Surg Am 2013;38:1137–44.
9. Cain S, Gohritz A, Fridén J, et al. Review of upper extremity nerve transfer in cervical spinal cord injury. J Brachial Plex Peripher Nerve Inj 2015;10: e34–42.
10. Wangdell J, Fridén J. Activity gains after reconstructions of elbow extension in patients with tetraplegia. J Hand Surg Am 2012;37:1003–10.
11. Wangdell J, Carlsson G, Fridén J. Enhanced independence: experiences after regaining grip function in people with tetraplegia. Disabil Rehabil 2013;35: 1968–74.
12. Hentz VR, Leclercq C. The management of the upper limb in incomplete lesions of the cervical spinal cord. Hand Clin 2008;24:185–201.
13. Maynard FM, Karunas RS, Waring WP 3rd. Epidemiology of spasticity following traumatic spinal cord injury. Arch Phys Med Rehabil 1990;71:566–9.
14. Sköld C, Levi R, Seiger A. Spasticity after traumatic spinal cord injury: nature, severity, and location. Arch Phys Med Rehabil 1999;80:1548–57.
15. Fridén J, Reinholdt C, Wangdell J, et al. Upper extremity reconstruction in non-traumatic spinal cord injuries: an under-recognized opportunity. J Rehabil Med 2014;46:33–8.
16. Van Heest A. Tetraplegia. In: Wolfe SW, Pederson WC, Hotchkiss RN, et al, editors. Green's operative hand surgery. 6th edition. Philadelphia: Elsevier Churchill Livingstone; 2011. p. 2009–34.
17. Fridén J, Reinholdt C. Current concepts in reconstruction of hand function in tetraplegia. Scand J Surg 2008;97:341–6.
18. Adams MM, Hicks AL. Spasticity after spinal cord injury. Spinal Cord 2005;43:577–86.
19. Elbasiouny SM, Moroz D, Bakr MM, et al. Management of spasticity after spinal cord injury: current techniques and future directions. Neurorehabil Neural Repair 2010;24:23–33.

20. Fridén J, Lieber RL. Spastic cells are stiffer than normal cells. Muscle Nerve 2003;27:157–64.

21. Gracies JM. Pathophysiology of spastic paresis. I: Paresis and soft tissue changes. Muscle Nerve 2005;31:535–51.

22. AllieuY. General indications for functional surgery of the hand in tetraplegic patients. Hand Clin 2002;18: 233–55.

23. Keenan MA. Management of the spastic upper extremity in the neurologically impaired adult. Clin Orthop Relat Res 1988;233:116–25.

24. Keenan MA, Mehta S. Neuro-orthopedic management of shoulder deformity and dysfunction in brain-injured patients: a novel approach. J Head Trauma Rehabil 2004;19:143–54.

25. Namdari S, Horneff JG, Baldwin K, et al. Muscle releases to improve passive motion and relieve pain in patients with spastic hemiplegia and elbow flexion contractures. J Shoulder Elbow Surg 2012;21: 1357–62.

26. Anakwenze OA, Namdari S, Hsu JE, et al. Myotendinous lengthening of the elbow flexor muscles to improve active motion in patients with elbow spasticity following brain injury. J Shoulder Elbow Surg 2013;22:318–22.

27. Abrams GD, Ward SR, Fridén J, et al. Pronator teres in an appropriate donor muscle for restoration of wrist and thumb extension. J Hand Surg Am 2005; 30:1068–73.

28. Pomerance JF, Keenan MA. Correction of severe spastic flexion contractures in the non-functional hand. J Hand Surg Am 1996;21:828–33.

29. Treanor WJ, Moberg E, Buncke HJ. The hyperflexed seemingly useless tetraplegic hand: a method of surgical amelioration. Paraplegia 1992;30:457–66.

30. Brown SH, Hentzen ER, Kwan A, et al. Mechanical strength of the side-to-side versus Pulvertaft weave tendon repair. J Hand Surg Am 2010;35:540–5.

31. Bunnell S. Surgery of the hand. 2nd edition. Philadelphia: Lippincott; 1948.

32. Fridén J, Tirrell TF, Bhola S, et al. The mechanical strength of side-to-side tendon repair with mismatched tendon size and shape. J Hand Surg Eur Vol 2015;40:236–45.

33. Reinholdt C, Fridén J. Selective release of the digital extensor hood to reduce intrinsic tightness in tetraplegia. J Plast Surg Hand Surg 2011;45:83–9.

34. Gras M, Leclerq C. Spasticity and hyperselective neurectomy in the upper limb. Hand Surg Rehabil 2017;36:391–401.

35. Fridén J, Shillito MC, Chehab EF, et al. Mechanical feasibility of immediate mobilization of the brachioradialis muscle after tendon transfer. J Hand Surg Am 2010;35:1473–8.

36. Wangdell J, Bunketorp-Käll L, Koch-Borner S, et al. Early active rehabilitation after grip reconstructive surgery in tetraplegia. Arch Phys Med Rehabil 2016;97:S117–25.

37. Wangdell J, Fridén J. Rehabilitation after spasticity-correcting upper limb surgery in tetraplegia. Arch Phys Med Rehabil 2016;97:S136–43.

38. Law M. The Canadian occupational performance measure. Ottawa (Canada): CAOT Publications; 1998.

39. Carswell A, McColl MA, Baptiste S, et al. The Canadian occupational performance measure: a research and clinical literature review. Can J Occup Ther 2004;71:210–22.

40. Wangdell J, Reinholdt C, Fridén J. Activity gains after upper limb surgery for spasticity in patients with spinal cord injury. J Hand Surg Eur Vol 2018;43(6): 613–20.

Rehabilitation Strategies Following Surgical Treatment of Upper Extremity Spasticity

Janese Petuchowksi, MS, OTR/L, CHT[a,1],
Kaitlin Kieras, MS, OTR/L[b], Kristina Stein, MS, OTR/L[c,*]

KEYWORDS

- Occupational therapy • Hand therapy • Postsurgical guidelines • Spasticity • Upper extremity
- Postsurgical treatment • Upper extremity transfers

KEY POINTS

- A comprehensive occupational therapy program is essential following surgical treatment of upper extremity spasticity.
- Variations in protocols are dependent on surgeon preference, skill of therapist, and function of the patient.
- Patient and/or family training is critical for successful postoperative outcomes.
- Therapy that is meaningful and functional is likely to promote better results.

INTRODUCTION

Upper motor neuron injuries, such as that seen in cerebral palsy (CP), cerebrovascular accidents (ie, stroke), and traumatic brain injury, often result in substantial challenges with motor function. Individuals may have underlying weakness and difficulty with motor control. This condition may result in static or dynamic restrictions of movement causing pain, skin breakdown, and impaired function. Multiple surgical options are available to improve upper extremity positioning and, in some cases, volitional control of the upper extremity.

Postoperative management with therapy is imperative to assist patients/caregivers in maximizing the potential functional gains. Techniques to improve motor control and functional training are important to incorporate into the therapy program.

As with all postoperative referrals to physical or occupational therapy, communication between the therapist and surgeon is critical. Surgical procedures vary based on surgeon preference, goals of surgery, restrictions of neurovascular structures or skin, and patient cognition/function. Postoperative joint immobilization and

Disclosure: The authors have no affiliations with or involvement in any organization or entity with any financial interest (eg, honoraria; educational grants; participation in speakers' bureaus; membership, employment, consultancies, stock ownership, or other equity interest; and expert testimony or patent-licensing arrangements) or nonfinancial interest (eg, personal or professional relationships, affiliations, knowledge, or beliefs) in the subject matter or materials discussed in this article.

[a] Occupational Therapy, Solace Health Care, 4500 Cherry Creek South Drive Suite 710, Denver, CO 80246, USA; [b] Occupational Therapy, Ann & Robert H. Lurie Children's Hospital of Chicago, 225 East Chicago Avenue, Box 142, Chicago, IL 60611-2605, USA; [c] Occupational Therapy, Ann & Robert H. Lurie Children's Hospital of Chicago, 225 East Chicago Avenue, Box 142, Chicago, IL 60611-2605, USA
[1] 3498 East Ellsworth Avenue Unit 801C, Denver, CO 80209.
* Corresponding author.
E-mail address: kstein@luriechildrens.org

Hand Clin 34 (2018) 567–582
https://doi.org/10.1016/j.hcl.2018.06.013
0749-0712/18/

progression of motion should take into account all concomitant upper limb procedures. As with many upper extremity procedures, postoperative rehabilitation for patients with upper extremity spasticity must balance necessary immobilization to prevent tendon rupture and/or attenuation with the risk of potential adhesions and/or contractures from delayed initiation of movement.

This article presents contemporary guidelines for immobilization and initiation of therapy after commonly performed surgeries for patients with upper extremity spasticity. In addition, it discusses a variety of therapy techniques that can be used to maximize functional outcomes.

Management of Shoulder Spasticity

The most common shoulder deformity for patients with hemiplegia is a position of adduction, internal rotation, and forward flexion. Muscles that contribute to this deformity include the pectoralis major, latissimus dorsi, subscapularis, and teres major. Shoulder releases are indicated for pain, skin breakdown, or difficulties with hygiene and dressing. Operative management in these patients may consist of release or lengthening of the spastic muscles/tendons (**Table 1**).[1,2]

Management of Elbow and Forearm Spasticity

Surgical intervention may be indicated in the setting of significant elbow flexion and forearm pronation deformities. These deformities may cause pain, difficulties with hygiene/self-care, poor cosmesis, and impaired motor function.

Elbow correction
Correction for an elbow flexion contracture is typically not required unless the deformity is greater than 30°. Flexion contractures between 30° and 60° may be treated with soft tissue lengthening procedures. Contractures greater than 60° may require aggressive soft tissue/tendon releases, with possible release of the anterior elbow capsule (**Table 2**).[3–7]

Pronator teres release/rerouting
Many patients with spasticity present with a severe pronation posture of the forearm that can severely impede function. A pronator teres rerouting improves resting posture of the forearm and may unmask active supination. However, a pronator teres rerouting improves both active supination and dynamic forearm positioning. Per Oishi and Butler,[8] the ideal candidate for a PT rerouting has no active supination but a near-full arc of passive supination. The primary indication for surgery is a pronation deformity of 25° or greater because this positioning precludes effective grasp of large objects (**Table 3**).[6,9–11]

Management of Wrist Spasticity

Flexion of the wrist with pronation of the forearm is common in patients with spasticity. These deformities can hinder function, cause pain, and interfere with caregiver assistance for activities of daily living. Range of motion (ROM) deficits at the wrist are commonly interrelated with elbow and hand/finger deformities. Depending on the degree and duration of deformity, management of the wrist can include both bone and soft tissue procedures (**Table 4**).

Proximal row carpectomy
An advantage of proximal row carpectomy (PRC) compared with wrist arthrodesis is the ability to maintain motion. The immobilization period is shorter and there is no need for internal hardware or concern regarding bone union. This procedure

---

Table 1
Postoperative management of the shoulder

Surgical Procedures	Week After Surgery	Postoperative Guideline	Immobilization/Orthosis
Shoulder releases: may include single or multiple musculotendinous lengthening, fractional lengthening, z lengthening, or complete tendon release	0–4	Wear pillow/wedge at all times except for sponge bathing Day 1 initiation of AAROM in supine for shoulder flexion, ER, horizontal abduction/adduction, and in standing for IR No PROM or resistance until after 3 wk	Limb positioned in abduction and external rotation with pillows while at rest for several months

Abbreviations: AAROM, active-assisted range of motion; ER, external rotation; IR, internal rotation; PROM, passive range of motion.

Table 2
Postoperative management of the elbow

Surgical Procedure	Week After Surgery	Postoperative Guidelines	Immobilization/Orthosis
Fractional lengthening of the long and short heads of biceps tendons, the brachialis, and brachioradialis	0–3	Immediate mobilization with AROM No resistive activities for 3 wk to prevent overstretch of muscles	—
Release of brachialis, brachioradialis, biceps (with or without joint capsule)	0–6	Early mobilization of self-assisted passive ROM in extension If frail skin, serial casting in extension completed for 2–4 wk before PROM is initiated to prevent excessive stretching of neurovascular/skin structures	Elbow orthosis worn at all times except in therapy for 6 wk
	6+		Discontinue orthosis
Lengthening of elbow flexors (typically brachioradialis and brachialis, but may include biceps in severe spasticity)	0–3 to 4	Immobilization	Casted at end-range elbow extension and supination or as advised by physician
	4–6	Begin AROM	Static elbow orthosis at all times except during ADLs and exercises
	Wek 6–12	Initiate strengthening of elbow extension; initiate PROM of elbow	Daytime splint as needed based on tone/reflexive responses Continue nighttime orthosis
	12+	Initiation strengthening of elbow flexion	May consider discontinuing night orthosis based on clinical judgment

Abbreviations: ADLs, activities of daily living; AROM, active range of motion; ROM, range of motion.

converts a more complex wrist joint into a hinge joint and causes a relative lengthening of the tendon that crosses the wrist. Patients and families should be educated on postoperative ROM expectations; all patients have a limited flexion-extension arc of motion. Digital flexion may also be limited because of the altered length-tension relationship of the flexor tendons.[12]

Table 3
Postoperative management of the forearm

Surgical Procedure	Week	Postoperative Guidelines	Immobilization/Orthosis
Pronator lengthening/ release or rerouting	0–4	ROM of uninvolved joints, edema management	Casting at 30° supination; if PT to ECRB long-arm cast 90° elbow flexion, forearm in maximum supination, wrist in maximum extension[10]
	4–6	Initiate AROM and home program	Transition to removable supination orthosis to be worn at all times except therapy/HEP
	6–8	Initiate PROM	Orthosis may be adjusted to improve supination
	8–12	Initiate strengthening and functional ADL retraining	Transition to nighttime orthosis until exercises are completed pain free
	12+	Continue with functional ADL retraining	Discontinue night orthosis

Abbreviations: ECRB, extensor carpi radialis brevis; HEP, home exercise program.

Table 4
Postoperative management of the wrist

Surgical Procedure	Week After Surgery	Postoperative Guidelines	Immobilization/Orthosis
Proximal row carpectomy	0–4	Complete immobilization of wrist; encourage AROM of all other joints with focus on active digital/thumb ROM; edema management	Casted in 0°–10° extension, digits free
	4–6	Gentle isolated AROM of the wrist for flexion/extension and radial/ulnar deviation Composite wrist and digital ROM should be avoided to prevent elongation of the extrinsic muscles	Transition to thermoplast orthosis wrist in neutral; worn full time except hygiene, therapy, and HEP
	6–8	AAROM, isometrics, and light functional use of the hand as patient is able; forceful manipulations/joint mobilizations are not appropriate	Orthosis weaned to nighttime, consider daytime neoprene orthosis
	8+	Gentle grip strengthening: isotonic exercises and progressive resistive exercises	Continue nighttime orthosis and daytime functional orthosis as clinically appropriate
Total wrist arthrodesis	0–4	Immobilization until healing confirmed on radiographs; AROM of the uninvolved joints, gentle ROM of digits; edema management	Short-arm cast; typically fusion at 10°–20° extension
	4–6	A/PROM of the digits continues, and can initiate A/PROM for forearm rotation; scar management, desensitization can be initiated; fine-motor manipulation tasks can be added as patient is able Therapy should continue to address any edema, pain/hypersensitivity, or ROM limitation of the noninvolved joints	Once healed, patient can transition to a removable wrist orthosis, which can include digits in extension
	6–8	Continue, with HEP focus on A/PROM of digits and forearm, 10 times every hour	Begin to reduce protective orthosis
	8+	Typically 2.3 kg (5 pound) weight limit for the first 8 wk Isometric grip strengthening exercises initiated; ADL adaptations/modifications	

Surgery	Week		
Flexor carpi ulnaris to the extensor carpi radialis brevis transfer	0–5	Patient is immobilized in a long-arm cast (may be bivalved), with wrist in neutral, forearm in maximum available and comfortable supination, and elbow in near-full extension; focus on edema management	Long-arm cast
	5–8	Scar management initiated; begin gentle active and passive wrist extension and forearm supination Passive wrist flexion should not be completed	Transition to short-arm, volar removable orthosis with wrist in neutral to be worn at all times except during supervised exercises
	8+	Gentle active wrist flexion activities initiated and light functional activities encouraged Progressive strengthening of wrist extension can be initiated	Orthosis discontinued during the day, transition to nighttime for at least 12 wk postsurgery
Flexor carpi radialis to extensor digitorum communis	0–2	Immobilization; edema management and ROM of noninvolved joints	Cast or orthosis, forearm in 15°–30° pronation, wrist in extension, MCPs in slight flexion, thumb in maximal radial abduction; IP joints free
	2	Passive tenodesis can be initiated with wrist in extension and full supination to wrist in neutral and pronation	
	3	Flex the wrist with slight radial deviation while simultaneously extending the digits	
	4	Begin active flexion of the digits with wrist in extension	Can begin to wean orthosis during the day
	5	Full active extension/flexion of digits in wrist extension; full AROM of wrist with digits/thumb relaxed	
	6	Gentle PROM initiated individually to wrist/digits	
	7	Composite wrist and digital flexion to reduce extensor tightness	
	8–10	Initiate gentle strengthening	Nighttime orthosis only

Abbreviations: IP, interphalangeal; MCP, metacarpophalangeal.

Total wrist arthrodesis

Total wrist arthrodesis is generally considered to be a salvage procedure, given that all motion (flexion/extension and radioulnar deviation) is sacrificed for stability and improved posture of the wrist; however, forearm supination/pronation is preserved. Consideration should be given to preoperative casting of the affected wrist, which may help determine the best functional position post-surgery and may also allow the patient and caregiver to adjust to an immobile wrist. The wrist is often fused at 10° to 20° of extension and slight ulnar deviation, because this position increases hand function.[13] Postoperative ROM of the digits should emphasize gliding of the extensor digitorum communis to prevent scar adherence to the underlying hardware and surrounding soft tissues.[12]

Flexor carpi ulnaris to the extensor carpi radialis brevis tendon transfer

A position of wrist and thumb flexion is common and limits grasp and overall function. If the fingers can still be extended in a wrist-neutral posture, the patient may be a good candidate for surgery, which may produce a neutral wrist posture and improved function and appearance.[14,15]

Flexor carpi radialis to extensor digitorum communis

This procedure can improve wrist and finger extension while maintaining finger flexion.[14,16] The flexor carpi radialis provides adequate excursion and strength without sacrificing wrist flexion and ulnar deviation, which is critical for the dart thrower's motion and power grip.

Management of Hand Spasticity

Commensurate with more proximal impairments, patients with spasticity experience limitations in hand/digit function. Common presentations include a thumb-in-palm deformity (adduction and flexion of the thumb) and flexed digits (ie, clenched fist). These deformities may result in fixed contractures of the muscles/joints.[17-26] The following are procedures that may be used to address these impairments. Typically, several procedures are performed in combination to address spasticity of the hand. As with the wrist, surgical management can include both bone and soft tissue procedures (**Table 5**).

Flexor digitorum superficialis/flexor digitorum profundus fractional lengthening or flexor digitorum superficialis to flexor digitorum profundus (superficialis to profundus transfer) transfer

Flexor tendon fractional lengthening can be advantageous in patients who have some active use of their hands. If active motion is not present, an STP (superficialis to profundus) transfer is preferred to release the digits from the palm and improve access for hand hygiene. Patients may be able to compensate for the resulting decrease in digital flexion strength by using wrist tenodesis to increase excursion of the extrinsic flexors.[25,27]

Flexor pollicis longus fractional or z lengthening

These procedures are indicated for patients with flexor pollicis longus (FPL) spasticity. Z lengthening results in a more substantial release and is indicated is severe flexion contractures of the interphalangeal joint of the thumb.[15,23,25]

Extensor pollicis longus rerouting and thenar intrinsic release

Extensor pollicis longus rerouting is commonly performed to improve thumb extension in patients with a passively correctable thumb-in-palm deformity. Thenar intrinsic release (ie, the adductor pollicis) may be spastic and is often the primary component of the spastic thumb.

Interosseous muscle slide

This procedure is performed to decrease metacarpophalangeal (MCP) joint flexion contractures resulting from intrinsic spasticity or contracture. In patients with upper extremity spasticity, it may be difficult to determine the extent of intrinsic spasticity until the extrinsic flexors are surgically addressed. Alternatively, in patients with absent volitional control, an ulnar motor neurectomy may lead to sufficient denervation of the intrinsics to allow digital opening.[28]

Central slip tenotomy

This procedure is a common option to address a swan-neck deformity secondary to extrinsic extensor tightness. This deformity limits digit flexion/functional grasp and, in severe cases, may cause pain with hand use.[25] Per Carlson and colleagues,[26] patients with proximal interphalangeal (PIP) joint contractures of greater than 20° and without MCP flexion deformity are candidates for this surgery. The PIP joint is typically pinned in 10° of flexion after the central slip has been released. After the splint/cast and pins are removed, care should be taken to limit extension to −10° (oval figure-of-eight splints are commonly used).

General Postoperative Care

The timing of postoperative therapy is based on a detailed discussion between the therapist and the surgeon. Even if the patient is immobilized and the surgical dressings are in place, important factors may still be addressed. Initiating therapy

Table 5
Postoperative management of the hand

Surgical Procedure	Week	Postoperative Guidelines	Immobilization/Orthoses
FDS/FDP fractional lengthening or FDS to FDP transfer (STP)	0–4	Complete immobilization, encourage AROM of all noninvolved joints	Casted with wrist neutral, MCP joints flexed to 90°, and IP joints in extension
	4–8	Begin PROM of wrist and digits. Can also begin active digit movement and functional use with tenodesis. Initiate scar management, desensitization, and edema management as needed	Transitioned to thermoplast resting hand orthosis
	8+	Continue with ROM and functional activities as able	May discontinue orthosis if clinically appropriate or as advised by physician. Some patients may require long-term orthosis usage
FPL fractional or z lengthening	0–4	Complete immobilization, encourage AROM of all noninvolved joints	Casted with wrist in slight flexion and thumb neutral
	4–8	Active and passive exercises initiated. Initiate scar management and desensitization as needed	Transition to short opponens or thumb spica thermoplast orthosis; worn full time except for hygiene, therapy, and HEP
	8+	Continue ROM, add functional activities and strengthening exercises as tolerated	Discontinue orthosis
Opponensplasty (fourth digit FDS to FPL)	0–3	Complete immobilization, encourage AROM of all noninvolved joints	Casted with wrist neutral and thumb in full opposition
	3–6	A/PROM initiated to thumb within dorsal blocking orthosis. Focus on individual joint movement. Initiate scar management and desensitization as needed	Transitioned to thermoplast dorsal blocking orthosis with wrist in 20° flexion, thumb abducted with MCP and IP joints in 20° flexion
	6	Passive extension of wrist and thumb in a slow progression to limit stretching of the transfer	Blocking orthosis discontinued. Nighttime wrist/thumb extension orthosis may be fabricated if extrinsic flexor tightness is present
	7–8	Continue with ROM and initiate progressive strengthening of thumb	Extension orthosis may be continued until tightness is resolved

(continued on next page)

Table 5
(continued)

Surgical Procedure	Week	Postoperative Guidelines	Immobilization/Orthoses
EPL rerouting and thenar release	0–5	Complete immobilization, encourage AROM of all noninvolved joints	Short-arm thumb spica cast with wrist in 30° extension and thumb positioned in maximal thumb extension and 15°–20° thumb abduction
	5–8	Gentle thumb extension and abduction AROM and nonresistive activities may be initiated with progression to passive thumb extension and abduction as tolerated Passive thumb flexion should be avoided Initiate scar management, desensitization and edema management as needed Thumb flexion and opposition active exercises are initiated	Transitioned to volar-based thermoplast thumb spica or long opponens orthosis with wrist in 15° extension, thumb in extension; worn full time except for hygiene, therapy, and HEP Care should be taken during orthosis fabrication to avoid MCP and IP joint hyperextension
	8+	Can begin a progressive strengthening program for thumb extension/abduction and participation in light functional activities is allowed as tolerated	Daytime use of orthosis is typically discontinued, pending patient's progress, cognitive awareness, and the extent of surgery The orthosis is continued during nighttime for 3 mo
FPL to EPL	0–4	Complete immobilization Focus on edema management and positioning Encourage AROM of all noninvolved joints	Immobilize in short-arm cast
	4–6	Focus on AROM and muscle reeducation Light tenodesis activities may be initiated Scar management, desensitization, and edema management as needed	Transition to volar wrist orthosis with wrist in 20° extension, to be worn at all times except for hygiene, therapy, and HEP
	7–11	Light resistive activities initiated with focus on functional tasks; resistive/strengthening slowly progressed as tolerated	Orthosis discontinued during daytime, continued at nighttime
	12+	Continue strengthening	Orthosis discontinued

Procedure	Week		
Thumb CMC arthrodesis	0–3 wk	Immobilization until healing confirmed on radiograph; AROM of the noninvolved joints, gentle ROM of digits; edema management	Immobilized in thumb spica cast with thumb in ~30° abduction, extension and pronation/opposition. May be immobilized for 4 wk or as advised by physician
	3–6	If healing is detected, begin AROM with focus on thumb abduction and extension. Scar management, desensitization can be initiated as needed	Thermoplast thumb spica orthosis worn at all times except for hygiene, therapy, and HEP
	6	Continue thumb AROM. Incorporate manipulative activities that require lateral and 3 jaw chuck pinch	Orthosis gradually weaned from daytime wear; continue at night and for protection during day as advised by physician
Central slip tenotomy	0–4	Complete immobilization, encourage AROM of all noninvolved joints	PIP joints pinned in 10° flexion and patient is immobilized in short-arm cast
	4–8	Active PIP flexion and extension may be initiated with extension to lacking 10°. Progress to PROM as tolerated. Splints may not limit end-range extension; ensure patient is educated on ROM restrictions. Monitor for edema and address as needed	Transitioned to wearing Oval-8 splints during day, or patient is placed in volar wrist orthosis with wrist in neutral position and digits in surgically corrected position (typically PIP joints in 20° flexion) per surgeon's protocol. Nighttime resting hand orthosis with digits maintained in optimal position. Worn for 3 mo
	8–12	Full ROM permitted. Progressive strengthening activities integrated into therapy and home program with careful monitoring of edema/joint inflammation and pain	Nighttime splint continued for 3 mo postsurgery. Oval-8 splints worn during day as recommended by surgeon
Interosseous muscle slide	0–3	Complete immobilization. Encourage AROM of all noninvolved joints	Short-arm cast with MCPs immobilized in full extension or slight hyperextension and PIP joints flexed. May be immobilized for 4 wk or as advised by physician
	3–8	AROM of wrist and digits. Begin AROM with focus on IP joint flexion exercises and functional activities	Transitioned to thermoplast resting hand orthosis; worn at all times except hygiene, therapy, and HEP
	8+	Continue AROM and begin progressive strengthening as appropriate	Orthosis discontinued. Nighttime orthosis continued if there is a concern for recurrence of preoperative position

Abbreviations: CMC, carpometacarpal; EPL, extensor pollicis longus; FDS, flexor digitorum superficialis; FPL, flexor pollicis longus; IP, interphalangeal; MCP, metacarpophalangeal; PIP, proximal interphalangeal; STP, superficialis to profundus.

immediately also serves to establish trust in the therapist. Emphasis on ROM of non–surgically involved joints is essential and also allows the therapist to assess the potential for the patient to follow single-step directions and to assess motor planning/execution of movements. If possible, preoperative assessment will have occurred; this involves an evaluation of active and passive ROM, functional skills, muscle tone, sensibility, and posture. Surgical expectations and goals should be clearly delineated to the therapist to allow for appropriate planning of therapy objectives. For example, therapy following surgery for hygiene, posture, pain relief, or ease of caregiving would clearly be different than therapy following functional surgery.

Treatment options vary depending on surgical goals, clinician skill, and the cognition and motor/sensory function of the patient. Potential options most frequently used by the authors include motor reeducation, constraint-induced movement therapy (CIMT), mirror therapy, and functional skill retraining. Supportive modalities may include therapeutic taping and functional electrical stimulation. Neuromuscular electrical stimulation, in conjunction with conventional occupational therapy, has been shown to improve ROM, spasticity, and hand function in children with CP.[29]

Edema Control

In the immediate postoperative phase, limb elevation should be initiated to prevent distal fluid accumulation. Acute postsurgical edema typically lasts approximately 72 hours and responds well to elevation; this reduces hydrostatic pressure, decreasing the flow of electrolytes and water into the surgical area. Exercise of uninvolved joints proximal to the surgical site may also assist in prevention of edema, and, when possible, light retrograde massage and icing of the limb are performed. Active motion of the noninvolved areas should be combined with elevation for the most effective results.[30] Subacute edema is defined as swelling lasting greater than 72 hours. To combat this sequela of surgery, the lymphatic system must be stimulated. Compression garments or low-stretch bandages, chip bags, edema management, taping techniques, and manual edema mobilization are more effective during this stage. Manual edema mobilization uses a combination of diaphragmatic breathing, light skin traction, massage, and exercise to stimulate the lymphatic system.[31] Various types of compression garments are available for use, including compressive stockinettes, finger sleeves/wraps, isotoner gloves, pressure garments, and tubular elastic bandages. Of note, any type of circular bandage has the potential for a tourniquet effect and should be used with caution and continuous monitoring.

Scar Management

Scar mobilization and management techniques are critical components of postoperative therapeutic intervention and should be initiated immediately following suture removal and wound closure. Hypertrophic scars following surgery can be associated with physical and psychological dissatisfaction. Various noninvasive techniques exist to prevent the formation of hypertrophic scars.[32–34] General protective measures include sun protection and the use of moisturizing creams. More targeted methods include use of moisture-retentive dressings such as silicone gel, taping, and manual massage. The safety and efficacy of silicone gel and sheets have been confirmed by several studies.[35] These studies recommend massage therapy in conjunction with silicone and pressure therapy. Although silicone gel sheets and topical silicone gel are both effective, topical sheets may be more convenient for patient use.[36]

Meaume and colleagues[35] provide practical guidelines for management of linear scars, keloids, and widened scars. They recommend that silicone sheets be worn over the scar for 12 to 24 h/d for 3 to 6 months. The sheets can be worn until they lose integrity but should be washed each day with mild soap and warm water. Silicone sheets may not be suitable for use on large areas of skin, in which case silicone gel can be applied to the skin in a thin layer. Education regarding use is essential to ensure compliance with gel and sheets. Additional measures may be required to prevent premature removal or mouthing of gel sheets in certain populations; noncompressive wraps or socks/gloves on the involved upper extremity are useful strategies.

Pressure garments may be applied once the wound is closed and stable. Edema reduction is an additional benefit with the use of pressure garments. Compression therapy can be used in combination with silicone.[35] However, garments can be expensive and long-term compliance may be poor. An alternative method to apply pressure to a scar is through the use of an elastomer scar mold. Paper tape may also be effective for prevention of hypertrophic scarring by reducing the tension on the wound edge.[37] It should be applied longitudinally along an incision line as soon as epithelialization has occurred (**Fig. 1**).

Motor Learning

Motor learning is "defined as internal neural and cognitive processes concerning practice or

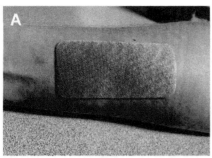 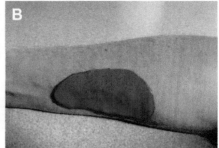

Fig. 1. (*A*) Silicone scar sheet. (*B*) Elastomer scar mold.

experience leading to a relatively permanent change in performance."[38] Motor learning is affected by cognition, active participation, area of brain affected/injured, frequency of feedback during new motor task, and working memory ability.[38–40] Burnter and colleagues[39] found that, for younger individuals, consistent feedback regarding accuracy of a task is helpful in skill attainment and retention, whereas adults benefit from less consistent feedback. For patients with lower cognition and/or poor working memory, it is recommended that tasks be modified to limit the amount of attention/awareness needed to complete the task.[40] Overall, it is essential to consider the individual, as well as quality rather than quantity. Multiple trials with poor motor patterns are not as effective as fewer trials performed with proper positioning and biomechanics. Clinicians cannot solely focus on gaining passive and active ROM but must consider practice and muscle activation in order to perform tasks using motion gained through surgery.[38–42]

Activation of the Transfer

Mobilization of a tendon transfer requires the patient to learn to activate the muscle-tendon unit for a new role. Movement patterns need to be relearned because the balance between the muscles has changed. Initial rehabilitation focuses on triggering the muscles to activate their original functions. Additional techniques include using the former function of a transferred tendon and the new function simultaneously, use of electrical stimulation or biofeedback, vibration/tapping techniques, and intentional focus on the use of the transferred muscle during functional daily tasks. The therapist also directs the patient in many other techniques for transfer activation, such as place and hold (passively placing the joints in the desired position and directing the patient to maintain that position); working in a gravity-eliminated position for easier activation of isolated motion; and performing the desired motion with

the uninvolved limb first, followed by the involved limb. Patients should be encouraged to use small movements rather than forceful muscle loading, which can trigger spasticity. In addition, training for relaxation of the whole upper limb should be included in the rehabilitation program; a relaxed arm makes it easier to isolate desired movements.[3,14,43]

Functional Training

Data show that meaningful task-specific training using functional activities results in greater functional improvement compared with a control group.[44] Functional retraining requires a high level of repetition and should include meaningful activities with task completion. The program begins with large movements requiring less skill, and then progresses to increasingly refined control. The exercises may include placement of objects in space; using reach; and lifting to variable levels, including overhead activities, if possible.[2] Therapists should also incorporate gravity-assisted, static-hold, or gravity-eliminated positions advancing to gravity-resisted movements. Use of adaptations with orthoses or modified equipment, such as built-up handles or Velcro on a glove to hold large objects, may allow greater success in an effort to build confidence. Therapy should focus first on bimanual tasks with gross motor activities and advance to more refined skills. High-interest activities with meaningful content for the patient increases intrinsic motivation (**Fig. 2**).

Sensibility of the extremity is essential to usage.[2,45] Dahlin and Komoto-Tufvesson[46] found improved stereognosis after reconstructive surgery, highlighting the importance of incorporating activities that emphasize functional hand sensation and motor control. Activities to promote increased sensibility may include movement of the hand/wrist while in tactile media, such as oatmeal/rice, tactile boards, and stereognosis tasks. To optimize outcomes, therapists offer tasks with progressive difficulty. These tasks

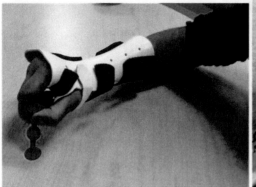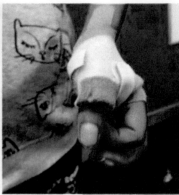

Fig. 2. Functional orthoses to improve grasp patterns.

range from the familiar to novel, bilateral to unilateral, and vision assisted to vision occluded (**Fig. 3**).

Self-Care

Goldenberg and colleagues[47] reported that direct training of self-care increases performance with less need for assistance. Self-care training should be patient specific and have a significant value to the patient. In a study by Arya and colleagues,[44] meaningful task-specific training produced significant improvements in the upper extremity in post-stroke patients. Practice of task-specific activities may be used in the clinic setting and as part of the home program. Breaking down self-care tasks into manageable and achievable objectives allows the patient to gain confidence and the fortitude to persist with the task, even when difficult.

Therapeutic Taping

Over the past few decades, therapeutic taping has become an increasingly popular adjunct for the management of upper extremity conditions.[48–53] Although, there are a variety of elastic taping brands, our experience has been primarily with Kinesio Tex Tape. According to The Kinesio Taping Method, the tape may be used to treat conditions involving the skin, lymphatics, muscles, and joints. Functional outcomes include decreased

pain, edema control, increased ROM, management of scar, inhibition of overactive muscles, correction of joint malalignment, decreased compensatory movement patterns, and enhancement of kinesthetic awareness.[48–56]

There are numerous resources regarding specific taping applications and it is recommended that therapists receive some training before using tape with their patients. Common upper extremity applications include those that promote elbow flexion and/or extension, forearm supination, wrist extension or stabilization, thumb extension and/or stabilization, and digit flexion and extension.[48,49,52] Regardless of the specific areas taped, clinicians must always be cognizant of taping precautions and application techniques.[53] Taping is not typically initiated until all incision sites are fully healed and the patient is cleared for active ROM. In general, taping is used until the desired result has been achieved, whether it be a specific motor pattern, resolution of pain, or improved alignment.[53,56] Although helpful to encourage desired movement patterns, Kinesio Tex Tape should be considered a treatment strategy that enhances therapeutic intervention rather than a primary treatment method.[48,50–52] Outcomes studies indicate that tape leads to pain relief,[51] improved grip strength,[49] and improved hand function.[48] Importantly, as with surgical

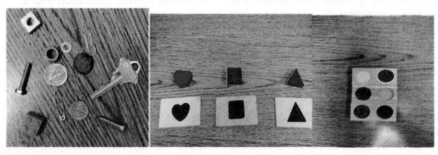

Fig. 3. Items for stereognosis and sensibility training.

intervention, taping is more effective in patients with higher cognition and those with better volitional control over movement[53,57] (**Fig. 4**).

Mirror Therapy

Mirror therapy has gained interest in recent years and has shown great promise in patients with neurologic disorders.[58–60] The technique is as follows: the affected arm/hand is hidden behind a mirror and the uninvolved arm/hand is positioned on the visible side of the mirror. While completing simple movements with the unaffected arm, the patient continues to observe the mirror image and visualizes it as the affected extremity.

In a review of the literature, Ezendam and colleagues[61] found that mirror therapy is effective in patients after stroke. They also suggested, for maximum benefit, that intervention should "consist of 20-minute sessions, delivered 5 days per week for 4 weeks."[61] Other groups have proposed variations of a mirror therapy protocol. The Royal National Hospital for Rheumatic Diseases protocol includes prescribed activities 5 to 6 times a day, for no more than 5 minutes at a time (or less if concentration is lost).[59] Rothgangel and Braun[62] recommend therapy once daily for 10 to 30 minutes. Visual imagery is also an important component of this program, starting with simple ROM activities, progressing to object manipulation after simple exercises have been mastered.

Constraint-Induced Movement Therapy

CIMT has gained recognition for the treatment of patients with neurologic disorders. CIMT is a therapeutic strategy used to increase the function of a paretic upper extremity through repetitive and adaptive task practice while the nonparetic arm is restrained.[63,64] As with other protocols, CIMT includes repetitive practice and shaping. Shaping involves breaking down a task into several smaller more manageable components to improve the person's overall efficiency in learning the task. CIMT may be considered after the postoperative acute rehabilitation program.

Discharge Considerations

The duration of treatment of patients who have undergone surgery for upper extremity spasticity is patient specific; discharge is dependent on functional gains. Home programs for all patients should be included from the beginning and should continue after formal therapy has concluded. These home programs may be as basic as passive ROM and positioning, including the use of orthoses or adaptive equipment, as needed. In the case of patients with higher cognitive ability, activities should include ROM, strengthening, and activities directed at sensibility along with functional activities to maintain and improve function.

Outcomes

Previous research regarding patients with upper extremity spasticity underscores the importance of patient-centered outcomes measures that assess meaningful changes in function. Skold and colleagues[65] showed common themes of satisfaction: improved appearance of the hand/arm, greater ease and efficiency with the use of the hand, improved ability to grasp items, and improvements and greater ease in completion of activities of daily living. When achieved, these

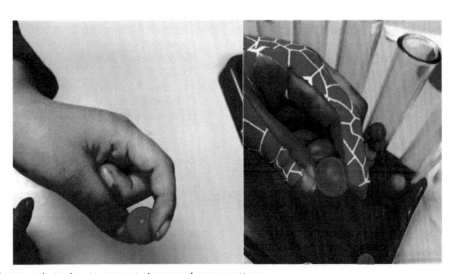

Fig. 4. Therapeutic taping to promote improved grasp patterns.

outcomes facilitate continued learning of new skills and greater independence.

SUMMARY

Rehabilitation following surgical treatment of upper extremity spasticity is a comprehensive process requiring a multidisciplinary team effort and incorporation of various strategies. A close working relationship between the surgeon, therapist, patient, and parents/caregivers is needed for optimal success. A personalized rehab program is required as each patient is unique and presents with individual patient specific goals of treatment. Rehabilitation of this population presents distinct challenges but can be a rewarding experience for both therapists and patients.

ACKNOWLEDGMENTS

Thank you to Dr Joshua Adkinson, who invited us to participate in this article. Thank you to our colleagues and coworkers. The drive to achieve a higher standard of clinical expertise is facilitated through our shared interest and willingness to support each other. Thank you to Aaron Petuchowski for his editing assistance.

REFERENCES

1. Namdari S, Hassan A, Baldwin K, et al. Outcomes of tendon fractional lengthenings to improve shoulder function in patients with spastic hemiparesis. J Shoulder Elbow Surg 2012;21:691–8.

2. Botte M, Kivirahk D, Kinoshita Y, et al. Hemiplegia. In: Skirven TM, Osterman AL, Fedorczyk JM, et al, editors. Rehabilitation of the hand and upper extremity. 6th edition. Philadelphia: Elsevier Mosby; 2011. p. 1659–83.

3. Koman LA, Zhongyu L, Smith BP, et al. Upper extremity musculoskeletal surgery in the child with cerebral palsy: surgical options and rehabilitation. In: Skirven TM, Osterman AL, Fedorczyk JM, et al, editors. Rehabilitation of the hand and upper extremity. 6th edition. Philadelphia: Elsevier Mosby; 2011. p. 1651–8.

4. Anakwenze OA, Namdari S, Hsu JE, et al. Myotendinous lengthening of the elbow flexor muscles to improve active motion in patients with elbow spasticity following brain injury. J Shoulder Elbow Surg 2013;22:318–22.

5. Namdari S, Horneff JG, Baldwin K, et al. Muscle releases to improve passive motion and relieve pain in patients with spastic hemiplegia and elbow flexion contractures. J Shoulder Elbow Surg 2012;21:1357–62.

6. Bunata R, Icenogle K. Cerebral palsy of the elbow and forearm. J Hand Surg Am 2014;39:1425–32.

7. Barus D, Kozin S. The evaluation and treatment of elbow dysfunction secondary to spasticity and paralysis. J Hand Ther 2006;2:192–205.

8. Oishi S, Butler L. Technique of pronator teres rerouting in pediatric patients with spastic hemiparesis. J Hand Surg Am 2016;41:389–92.

9. Bunata RE. Pronator teres rerouting in children with cerebral palsy. J Hand Surg 2006;31(3):474–82.

10. Ho JJ, Wang TM, Shieh JY, et al. Pronator teres transfer for forearm and wrist deformity in cerebral palsy children. J Pediatr Orthop 2015;35:412–8.

11. De Roode CP, James MA, Van Heest A. Tendon transfers and releases for the forearm, wrist, and hand in spastic hemiplegic cerebral palsy. Tech Hand Up Extrem Surg 2010;14(2):129–34.

12. Cannon NM, Beal B, Walters K. Diagnosis and treatment manual for physicians and therapists. Indianapolis (IN): Hand Rehabilitation Center of Indiana; 2001.

13. Bednar JM, Feldscher SB, Seftchick J. Wrist reconstruction: salvage procedures. In: Skirven TM, Osterman AL, Fedorczyk JM, et al, editors. Rehabilitation of the hand and upper extremity. 6th edition. Philadelphia: Elsevier Mosby; 2011. p. 1024–33.

14. Duff SV, Humpl D. Therapists management of tendon transfers. In: Skirven TM, Osterman AL, Fedorczyk JM, et al, editors. Rehabilitation of the hand and upper extremity. 6th edition. Philadelphia: Elsevier Mosby; 2011. p. 781–91.

15. Bansal A, Wall LB, Goldfarb CA. Cerebral palsy tendon transfers: flexor carpi ulnaris to extensor carpi radialis brevis and extensor pollicis longus reroutement. Hand Clin 2016;32:423–30.

16. Giuffre JL, Bishop AT, Spinner RJ, et al. The best tendon and nerve transfers in the upper extremity. Plast Reconstr Surg 2015;135:617–30.

17. Tawde PN, Athani BD, Rege PV. Pre and post surgical functional analysis of spastic hand. Indian J Occup Ther 2002;34(3):3–7.

18. Davids JR, Sabesan VJ, Ortmann F, et al. Surgical management of thumb deformity in children with hemiplegic-type cerebral palsy. J Pediatr Orthop 2009;29(5):504–10.

19. Van Heest AE, Ramachandran V, Stout J, et al. Quantitative and qualitative functional evaluation of upper extremity tendon transfers in spastic hemiplegia caused by cerebral palsy. J Pediatr Orthop 2008;28(6):679–83.

20. Basu AP, Pearse J, Kelly S, et al. Early intervention to improve hand function in hemiplegic cerebral palsy. Front Neurol 2014;5:281.

21. Pappas N, Baldwin K, Keenan MA. Treatment of the non-functional contracted hand. UPOJ 2011;21:90–2.

22. Fridén J, Reinholdt C, Turcsányii I, et al. A single-stage operation for reconstruction of hand flexion, extension, and intrinsic function in tetraplegia: the

alphabet procedure. Tech Hand Up Extrem Surg 2011;15(4):230–5.

23. Tonkin MA. Thumb deformity in the spastic hand: classification and surgical techniques. Tech Hand Up Extrem Surg 2003;7(1):18–25.

24. Tonkin MA, Freitas A, Koman A, et al. The surgical management of thumb deformity in cerebral palsy. J Hand Surg Eur Vol 2008;33:77–82.

25. Koman LA, Sarlikiotis T, Smith BP. Surgery of the upper extremity in cerebral palsy. Orthop Clin North Am 2010;41:519–29.

26. Carlson MG, Gallagher K, Spirtos M. Surgical treatment of swan-neck deformity in hemiplegic cerebral palsy. J Hand Surg 2007;32(9):1418–22.

27. Wolfe SW, Pederson WC, Hotchkiss RN, et al. Green's operative hand surgery: the pediatric hand E-book. Philadelphia: Elsevier Health Sciences; 2010.

28. Danikas D. Intrinsic hand deformity treatment and management. Medscape (serial online). 2015. Available at: Medscape with full test. Available at: https://doi.org/10.1080/09638288.2017.1360403. Accessed July 14, 2017.

29. Yildizgoren MT, Yuzer GFN, Ekiz T, et al. Effects of neuromuscular electrical stimulation on the wrist and finger flexor spasticity and hand functions in cerebral palsy. Pediatr Neurol 2014;51:360–4.

30. Guideice ML. Effects of continuous passive motion and elevation on hand edema. Am J Occup Ther 1990;44:914–20.

31. Artzberger SM, Priganc VW. Manual edema mobilization: an edema reduction technique for orthopedic patient. In: Skirven TM, Osterman AL, Fedorczyk JM, et al, editors. Rehabilitation of the hand and upper extremity. 6th edition. Philadelphia: Elsevier Mosby; 2011. p. 868–81.

32. Iddelkoop E, Monstrey S, Teot L, et al, editors. Scar management: practical guidelines. Elsene (Belgium): Maca-Cloetens; 2011. p. 1–109.

33. Reiffel RS. Prevention of hypertrophic scars by long term paper tape application. Plast Reconstr Surg 1995;96:1715–8.

34. Shin TM, Bordeaux JS. The role of massage in scar management: a literature review. Dermatol Surg 2012;38:414–23.

35. Meaume S, Le Pillouer-Prost A, Richert B, et al. Management of scars: updated practical guidelines and use of silicones. Eur J Dermatol 2014; 24(2):435–43.

36. Kim SM, Lee JH, Kim YJ, et al. Prevention of postsurgical scars: comparison of efficacy and convenience between silicone gel sheet and topical silicone gel. J Korean Med Sci 2014;29:S249–53.

37. Guideice JA, McKenna KT, Barnett AG, et al. A randomized control trial to determine the efficacy of paper tape in preventing hypertrophic scar formation in surgical incisions that traverse Langer's skin tension lines. Plast Reconstr Surg 2005;116:1648–56.

38. Robert MT, Guberek R, Sveistrup H, et al. Motor learning in children with hemiplegic cerebral palsy and the role of sensation in short-term motor training of goal-directed reaching. Dev Med Child Neurol 2013;55(12):1121–8.

39. Burtner PA, Leinwand R, Sullivan KJ, et al. Motor learning in children with hemiplegic cerebral palsy: feedback effects on skill acquisition. Developmental Med Child Neurol 2014;56(3):259–66.

40. Van abswoude van Abswoude F, Santos-Vieira B, van der Kamp J, et al. The influence of errors during practice on motor learning in young individuals with cerebral palsy. Res Dev Disabil 2015;45:353–64.

41. van der Kamp J, Steenbergen B, Masters RS. Explicit and implicit motor learning in children with unilateral cerebral palsy. Disabil Rehabil 2017;1–8.

42. Keller JW, van Hedel HJ. Weight-supported training of the upper extremity in children with cerebral palsy: a motor learning study. J Neuroeng Rehabil 2017;14(1):87.

43. Wangdell J, Friden J. Rehabilitation after spasticity-correcting upper limb surgery in tetraplegia. Arch Phys Med Rehabil 2016;97:S316–43.

44. Arya KN, Verma R, Garg RK, et al. Meaningful task-specific training (MTST) for stroke rehabilitation: a randomized controlled trial. Top Stroke Rehabil 2012;19(3):193–211.

45. Krumlinde-Sundholm L, Eliasson AC. Comparing tests of tactile sensibility: aspects relevant to testing children with spastic hemiplegia. Developmental Med Child Neurol 2002;44(9):604–12.

46. Dahlin LB, Komoto-Tufvesson Y, Salgeback S. Surgery of the spastic hand in cerebral palsy: improvement in stereognosis and hand function after surgery. J Hand Surg 1998;23B(3):334–9.

47. Goldenberg G, Daumüller M, Hagmann S. Assessment and therapy of complex activities of daily living in apraxia. Neuropsychol Rehabil 2001; 11(2):147–69.

48. Yasukawa A, Patel P, Sisung C. Pilot study: investigating the effects of Kinesio Taping® in an acute pediatric rehabilitation setting. Am J Occup Ther 2006; 60(1):104–10.

49. Kim JY, Kim SY. Effects of Kinesio tape compared with non-elastic tape on hand grip strength. J Phys Ther Sci 2016;28(5):1565–8.

50. dos Santos GL, Souza MB, Desloovere K, et al. Elastic tape improved shoulder joint position sense in chronic hemiparetic subjects: a randomized sham-controlled crossover study. PLoS One 2017; 12(1):e0170368.

51. Morris D, Jones D, Ryan H, et al. The clinical effects of Kinesio® Tex taping: a systematic review. Physiother Theory Pract 2013;29(4):259–70.

52. Shamsoddini A, Rasti Z, Kalantari M, et al. The impact of Kinesio taping technique on

children with cerebral palsy. Iran J Neurol 2016; 15(4):219–27.

53. Coopee RA. Elastic taping (Kinesio Taping Method). In: Skirven TM, Osterman AL, Fedorczyk JM, et al, editors. Rehabilitation of the hand and upper extremity. 6th edition. Philadelphia: Elsevier Mosby; 2011. p. 1529–38.

54. Keklicek H, Uygur F, Yakut Y. Effects of taping the hand in children with cerebral palsy. J Hand Ther 2015;28(1):27–33.

55. Shah D, Balusamy D, Verma M, et al. Comparative study of the effect of taping on scapular stability and upper limb function in recovering hemiplegics with scapular weakness. CYS Journal 2013;4(2): 121–9.

56. Kase K, Wallis J, Kase T. Clinical therapeutic applications of the Kinesio taping method. Albuquerque (NM): Kinesio Taping Association; 2003.

57. Footer CB. The effects of therapeutic taping on gross motor function in children with cerebral palsy. Pediatr Phys Ther 2006;18(4):245–52.

58. Deconinck FJ, Smorenburg AR, Benham A, et al. Reflections on mirror therapy: a systematic review of the effect of mirror visual feedback on the brain. Neurorehabil Neural Repair 2015;29(4):349–61.

59. McCabe C. Mirror visual feedback therapy. A practical approach. J Hand Ther 2011;24(2):170–8.

60. Yavuzer G, Selles R, Sezer N, et al. Mirror therapy improves hand function in subacute stroke: a randomized controlled trial. Arch Phys Med Rehabil 2008;89:393–8.

61. Ezendam D, Bongers RM, Jannink MJ. Systematic review of the effectiveness of mirror therapy in upper extremity function. Disabil Rehabil 2009;31(26): 2135–49.

62. Rothgangel AS, Braun SM. Mirror therapy: practical protocol for stroke rehabilitation. Research Gate 2013.

63. Wolf SL, Lecraw DE, Barton LA, et al. Forced use of hemiplegic upper extremities to reverse the effect of learned nonuse among chronic stroke and head-injured patients. Exp Neurol 1989;104(2): 125–32.

64. Taub E, Miller NE, Novak TA, et al. Technique to improve chronic motor deficit after stroke. Arch Phys Med Rehabil 1993;74:347–54.

65. Skold A, Josephsson S, Fitinghoff H, et al. Experiences of use of the cerebral palsy hemiplegic hand in young persons treated with upper extremity surgery. J Hand Ther 2007;20:262–73.

Outcomes After Surgical Treatment of Spastic Upper Extremity Conditions

Geneva V. Tranchida, MD, Ann E. Van Heest, MD*

KEYWORDS

- Surgical outcomes • Cerebral palsy • Spastic hemiplegia • Treatment • Upper extremity

KEY POINTS

- Surgical outcomes include motor function and limb positioning, sensory function, and effects on self-esteem.
- Single-event multilevel surgery for wrist flexion and ulnar deviation, forearm pronation, elbow flexion, and thumb-in-palm deformity yield improved limb positioning, motor function, and hygiene.
- Sensory dysfunction exists with high prevalence in children with cerebral palsy. It is unclear whether or not surgery improves sensory dysfunction and further investigation is necessary.
- The position of the upper limb is linked to self-esteem, with elbow flexion contracture deformity having the greatest impact. Surgical outcomes have been reported to have higher patient satisfaction when they address not only functional limitations but also aesthetics.

INTRODUCTION

In general, surgical management for spastic upper extremity conditions focuses on improving muscle balance to maximize hand function.[1] The goals of surgical management must be based on shared decision-making with the child and family, taking into account the child's level of function. For example, the goals of operative management for a high-functioning child are improved joint position, improved grasp, release, and pinch, as well as improved cosmesis. In a lower functioning child, the goals are improved joint positioning and hygiene.[1] This article discusses surgical outcomes as they relate to function, stereognosis, and self-esteem or self-concept.

OUTCOMES MEASURES

Validated outcome measures based on the World Health Organization's *International Classification of Functioning, Disability and Health (ICF)*[2] focus on bodily impairment, activity limitation, and participation restriction. The following assessment tools measure constructs of the *ICF*:

- The Assisting Hand Assessment (AHA) video-based tests grade interaction with 22 test items on a 4-point scale.[3]
- The Shriners Hospital Upper Extremity Evaluation (SHUEE) includes dynamic positional analysis (DPA) and spontaneous functional assessment (SFA). DPA is a video-based test in which completion of 16 tasks is measured in terms of alignment of the elbow, forearm, wrist, thumb, and fingers.[4] The SFA rates spontaneous use and incorporation of the hemiplegic hand into bimanual activities based on 9 selected tasks.[4]
- The Box and Blocks Test measures the number of blocks that can be transferred over a barrier in 1 minute.[5]
- Grip and pinch strength is measured.

Department of Orthopaedic Surgery, University of Minnesota, 2450 Riverside Avenue South, Suite R200, Minneapolis, MN 55455, USA
* Corresponding author.
E-mail address: vanhe003@umn.edu

Hand Clin 34 (2018) 583–591
https://doi.org/10.1016/j.hcl.2018.06.014
0749-0712/18/© 2018 Elsevier Inc. All rights reserved.

Validated questionnaires include the following[6]:

- The Pediatric Outcomes Data Collection Instrument (PODCI) measures the percent of function on the 6 different scales of upper extremity function, mobility or transfers, sports or physical function, pain or comfort, happiness, and global function. A score of less than 80% is abnormal.[6]
- The Pediatric Quality of Life Inventory (PedsQL) parent version and the PedsQL cerebral palsy (CP) module reports percentage results of 4 and 5 domains, respectively.[6]
- For the Canadian Occupational Performance Measure (COPM), an occupational therapist administers a questionnaire to obtain performance and satisfaction scores based on an activity selected by the patient.[6]

SURGICAL OUTCOMES
Motor Function and Limb Positioning Concepts

Surgical outcomes include motor function, limb positioning, sensory function, and self-esteem. This section reviews postoperative motor function and limb positioning outcomes.

Single-Event Multilevel Surgery

Most children undergo multiple, concomitant procedures in a single setting to correct the combined deformities of elbow flexion, forearm pronation, wrist flexion, and thumb-in-palm deformity (**Fig. 1**). Therefore, functional outcomes studies report on groups of subjects who have undergone a variety of procedures. Some studies show improved limb

positioning but no improvement in functional outcomes, whereas other studies demonstrate improved postoperative functional outcomes. Smitherman and colleagues[7] found that single-event multilevel surgery for children with hemiplegic CP can significantly improve thumb, finger, wrist, and forearm segmental positioning, as well as spontaneous function; however, it does not significantly change their grasp–release ability.[7,8]

van Munster and colleagues[9] reviewed 8 studies and found that, although there was improvement in supination and wrist extension with tendon transfer surgery, there were no definitive improvements in hand function. Similarly, using the Jebsen-Taylor Hand Function Test at 3.6-year follow-up to assess function, hemiplegic subjects demonstrated statistically significant improvements in wrist, finger, and elbow positioning; however, this did not translate into a shorter time to test completion.[9]

During a 25-year period, Van Heest and colleagues[10] reported preoperative and postoperative functional outcomes of 134 subjects who underwent 180 operations (this represented 718 procedures individually tailored for each subject). The most common procedures performed during a single surgical intervention were pronator teres (PT) and biceps aponeurosis release; flexor carpi ulnaris (FCU), brachioradialis (BR), or extensor carpi ulnaris transfer to extensor carpi radialis brevis (ECRB) and first web space Z-plasty plus adductor and/or first dorsal interosseous tendon release, and a tendon transfer to abductor pollicis longus. The House functional assessment tool revealed that subjects had an average score of 2.3 preoperatively and 5.0 postoperatively, indicating an average improvement of 2.7 levels. In other words, operated hands went from a fair passive assist to a fair active assist that could grasp an object well[10] (**Fig. 2**).

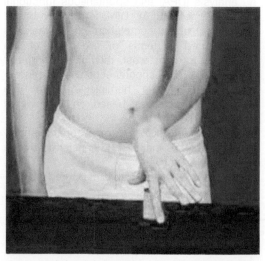

Fig. 1. Multilevel deformity in CP with elbow flexion, forearm pronation, wrist flexion with ulnar deviation, and thumb-in-palm deformity.

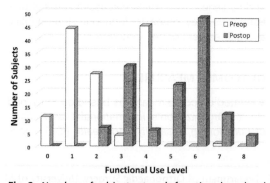

Fig. 2. Number of subjects at each functional use level before (Preop) and after (Postop) surgery. (*Data from* Van Heest AE, House JH, Cariello C. Upper extremity surgical treatment of cerebral palsy. J Hand Surg Am 1999;24(2):323–30.)

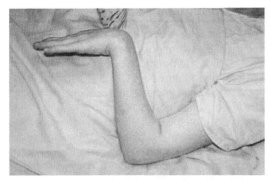

Fig. 3. Preoperative wrist flexion deformity in CP.

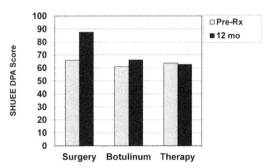

Fig. 5. Comparison of the 3 treatment groups (surgery, botulinum toxin injections, physical therapy), pretreatment (Pre-Rx) and 12 months posttreatment based on SHUEE DPA scores. (*From* Van Heest AE, Bagley A, Molitor F, et al. Tendon transfer surgery in upper-extremity cerebral palsy is more effective than botulinum toxin injections or regular, ongoing therapy. J Bone Joint Surg Am 2015;97(7):534; with permission.)

They conclude that similar functional improvement (2 levels) can be achieved in highly motivated patients, regardless of preoperative mentation, sensibility, and type of CP. However, subjects with good voluntary motor control had significantly greater improvement in functional levels than those with poor voluntary control[10] (**Figs. 3** and **4**).

In 27 subjects who underwent single-event multilevel upper extremity surgery, with an average of 5.9 procedures per subject, Gong and colleagues[11] found that subjects with a higher baseline Manual Abilities Classification System (MACS) level had greater improvement in function and overall satisfaction.[8] Finally, a recent randomized trial compared tendon transfer surgery (group I) with 3 serial botulinum toxin injections plus therapy (group 2) and with treatment with occupational therapy alone (group 3) in 29 subjects. If subjects had a pronation deformity, wrist flexion deformity with FCU as the primary deforming force, adequate digital control, and adduction of the thumb with flexion at the metacarpophalangeal (MCP) joint, they received tendon transfer surgery (FCU transfer to ECRB, pronator teres release, adductor pollicis release, plus extensor pollicis longus [EPL] rerouting). Outcomes for bodily impairments, activity limitations, and participation restriction were reported. Subjects managed with surgery exhibited a statistically significant increase in forearm supination ($P = .03$), wrist extension

($P = .007$), and grip and pinch strength ($P = .006$ and $P = .003$, respectively). The surgical group demonstrated much greater improvement on the SHUEE DPA, improving from 66% to 88% at 12 months ($P<.001$). Subjects in group II improved from 61% to 66% and group III declined from 64% to 63%. Group I had a greater increase in pinch strength compared with groups II and III. Although subjects in group I had no improvement in the 4 domains of the PedsQL CP module, they did exhibit an increase in the movement domain of 26.4%, whereas subjects in groups II and III had a mean decrease of 3.3%. They conclude that, for those who meet specific inclusion criteria, tendon transfer surgery is more effective than serial botulinum toxin injections or therapy alone. For this subset of patients, they no longer recommend botulinum toxin injections[6] (**Fig. 5**).

Elbow Flexion Contracture Release

A well-executed elbow flexion contracture release, guided by the extent of preoperative contracture, can yield improvements in elbow

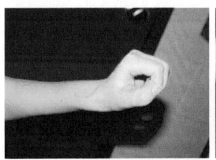
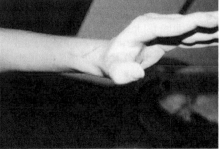

Fig. 4. Results (*left* and *right*) after flexor carpi ulnaris to extensor carpi radialis tendon transfer.

posture with ambulation, active and passive extension, and total range of motion. In general, fixed contractures less than 45° are treated by partial flexor lengthening, whereas contractures greater than 45° are treated with a full release.[8,12] Partial lengthening consists of lacertus fibrosis transection, lengthening of the brachialis with 2 parallel incisions in the brachialis fascia, release of the proximal half of the BR origin off the humerus, and lengthening of the biceps tendon by dividing the medial half distally and the lateral half proximally and securing this with sutures in the medial aspect of the tendon. Full release consists of lacertus fibrosis transection, myotomy of the anterior half of the brachialis, release of BR origin off the humerus, Z-lengthening of biceps tendon, and release of anterior elbow capsule.[12]

Carlson and colleagues[12] reported short-term (18–22 months) results on 90 elbows that underwent either partial or full elbow release using these surgical guidelines. In the partial release group, elbow flexion posture at ambulation improved by 57° and active extension improved by 17°. In the full-release group, elbow flexion posture at ambulation improved by 51° and active extension improved by 38°.

A subsequent study by Dy and colleagues[13] reported 5-year follow-up on 23 elbows that underwent partial release. All subjects showed improvement from baseline, with an average improvement in elbow flexion posture angle of 63°, a 12° improvement in active extension, with an 8° decrease in active flexion.

Forearm Pronation

A forearm pronation deformity can be addressed with a PT release. Active forearm supination can also be achieved when the released PT tendon is rerouted around the radius. In a cadaveric model, rerouting the PT through a window in the interosseous membrane around the dorsal aspect of the radius and then inserting it on the volar surface of the radius (360° wraparound) provided greater supination (47°) than any of the following transfers: (1) inserting it on the volar surface of the radius, (2) inserting it on the interosseous ligament, (3) inserting it on the dorsal surface of the radius, or (4) rerouting it through a window in the interosseous ligament and attaching it to its native insertion on the lateral surface of the radial shaft.[14] Other studies have assessed outcomes after PT rerouting with tendon docking in the native insertion site and found postoperative active supination to be 46° to 48°.[14,15]

Wrist Tendon Transfers

The FCU to ECRB tendon transfer is the most commonly performed procedure to address a wrist flexion deformity secondary to spasticity. The primary goal of the FCU to ECRB transfer is to move the wrist into a neutral or slightly extended posture or, when possible, to provide active wrist extension. The FCU to ECRB transfer can also augment forearm supination. Although wrist extension can be achieved by releasing only one-third of the FCU ulnar origin and transferring to either ECRL or ECRB, supination can be achieved by releasing and transferring at least two-thirds of the FCU ulnar origin. This additional release augments the tendon pull vector and imparts a greater supination moment across the forearm. In a cadaver model, the additional release has been shown to achieve 51° of supination, compared with −3° supination when only releasing one-third of the FCU ($P<.001$).[16] Although the additional release of the FCU muscle is technically straightforward, the cadaveric model does not take into account any underlying muscle dysfunction.

On motion and electromyography analysis, the FCU can fire phasically or continuously. A patient is considered to have phasic control of their FCU if the FCU relaxes during grasp and contracts during release of an object. This means that wrist extension is synergistic with finger flexion and wrist flexion is synergistic with finger extension. The best surgical candidates for tendon transfer are those that have phasic contraction of the FCU, whereas those that are poor candidates fire the FCU continuously. Some hemiplegic patients exhibit phasic FCU activation, whereas in others FCU activity is not synergistic with finger motion at baseline and the FCU is continuously firing.

Knowing this relationship of FCU relaxation and contraction to finger flexion and extension, respectively, Van Heest and colleagues[17] investigated whether the FCU changes phase of activation after FCU to ECRB tendon transfer. Using the Jebsen-Taylor Hand Function Test to measure outcomes, a sample of 7 subjects who exhibited phasic activation of the FCU between grasp and release tasks were assessed. Preoperatively, 4 out of 7 subjects activated their FCU during grasp and relaxed the FCU during release. Postoperatively, 5 subjects showed improvement of wrist position from wrist flexion to wrist extension. Following FCU to ECRB tendon transfer, 6 subjects activated their FCU during grasp (aiding in wrist extension) and relaxed their FCU during release (allowing wrist flexion). These results indicate that these subjects did not exhibit change of phase and, therefore, continued to activate the FCU with grasp (which is beneficial because after FCU to ECRB transfer, FCU acts as a wrist extensor) and relax the FCU with release (allowing for wrist flexion). As is common with spasticity surgery, improved limb position did not reliably improve functional outcomes.

Wrist Arthrodesis

In the setting of a skeletally mature adolescent or adult with a long-standing wrist flexion deformity unlikely to be helped with soft tissue procedures alone, wrist arthrodesis is the preferred option.[18] Although this is generally viewed as a salvage procedure, patients with poor volitional control of the upper extremity may benefit from the improved cosmesis, hygiene, and paperweight hand function.

Rayan and Young[19] reviewed outcomes after wrist arthrodesis in 11 subjects with spastic wrist flexion deformities. They report that, regardless of cognitive function, all subjects had some improvement in appearance, hygiene, and function. They obtained an average correction of 85°, resulting in a final wrist position in 15° of flexion. All subjects achieved union at 9 weeks postoperatively and 0% of subjects reported skin breakdown or maceration after surgery (compared with 45% before surgery). All caretakers reported that wrist fusion facilitated hygiene and was more aesthetically pleasing. Functional improvement in tasks such as independent dressing, face washing, propelling a wheelchair, and picking up objects was reported in 91% of subjects.

Van Heest and Strothman[18] performed wrist arthrodesis with dorsal plating in 41 wrists and achieved an average correction of 89° with an average final wrist position of 5° of extension (**Figs. 6–8**). They reported a 98% union rate, as well as postoperative satisfaction with outcome

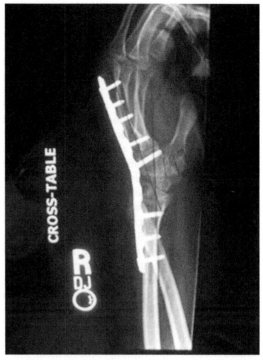

Fig. 7. Radiograph of postoperative wrist arthrodesis with a dorsal plate.

in 94% of subjects. Subject disability decreased significantly, with a mean preoperative disability assessment scale score of 9.6 decreasing to 5.5 postoperatively. The investigators also report a 10% rate of periimplant fractures. Additionally, 36% had elective plate removal for symptomatic and asymptomatic reasons. As a result of these reported complications, when there is evidence of solid arthrodesis, the authors recommend elective plate removal in all cases.

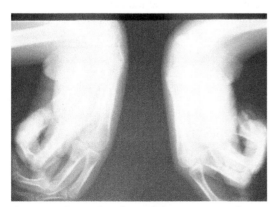

Fig. 6. Radiograph of preoperative wrist flexion deformity before wrist arthrodesis.

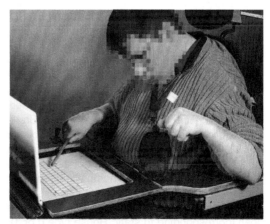

Fig. 8. A 25-year-old spastic quadriplegic man with postoperative bilateral wrist arthrodesis for wrist flexion deformity.

Thumb-in-Palm Deformity

The overall goal in surgical correction of thumb-in-palm deformity is to counteract the spastic thumb adductor and flexor muscles that overpower the abductor and extensor muscles. In long-standing deformities, the subject may also develop MCP joint hyperextension and instability. Surgical correction involves muscle release to correct adduction and flexion, tendon transfer to augment abduction and extension, and joint stabilization to optimize function.[20] Although the concept is straightforward, thumb-in-palm deformity may be difficult to treat and methods of surgical correction, as well as outcomes, are variable.

A Cochrane review, performed on 14 prospective studies from 1976 to 2002, assessed outcomes greater than 6 months after surgical correction of thumb-in-palm deformity. Unfortunately, the review was limited by inconsistent methodology and lack of functional outcomes testing. However, outcomes after thumb-in-palm deformity surgery were considered satisfactory by subjects and caregivers, and subjects demonstrated modest improvement in movement.[21]

More recently, Davids and colleagues[20] used the SHUEE to assess spontaneous functional use, static alignment, and dynamic positional alignment of the thumb after surgical correction of thumb-in-palm deformity at a mean 2-year follow-up. For a contracted first web space, the first dorsal interosseous and the adductor pollicis were released from their insertion; a Z-plasty was not performed. MCP joint hyperextension instability was addressed with standard or sesamoid arthrodesis. Deficient thumb extension and abduction was treated with EPL rerouting. Thumb-in-palm deformity correction was always performed in combination with surgery to address wrist and forearm deformities. Scoring for static thumb alignment was based on the static House scale (type 0 is normal alignment, type 1 is simple metacarpal adduction contracture, type 2 is metacarpal adduction plus MCP joint flexion contracture, type 3 is metacarpal adduction plus MCP joint hyperextension or instability, and type 4 is metacarpal adduction plus MCP joint and interphalangeal joint flexion contracture).[22] Static thumb alignment improved in 55% of subjects and 82% of subjects achieved an optimal outcome (ie, a static House score alignment of 0 or 1); 15% of subjects had worse static thumb alignment after surgery. Dynamic thumb alignment was assessed using the SHUEE DPA and was categorized as open (corresponding to static House type 0 or 1), closed (corresponding to static House type 2 or 3), and in palm (corresponding to House type 4).

Dynamic thumb alignment improved in 58% of subjects and 61% achieved an optimal outcome; 5% of subjects had worse dynamic thumb alignment after surgery. The investigators conclude that, no matter the degree of underlying neurologic impairment, surgical intervention can improve both static and dynamic thumb position; however, better results are seen in static alignment.

Alewijnse and colleagues[23] obtained a minimum of 5-year follow-up on subjects with the Gross Motor Function Classification System (GMFCS) I to III, who underwent surgical correction of thumb-in-palm deformity via the adductor pollicis muscle slide, EPL rerouting, and MCP joint capsulodesis. At 1-year follow-up, 13% of subjects developed recurrence of the deformity. At 5-year follow-up, 29% of subjects had deterioration of thumb position and 2 had full recurrence of deformity. Despite this, 74% of subjects were satisfied with their result and 87% would undergo surgery again. Based on these outcomes, it is clear that further investigation into surgical techniques to address thumb-in-palm deformity is warranted.[23]

SENSORY FUNCTION (STEREOGNOSIS)

Although neuroplasticity allows children to adapt to the initial central nervous system insult and exhibit greater recruitment of the ipsilateral brain for motor and sensory function of the affected limb,[8] 46% to 97% of children with spastic hemiplegia develop persistent sensory deficits.[24] Furthermore, there is a correlation between more profound motor dysfunction and greater sensory impairments.[25] Stereognosis testing is shown in **Fig. 9**.

Neurophysiology literature has shown that functional reorganization of the somatosensory cortex can occur as a result of changes in afferent input from the hand.[26–28] After surgical correction, improved hand position leads to greater contact between the palm and the fingertips and external stimuli, which may lead to functional cerebral

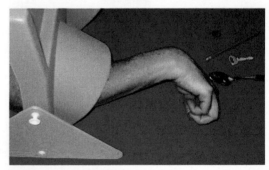

Fig. 9. Patient performing stereognosis testing. Patient is blinded by the blue barrier.

reorganization and perhaps improved recognition of tactile stimuli. Most studies have failed to show improved stereognosis following tendon transfer surgery.

However, in a sample of 38 subjects, Dahlin and colleagues[29] found improved stereognosis at 6 and 18 months following surgery. A recent study of 63 children assessed baseline stereognosis and compared it with stereognosis following tendon transfer surgery plus rehabilitation, botulinum toxin injection plus rehabilitation, or rehabilitation alone.[30] They found no statistically significant difference in stereognosis scores postintervention among the 3 different treatment groups and no difference when comparing results between surgical and nonsurgical groups.

Although surgery has not been shown to reliably improve stereognosis, some investigators postulate that longer follow-up may uncover improvement. Furthermore, older patient age at time of surgery may be associated with improved stereognosis.[30]

SELF-ESTEEM AND SELF-CONCEPT

Self-esteem defines how a person values himself or herself and it has a profound impact on personal development.[31–33] One component of self-esteem is self-concept, which refers to how one views himself or herself.[34] Unfortunately, reduced self-esteem is common among patients with CP, and female adolescents, in particular, have been found to have reduced self-concept. Russo and colleagues[35] found that hemiplegic children had lower quality of life and self-concept scores than their nondisabled peers, specifically in the domains of physical, athletic, and scholastic competence. Hemiplegic patients with mild-moderate functional impairments may be even more susceptible to low self-esteem and low-self-concept because they are expected to perform at the level of their peers and may perceive their level of function to be inadequate.

Upper extremity deformity, particularly in the subset of high-functioning subjects, can adversely affect self-esteem.[8] The position of the upper extremity is closely linked to self-esteem; the elbow flexion deformity is the main contributor to low self-esteem. Although gait profile scores and arm posturing scores are significantly impaired in patients with unilateral impairment, only the arm posturing score has demonstrated a correlation with self-esteem; less deviation in arm movement corresponds to higher self-esteem.[36]

Surgery results in higher patient satisfaction when it not only addresses functional limitations but also aesthetics. Some investigators have found cosmetic appearance after surgical correction to yield significantly higher patient satisfaction,[37] and there was no correlation between functional outcomes and patient satisfaction. Further, other researchers have found that a patient's perceived impact of their disability was a much greater predictor of self-esteem than their functional abilities.[38]

Although tendon transfer surgery may not lead to significant functional improvement, it is still reasonable to perform surgery for improved aesthetics and self-esteem.[8] Because of the significant role of self-esteem on patient-rated outcomes after upper extremity spasticity surgery, further investigation should use specific self-esteem or self-concept assessment tools, such as the I Think I Am,[39] the Self-Perception Profile for Children,[40] and the Pictorial Scale of Perceived Competence and Social Acceptance for Young Children,[41] to guide treatment.

SUMMARY

Surgical interventions for the spastic upper extremity aim to correct the common deformities of elbow flexion, forearm pronation, wrist flexion and ulnar deviation, and thumb-in-palm deformity. Single-event multilevel surgery can result in improved function, limb positioning, and hygiene. Further, recent data suggest that tendon transfers for wrist flexion deformity lead to better outcomes than botulinum toxin and/or ongoing physical or occupational therapy. Because aesthetics of the limb are extremely important and have a profound impact on self-esteem, self-concept, patient quality of life, and satisfaction, it is reasonable to perform surgery even without the hope of any functional improvement. Unfortunately, deformity correction, has not been shown to improve sensory function and further investigation is needed in this area.

REFERENCES

1. Van Heest A. Management of the upper extremity in children with cerebral palsy. In: University of California Davis Medical Centre, editor. Chapman's comprehensive orthopaedic surgery 4th edition. 13th edition. Philadelphia: Jp Medical Ltd; 2017. p. 3–15.
2. International Classifiation of Functioning Disability and Health (ICF). World Health Organization, classifications. Available at: http://www.who.int/classifications/icf/en/.
3. Krumlinde-Sundholm L, Holmefur M, Kottorp A, et al. The Assisting Hand Assessment: current evidence of validity, reliability, and responsiveness to change. Dev Med Child Neurol 2007;49(4):259–64.

4. Davids JR, Peace LC, Wagner LV, et al. Validation of the Shriners Hospital for Children Upper Extremity Evaluation (SHUEE) for children with hemiplegic cerebral palsy. J Bone Joint Surg Am 2006;88(2): 326–33.

5. Mathiowetz V, Federman S, Wiemer D. Box and block test of manual dexterity: norms for 6-19 year olds. Can J Occup Ther 1985;52:241–5.

6. Van Heest AE, Bagley A, Molitor F, et al. Tendon transfer surgery in upper-extremity cerebral palsy is more effective than botulinum toxin injections or regular, ongoing therapy. J Bone Joint Surg Am 2015;97(7):529–36.

7. Smitherman JA, Davids JR, Tanner S, et al. Functional outcomes following single-event multilevel surgery of the upper extremity for children with hemiplegic cerebral palsy. J Bone Joint Surg Am 2011;93(7):655–61.

8. Leafblad ND, Van Heest AE. Management of the spastic wrist and hand in cerebral palsy. J Hand Surg Am 2015;40(5):1035–40.

9. van Munster JC, Maathuis KG, Haga N, et al. Does surgical management of the hand in children with spastic unilateral cerebral palsy affect functional outcome? Dev Med Child Neurol 2007; 49(5):385–9.

10. Van Heest AE, House JH, Cariellol C. Upper extremity surgical treatment of cerebral palsy. J Hand Surg Am 1999;24(2):323–30.

11. Gong HS, Chung CY, Park MS, et al. Functional outcomes after upper extremity surgery for cerebral palsy: comparison of high and low manual ability classification system levels. J Hand Surg Am 2010; 35(2):277–83.e1-3.

12. Carlson MG, Hearns KA, Inkellis E, et al. Early results of surgical intervention for elbow deformity in cerebral palsy based on degree of contracture. J Hand Surg Am 2012;37(8):1665–71.

13. Dy CJ, Pean CA, Hearns KA, et al. Long-term results following surgical treatment of elbow deformity in patients with cerebral palsy. J Hand Surg Am 2013;38(12):2432–6.

14. Van Heest AE, Sathy M, Schutte L. Cadaveric modeling of the pronator teres rerouting tendon transfer. J Hand Surg Am 1999;24(3):614–8.

15. Strecker WB, Emanuel JP, Dailey L, et al. Comparison of pronator tenotomy and pronator rerouting in children with spastic cerebral palsy. J Hand Surg Am 1988;13(4):540–3.

16. Van Heest AE, Murthy NS, Sathy MR, et al. The supination effect of tendon transfer of the flexor carpi ulnaris to the extensor carpi radialis brevis or longus: a cadaveric study. J Hand Surg Am 1999;24(5): 1091–6.

17. Van Heest A, Stout J, Wervey R, et al. Follow-up motion laboratory analysis for patients with spastic hemiplegia due to cerebral palsy: analysis of the flexor carpi ulnaris firing pattern before and after tendon transfer surgery. J Hand Surg Am 2010; 35(2):284–90.

18. Van Heest AE, Strothman D. Wrist arthrodesis in cerebral palsy. J Hand Surg Am 2009;34(7):1216–24.

19. Rayan GM, Young BT. Arthrodesis of the spastic wrist. J Hand Surg 1999;24A:944–52.

20. Davids JR, Sabesan VJ, Ortmann F, et al. Surgical management of thumb deformity in children with hemiplegic-type cerebral palsy. J Pediatr Orthop 2009;29(5):504–10.

21. Smeulders M, Coester A, Kreulen M. Surgical treatment for the thumb-in-palm deformity in patients with cerebral palsy. Cochrane Database Syst Rev 2005;(4):CD004093.

22. House JH, Gwathmey FW, Fidler MO. A dynamic approach to the thumb-in palm deformity in cerebral palsy. J Bone Joint Surg Am 1981;63(2):216–25.

23. Alewijnse JV, Smeulders MJ, Kreulen M. Short-term and long-term clinical results of the surgical correction of thumb-in-palm deformity in patients with cerebral palsy. J Pediatr Orthop 2015;35(8): 825–30.

24. Van Heest AE, House J, Putnam M. Sensibility deficiencies in the hands of children with spastic hemiplegia. J Hand Surg Am 1993;18(2):278–81.

25. Kinnucan E, Van Heest A, Tomhave W. Correlation of motor function and stereognosis impairment in upper limb cerebral palsy. J Hand Surg Am 2010; 35(8):1317–22.

26. Allard T, Clark SA, Jenkins WM, et al. Reorganization of somatosensory area 3b representations in adult owl monkeys after digital syndactyly. J Neurophysiol 1991;66(3):1048–58.

27. Eliasson AC, Gordon AM, Forssberg H. Tactile control of isometric fingertip forces during grasping in children with cerebral palsy. Dev Med Child Neurol 1995;37(1):72–84.

28. Merzenich MM, Jenkins WM. Reorganization of cortical representations of the hand following alterations of skin inputs induced by nerve injury, skin island transfers, and experience. J Hand Ther 1993; 6(2):89–104.

29. Dahlin LB, Komoto-Tufvesson Y, Salgeback S. Surgery of the spastic hand in cerebral palsy. Improvement in stereognosis and hand function after surgery. J Hand Surg Br 1998;23(3):334–9.

30. Petersen E, Tomhave W, Agel J, et al. The effect of treatment on stereognosis in children with hemiplegic cerebral palsy. J Hand Surg Am 2016;41(1): 91–6.

31. Brooks RB. Self-esteem during the school years. Its normal development and hazardous decline. Pediatr Clin North Am 1992;39(3):537–50.

32. Harter S. Causes, correlates, and the functional role of global self-worth: a life-span perspective. In: Sternberg RJ, Kolligan J, editors. Competence

considered. New Haven (CT): Yale University Press; 1990. p. 67–97.

33. King GA, Shultz IZ, Steel K, et al. Self-evaluation and self-concept of adolescents with physical disabilities. Am J Occup Ther 1993;47(2):132–40.

34. Willoughby C, King G, Polatajko H. A therapist's guide to children's self-esteem. Am J Occup Ther 1996;50(2):124–32.

35. Russo RN, Goodwin EJ, Miller MD, et al. Self-esteem, self-concept, and quality of life in children with hemiplegic cerebral palsy. J Pediatr 2008; 153(4):473–7.

36. Riad J, Brostrom E, Langius-Eklof A. Do movement deviations influence self-esteem and sense of coherence in mild unilateral cerebral palsy? J Pediatr Orthop 2013;33(3):298–302.

37. Libberecht K, Sabapathy SR, Bhardwaj P. The relation of patient satisfaction and functional and cosmetic outcome after correction of the wrist flexion deformity in cerebral palsy. J Hand Surg Eur Vol 2011;36(2):141–6.

38. Manuel JC, Balkrishnan R, Camacho F, et al. Factors associated with self-esteem in pre-adolescents and adolescents with cerebral palsy. J Adolesc Health 2003;32(6):456–8.

39. Ouvinen-Birgerstam P. Jag tycker jag är: manual. [I think I am: a manual]. Stockholm (Sweden): Psykologiförlaget AB; 1999.

40. Hatrter S. Manual for the self-perception profile for children. Denver (CO): University of Denver; 1985.

41. Harter S, Pike R. The pictorial scale of perceived competence and social acceptance for young children. Child Dev 1984;55(6):1969–82.

The Future of Upper Extremity Spasticity Management

Mitchel Seruya, MD

KEYWORDS

• Spasticity • Upper extremity • Nerve transfers • Contralateral C7

KEY POINTS

- Treatment of upper limb spasticity has historically relied on rebalancing the affected musculotendinous units and joints.
- Future management of upper limb spasticity may focus on reestablishing a normal neuronal impulse pathway to the dysfunctional musculotendinous unit.
- Transfer of the contralateral C7 nerve root to the injured C7 nerve root may open the potential for simultaneously releasing flexor spasticity while improving extensor function for reach and grasp activities.
- On the nonsurgical frontier, robotic exoskeletons offer the potential to facilitate rehabilitation of upper extremity spasticity.

INTRODUCTION

Treatment of upper limb spasticity has historically relied on rebalancing the affected musculotendinous units and joints[1–8] by means of a wide variety of medical and surgical methods. Botulinum toxin A (Botox) therapy has been useful as a stand-alone or adjunctive modality for temporarily relaxing spasticity.[9–13] Tendon release, lengthening, or transfer procedures may help correct the resultant abnormal postures. Arthrodesis can address severe joint deformities, with static placement into a more functional position.

Although these approaches tackle the downstream effects of spasticity at the muscle, tendon, and joint levels, they do not address the primary pathologic condition within the nerve. Muscle tension is normally maintained by the γ-neuron circuit,[14–16] which is located in the spinal cord (Fig. 1). The activity of the γ-neuron circuit is normally inhibited by upper motor neurons within the cerebral cortex; this process regulates muscle

tension and prevents spasticity. When there is an insult to the cerebral cortex, the negative feedback loop between the upper motor neuron and γ-neuron circuit is disconnected. As a result, the γ-neuron circuit runs uninhibited and muscle spasticity ensues. Peripheral procedures to address the manifestations of upper extremity spasticity do not influence the disrupted feedback loop and, as such, the pathologic neuronal pathways persist. As a result, functional return is only temporary in the case of Botox or, with respect to tendon procedures, progressively less apparent over time.

When upper extremity spasticity develops, functional placement of the hand in space is no longer achievable. Hand dysfunction ensues due to the fact that the delicate balance between flexor, extensor, pronator, and supinator muscles is disrupted. Classically, patients with upper limb spasticity present with a flexed elbow, pronated forearm, flexed wrist, thumb in palm, and a flexed finger posture. This abnormal set of postures

Disclosure Statement: The author has no financial interest to declare in relation to the content of this article.
Division of Plastic and Maxillofacial Surgery, USC Keck School of Medicine, Children's Hospital Los Angeles, 4650 Sunset Boulevard, MS#96, Los Angeles, CA 90027, USA
E-mail address: mseruya@chla.usc.edu

Hand Clin 34 (2018) 593–599
https://doi.org/10.1016/j.hcl.2018.07.002

hand.theclinics.com

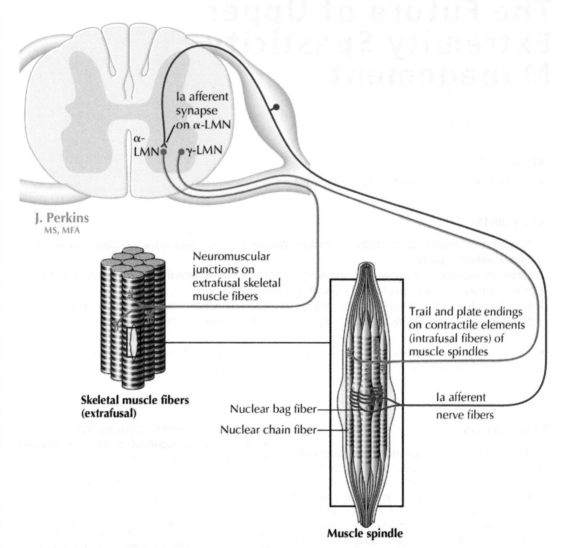

Fig. 1. Located in the spinal cord, the γ-neuron circuit maintains muscle tension and is modulated by a negative feedback loop from upper motor neurons in the CNS. (Netter illustration used with permission of Elsevier, Inc. All rights reserved. Available at: www.netterimages.com.)

limits the interaction of the upper limb with the environment (**Fig. 2**).[17,18]

Depending on the severity, the flexor spasticity may produce a hygienic, cosmetic, and/or functional deformity.[1,19] Severe flexion deformities can promote skin intertrigo and eventually lead to skin breakdown, thus requiring wound management. Physical appearance is also an important consideration, because the hyperflexion deformity represents one of the key stigmata of upper limb spasticity. The functional implications of flexor spasticity are also numerous and include limitations on reaching a wider radius of objects, 2-handed manipulation of objects away from the body, and grasp, pinch, and release activities.

NOVEL SURGICAL APPROACH FOR UPPER LIMB SPASTICITY

In 2011, Xu and colleagues[20] introduced a novel surgical approach for treating upper limb spastic hemiplegia. Rather than focusing on the downstream effects of spasticity on the muscle, tendon, and/or joint, the investigators argued for intervening at the nerve level. Because the flexor muscles are spastic while the extensor groups are weak in upper limb spasticity, the investigators proposed a nerve procedure that could partially release flexor spasticity while simultaneously improving extensor function.

The investigators based their approach on previous literature demonstrating the benefits of

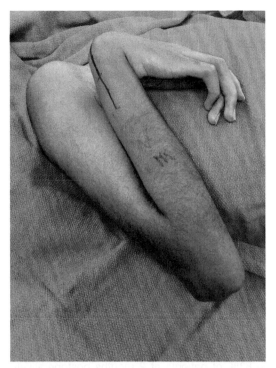

Fig. 2. Classic posture of patients with upper limb spasticity, marked by shoulder adduction, elbow flexion, wrist flexion, thumb in palm, and flexed fingers.

selective posterior rhizotomy (SPR) on lessening flexor spasticity, concurrent with the mounting evidence in support of contralateral C7 nerve root transfer for treating brachial plexus avulsion injuries. As popularized by Gros and colleagues,[21] SPR interrupts the γ-neuron circuit by selectively cutting off the affected posterior nerve roots responsible for spasticity. Although the body of literature in favor of posterior rhizotomy is more extensive for lower limb spasticity, outcomes studies on upper extremity treatment are also available.[22,23] In a series of 16 hemiplegic patients, spasticity was totally abolished in 5 cases (31.3%), markedly reduced in 9 patients (56.2%), and slightly diminished in 2 cases (12.5%).[23] Half of the patients also demonstrated an improvement in volitional control of the upper limb. In a study of 15 spastic upper limbs, dorsal root rhizotomy at 2 or more cervical levels yielded permanent spasticity relief in all but one limb.[22] Spasticity decreased to an Ashworth grade of 1 or 2 at the shoulder, elbow, and hand and remained stable over time in all but one limb. One recurrence was noted at 3 months after surgery; this was localized to the hand and attributed to an incomplete rhizotomy. Increased arc of motion was also appreciated at the shoulder and elbow, with the hand

only gaining range of motion if active finger extension was noted preoperatively.

Concurrent with the rising popularity of SPR in the 1990s, Gu and colleagues[24] introduced the concept of contralateral C7 nerve root transfer for treatment of brachial plexus avulsion injuries.[25,26] Since then, clinical and experimental studies have demonstrated both safety and efficacy for the procedure.[24,27–34] Chuang and colleagues[27] reported on the safety of the procedure for 21 patients with at least 2 years of follow-up. In 48% of patients, no significant sensory disturbance was reported, whereas the remaining 52% of patients reported dysesthesia at the distal phalangeal level mostly for the thumb, index, and long fingers. Most cases of dysesthesia improved by 1 month postoperatively; however, 1 patient needed up to 16 months for resolution of the sensory disturbance. Regarding motor function of the donor limb, 81% of patients did not notice any weakness on postoperative day 1. Transient weakness of the triceps and extensor digitorum communis resolved by the second month postoperatively. The only persistent donor deficit was a weak or absent triceps reflex.

Recently, a 2017 meta-analysis detailed the functional efficacy of contralateral C7 nerve root transfers, defined as scores on the British Medical Research Council greater than or equal to M3 and S3 for motor and sensory function, respectively.[34] The pooled muscle strength recovery rate was 0.57, whereas the sensory recovery rate was 0.52. More specifically, the muscle strength recovery rates were 0.50, 0.74, and 0.50 for the median, radial, and musculocutaneous nerves, respectively. Regarding sensation, the recovery rate for the median nerve was 0.56. Sensory recovery for the radial and ulnar nerves was not studied.

Largely borne out of these observations, Xu and colleagues[20] treated a 4-year-old girl with spastic hemiplegic cerebral palsy with a C7 nerve root rhizotomy and contralateral C7 nerve root transfer to the ipsilateral middle trunk of the brachial plexus, using an interpositional sural nerve graft passed through a chest subcutaneous tunnel. Transection of the affected C7 served as a rhizotomy, aiming to interrupt the γ-neuron circuit and lessen flexor spasticity. Nerve transfer to the middle trunk aimed to power up the radial nerve, with the potential for restoring extension power across the elbow, wrist, and fingers and improving reach and grasp. In a 2-year follow-up, the results showed a significant reduction in spasticity as measured by the Modified Ashworth Scale and improvement in extension power of the elbow, the wrist, and fingers as per the Quality of Upper Extremity Skills Test. This case provided preliminary evidence in support for "peripheral rewiring" in overcoming the untoward effects of a central nervous system injury.

LEVEL 1 EVIDENCE FOR CONTRALATERAL C7 NERVE ROOT TRANSFER

Making the case for contralateral C7 nerve root transfer in treatment of the hemiplegic upper extremity, Hua and colleagues[35] performed a randomized control trial (RCT). Twelve adult patients with spastic hemiplegia from central neurologic injury were randomly assigned to contralateral C7 nerve root surgery plus rehabilitation versus rehabilitation alone. Similar to their case report in 2011, the gap between the proximal cut end of the contralateral C7 nerve root and the distal cut end of the ipsilateral C7 nerve root was bridged with interpositional sural nerve grafts via a cross-neck subcutaneous tunnel.

Outcomes were evaluated at 6-month intervals to determine the effect on functional recovery per the Fugl-Meyer upper extremity scale, active range of motion (AROM), and spasticity per Modified Ashworth Scale scores. Fugl-Meyer scores significantly increased for surgery versus control groups and on comparison of preoperative and postoperative periods at both 18 and 24 months. Muscle strength of the affected extensor digitorum communis and extensor carpi radialis increased significantly by 18 and 24 months for the surgery group, with final scores at the M3 level. Spasticity scores clinically improved for the surgical group by 6 months postoperatively, including at the elbow, wrist, thumb, and fingers.

Building on this momentum, Zheng and colleagues[36] recently performed a higher-powered RCT to study the safety and efficacy of contralateral C7 nerve root transfer in treatment of spastic arm paralysis. Thirty-six patients with established cerebral injury and resultant spastic hemiplegia were randomized in a 1:1 fashion to undergo contralateral C7 nerve root transfer to the affected C7 nerve root followed by rehabilitation versus rehabilitation alone. To maximize neurotization of the recipient nerve, the investigators divided the donor C7 nerve root at the nerve division/cord junction and routed it between the spinal column and esophagus. Increasing the length of the donor nerve and using an alternate route avoided the need for a nerve graft and allowed for direct nerve coaptation (Fig. 3).

Outcomes were evaluated at 2-month intervals to determine the effect on functional recovery per the Fugl-Meyer upper extremity scale and AROM, spasticity per Modified Ashworth Scale scores, and functional MRI assessments. The

mean increase in Fugl-Meyer score was 17.7 ± 5.6 in the nerve transfer group and 2.6 ± 2.0 in the control, showing a significantly greater improvement for the surgery group. This significant increase was noted at months 10 and 12 in the surgery group, a more expedited time-frame for recovery than their previous RCT, possibly attributed to avoiding use of an interpositional nerve graft. Improvements in AROM from baseline to 12 months also significantly favored the surgical group over the control, with changes in AROM of 24 ± 19 versus 0 ± 3, 36 ± 19 versus 1 ± 5, 49 ± 21 versus 1 ± 5 at the elbow, forearm, and wrist, respectively. Spasticity scores from baseline to month 12 were significantly improved for the surgical group, encompassing elbow extension, forearm rotation, wrist extension, thumb extension, and finger extension. Transcranial magnetic stimulation and functional MRI confirmed connectivity between the ipsilateral (uninjured) hemisphere and the paralyzed arm.

Donor-site morbidity was also evaluated for the contralateral C7 nerve root transfer group. Although extensor muscle power was decreased in 83% of patients at 2 months postoperatively, donor site elbow, wrist, and finger extension fully recovered by 6 months postoperatively. In a similar fashion, the donor site demonstrated an increased tactile sensory threshold and diminished 2-point discrimination in 89% of patients at 2 months postoperatively. By 6 months postoperatively, these sensory disturbances fully resolved.

ROBOTIC EXOSKELETONS IN TREATMENT OF UPPER EXTREMITY SPASTICITY

On the nonsurgical frontier, robotic exoskeletons offer the potential to facilitate rehabilitation of upper extremity spasticity. Patients with spasticity often have a substantial level of stiffness; thus, exercise treatments involve a considerable physical burden to therapists. Over time, these burdens can pose real obstacles to providing sufficient rehabilitation. An exoskeleton, which is an external structural mechanism with joints and links corresponding to those of the human body, may offer the opportunity to overcome these obstacles.

The field of rehabilitation robotics began by using exoskeletons to passively mobilize patients' limbs during the first stage of recovery, when the patient was unable to move alone (passive mode). Initial studies demonstrated limited efficacy of such passive movements in stimulating recovery.[37] To truly spur recovery, rehabilitation robotics had to exhibit shared control of movement as soon as the patient recovered a minimal amount of motor capacity (active mode).

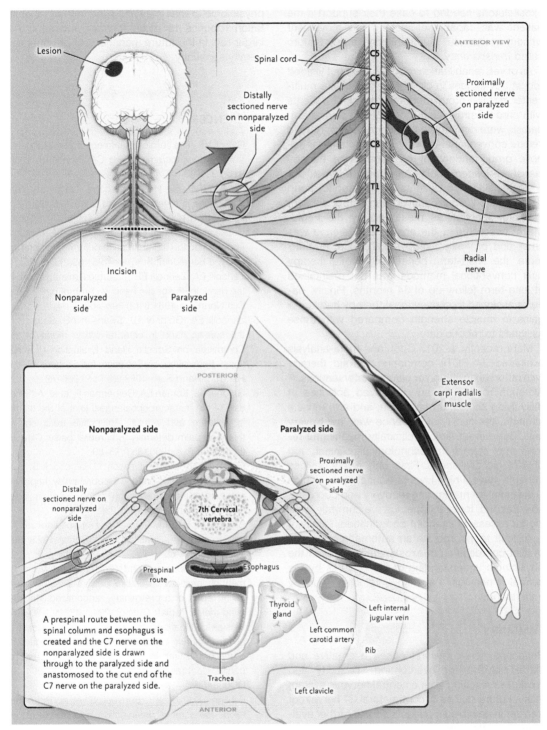

Fig. 3. Contralateral C7 nerve root transfer where the donor C7 nerve is transected at the division/cord junction and routed between the spinal column and esophagus, thus avoiding the need for an interpositional nerve graft. (*From* Zheng M, Hua X, Feng J, et al. Trial of contralateral seventh cervical nerve transfer for spastic arm paralysis. N Engl J Med 2018;378(1):25; with permission.)

Exoskeletons needed to ease their support if the patient was capable of making the movement without assistance, thus exhibiting a key feature called *transparency*.

As of yet, rehabilitation robotics have not yielded robust advantages in clinical trials.[38,39] In a multicenter, parallel-group randomized trial, 77 patients with chronic stroke and moderate to severe arm paresis were randomly assigned to receive robotic versus conventional therapy.[38] Patients in the robotic group underwent 45 minutes of therapy (*assist-as-needed mode*) 3 times a week for 8 weeks. Although patients in the robotic group demonstrated significantly greater improvement in motor function as measured by the Fugle-Meyer assessment, the absolute difference was small and of weak clinical significance. Furthermore, the short-term benefit of robotic therapy over conventional methods was not maintained at long-term follow-up of 34 months. Finally, patients assigned to conventional therapy had larger gains in muscle strength compared with those assigned to robotic care.

More recently, a 2015 Cochrane meta-analysis evaluated 34 RCTs comparing robotic therapy with other rehabilitation or placebo interventions.[39] Although robotic therapy improved activities of daily living scores, arm function, and arm muscle strength, the quality of evidence was low to very low. The current lack of clinically meaningful results may stem from technological, clinical, and physiologic challenges. First, only a few devices currently have a high level of transparency, which is essential for maximizing recovery and coordination. Second, tools and metrics are currently lacking for assessing interjoint coordination. Finally, it is difficult to incorporate an automatic generator of joint coordination in exoskeletons as even the physiologic understanding of the process by the central nervous system remains poorly understood.

SUMMARY

Peripheral nerve rewiring poses a creative and viable solution for overcoming spasticity and weakness resulting from a central nervous system injury. Future studies of contralateral C7 nerve root transfer in hemiplegic patients should further evaluate the effect of C7 nerve transection alone versus C7 nerve transection plus the contralateral C7 nerve transfer. Careful patient selection will be critical in avoiding compromise of existing wrist and digital extension. Presently, robotic exoskeletons have not shown a substantial benefit over conventional methods for rehabilitation. Advancements in the technological, clinical, and physiologic arenas may allow the field of rehabilitation robotics to move forward and secure a larger role in the future management of upper extremity spasticity.

REFERENCES

1. Carroll RE. The surgical treatment of cerebral palsy. I. The upper extremity. Surg Clin North Am 1950; 31(2):385–90.
2. Green WT, Banks HH. Flexor carpi ulnaris transplant and its use in cerebral palsy. J Bone Joint Surg Am 1962;44-A:1343–430.
3. House JH, Gwathmey FW, Fidler MO. A dynamic approach to the thumb-in palm deformity in cerebral palsy. J Bone Joint Surg Am 1981;63(2):216–25.
4. Zancolli EA, Zancolli ER Jr. Surgical management of the hemiplegic spastic hand in cerebral palsy. Surg Clin North Am 1981;61(2):395–406.
5. Zancolli EA, Goldner LJ, Swanson AB. Surgery of the spastic hand in cerebral palsy: report of the Committee on Spastic Hand Evaluation (International Federation of Societies for Surgery of the Hand). J Hand Surg 1983;8(5 Pt 2):766–72.
6. Goldner JL, Koman LA, Gelberman R, et al. Arthrodesis of the metacarpophalangeal joint of the thumb in children and adults. Adjunctive treatment of thumb-in-palm deformity in cerebral palsy. Clin Orthop Relat Res 1990;(253):75–89.
7. Dahlin LB, Komoto-Tufvesson Y, Salgeback S. Surgery of the spastic hand in cerebral palsy. Improvement in stereognosis and hand function after surgery. J Hand Surg 1998;23(3):334–9.
8. Braun RM, Botte MJ. Treatment of shoulder deformity in acquired spasticity. Clin Orthop Relat Res 1999;(368):54–65.
9. Koman LA, Mooney JF 3rd, Smith BP, et al. Management of spasticity in cerebral palsy with botulinum-A toxin: report of a preliminary, randomized, double-blind trial. J Pediatr Orthop 1994;14(3):299–303.
10. Wasiak J, Hoare B, Wallen M. Botulinum toxin A as an adjunct to treatment in the management of the upper limb in children with spastic cerebral palsy. Cochrane Database Syst Rev 2004;(3): CD003469.
11. Fehlings D, Novak I, Berweck S, et al. Botulinum toxin assessment, intervention and follow-up for paediatric upper limb hypertonicity: international consensus statement. Eur J Neurol 2010;17(Suppl 2):38–56.
12. Hoare BJ, Wallen MA, Imms C, et al. Botulinum toxin A as an adjunct to treatment in the management of the upper limb in children with spastic cerebral palsy (UPDATE). Cochrane Database Syst Rev 2010;(1):CD003469.

13. Hoare B. Rationale for using botulinum toxin A as an adjunct to upper limb rehabilitation in children with cerebral palsy. J Child Neurol 2014;29(8):1066–76.

14. Mori S. Pathogenesis of spasticity following spinal cord injury with special reference to the role of the gamma motor system. No To Shinkei 1966;18(10): 1023–32 [in Japanese].

15. Bishop B. Spasticity: its physiology and management. Part II. Neurophysiology of spasticity: current concepts. Phys Ther 1977;57(4):377–84.

16. Bishop B. Spasticity: its physiology and management. Part I. Neurophysiology of spasticity: classical concepts. Phys Ther 1977;57(4):371–6.

17. Van Heest AE, House JH, Cariello C. Upper extremity surgical treatment of cerebral palsy. J Hand Surg 1999;24(2):323–30.

18. Carlson MG, Athwal GS, Bueno RA. Treatment of the wrist and hand in cerebral palsy. J Hand Surg 2006; 31(3):483–90.

19. Hoffer MM. The use of the pathokinesiology laboratory to select muscles for tendon transfers in the cerebral palsy hand. Clin Orthop Relat Res 1993;(288): 135–8.

20. Xu WD, Hua XY, Zheng MX, et al. Contralateral C7 nerve root transfer in treatment of cerebral palsy in a child: case report. Microsurgery 2011;31(5): 404–8.

21. Gros C, Ouaknine G, Vlahovitch B, et al. [Selective posterior radicotomy in the neurosurgical treatment of pyramidal hypertension]. Neurochirurgie 1967; 13(4):505–18 [in French].

22. Bertelli JA, Ghizoni MF, Michels A. Brachial plexus dorsal rhizotomy in the treatment of upper-limb spasticity. J Neurosurg 2000;93(1):26–32.

23. Sindou M, Mifsud JJ, Boisson D, et al. Selective posterior rhizotomy in the dorsal root entry zone for treatment of hyperspasticity and pain in the hemiplegic upper limb. Neurosurgery 1986;18(5):587–95.

24. Gu YD, Chen DS, Zhang GM, et al. Long-term functional results of contralateral C7 transfer. J Reconstr Microsurg 1998;14(1):57–9.

25. Chen L, Gu YD. An experimental study of the treatment of root avulsion of brachial plexus using contralateral C7 nerve neurotization (nerve transfer). Zhonghua Wai Ke Za Zhi 1992;30(9):525–7, 570–1. [in Chinese].

26. Chen L, Gu YD. An experimental study of contralateral C7 root transfer with vascularized nerve grafting to treat brachial plexus root avulsion. J Hand Surg 1994;19(1):60–6.

27. Chuang DC, Cheng SL, Wei FC, et al. Clinical evaluation of C7 spinal nerve transection: 21 patients with at least 2 years' follow-up. Br J Plast Surg 1998;51(4):285–90.

28. Gu Y, Xu J, Chen L, et al. Long term outcome of contralateral C7 transfer: a report of 32 cases. Chin Med J (Engl) 2002;115(6):866–8.

29. Gu YD. Contralateral C7 root transfer over the last 20 years in China. Chin Med J (Engl) 2007;120(13): 1123–6.

30. Zhang CG, Gu YD. Contralateral C7 nerve transfer - our experiences over past 25 years. J Brachial Plex Peripher Nerve Inj 2011;6(1):10.

31. Chuang DC, Hernon C. Minimum 4-year follow-up on contralateral C7 nerve transfers for brachial plexus injuries. J Hand Surg 2012;37(2):270–6.

32. Gao K, Lao J, Zhao X, et al. Outcome of contralateral C7 transfer to two recipient nerves in 22 patients with the total brachial plexus avulsion injury. Microsurgery 2013;33(8):605–11.

33. Gao KM, Lao J, Zhao X, et al. Outcome of contralateral C7 nerve transferring to median nerve. Chin Med J (Engl) 2013;126(20):3865–8.

34. Li WJ, He LY, Chen SL, et al. Contralateral C7 nerve root transfer for function recovery in adults: a meta-analysis. Chin Med J (Engl) 2017;130(24):2960–8.

35. Hua XY, Qiu YQ, Li T, et al. Contralateral peripheral neurotization for hemiplegic upper extremity after central neurologic injury. Neurosurgery 2015;76(2): 187–95 [discussion: 195].

36. Zheng MX, Hua XY, Feng JT, et al. Trial of contralateral seventh cervical nerve transfer for spastic arm paralysis. N Engl J Med 2018;378(1):22–34.

37. Jarrasse N, Proietti T, Crocher V, et al. Robotic exoskeletons: a perspective for the rehabilitation of arm coordination in stroke patients. Front Hum Neurosci 2014;8:947.

38. Klamroth-Marganska V, Blanco J, Campen K, et al. Three-dimensional, task-specific robot therapy of the arm after stroke: a multicentre, parallel-group randomised trial. Lancet Neurol 2014;13(2):159–66.

39. Mehrholz J, Pohl M, Platz T, et al. Electromechanical and robot-assisted arm training for improving activities of daily living, arm function, and arm muscle strength after stroke. Cochrane Database Syst Rev 2015;(11):CD006876.

UNITED STATES POSTAL SERVICE®

Statement of Ownership, Management, and Circulation (All Periodicals Publications Except Requester Publications)

1. Publication Title	2. Publication Number	3. Filing Date
HAND CLINICS	000 – 709	9/18/2018

4. Issue Frequency	5. Number of Issues Published Annually	6. Annual Subscription Price
FEB, MAY, AUG, NOV	4	$422.00

7. Complete Mailing Address of Known Office of Publication (Not printer) (Street, city, county, state, and ZIP+4®)

ELSEVIER INC.
230 Park Avenue, Suite 800
New York, NY 10169

Contact Person: STEPHEN R. BUSHING
Telephone (Include area code): 215-239-3688

8. Complete Mailing Address of Headquarters or General Business Office of Publisher (Not printer)

ELSEVIER INC.
230 Park Avenue, Suite 800
New York, NY 10169

9. Full Names and Complete Mailing Addresses of Publisher, Editor, and Managing Editor (Do not leave blank)

Publisher (Name and complete mailing address)

TAYLOR E BALL, ELSEVIER INC.
1600 JOHN F KENNEDY BLVD. SUITE 1800
PHILADELPHIA, PA 19103-2899

Editor (Name and complete mailing address)

LAUREN BOYLE, ELSEVIER INC.
1600 JOHN F KENNEDY BLVD. SUITE 1800
PHILADELPHIA, PA 19103-2899

Managing Editor (Name and complete mailing address)

PATRICK MANLEY, ELSEVIER INC.
1600 JOHN F KENNEDY BLVD. SUITE 1800
PHILADELPHIA, PA 19103-2899

10. Owner (Do not leave blank. If the publication is owned by a corporation, give the name and address of the corporation immediately followed by the names and addresses of all stockholders owning or holding 1 percent or more of the total amount of stock. If not owned by a corporation, give the names and addresses of the individual owners. If owned by a partnership or other unincorporated firm, give its name and address as well as those of each individual owner. If the publication is published by a nonprofit organization, give its name and address.)

Full Name	Complete Mailing Address
WHOLLY OWNED SUBSIDIARY OF REED/ELSEVIER, US HOLDINGS	1600 JOHN F KENNEDY BLVD. SUITE 1800 PHILADELPHIA, PA 19103-2899

11. Known Bondholders, Mortgagees, and Other Security Holders Owning or Holding 1 Percent or More of Total Amount of Bonds, Mortgages, or Other Securities. If none, check box ▶ ☐ None

Full Name	Complete Mailing Address
N/A	

12. Tax Status (For completion by nonprofit organizations authorized to mail at nonprofit rates) (Check one)
The purpose, function, and nonprofit status of this organization and the exempt status for federal income tax purposes:
☒ Has Not Changed During Preceding 12 Months
☐ Has Changed During Preceding 12 Months (Publisher must submit explanation of change with this statement)

PS Form **3526**, July 2014 (Page 1 of 4 (see instructions page 4)) PSN: 7530-01-000-9931   PRIVACY NOTICE: See our privacy policy on www.usps.com.

---

13. Publication Title	14. Issue Date for Circulation Data Below
HAND CLINICS	MAY 2018

15. Extent and Nature of Circulation

		Average No. Copies Each Issue During Preceding 12 Months	No. Copies of Single Issue Published Nearest to Filing Date
a. Total Number of Copies (Net press run)		290	426
b. Paid Circulation (By Mail and Outside the Mail)	(1) Mailed Outside-County Paid Subscriptions Stated on PS Form 3541 (Include paid distribution above nominal rate, advertiser's proof copies, and exchange copies)	174	233
	(2) Mailed In-County Paid Subscriptions Stated on PS Form 3541 (Include paid distribution above nominal rate, advertiser's proof copies, and exchange copies)	0	0
	(3) Paid Distribution Outside the Mails Including Sales Through Dealers and Carriers, Street Vendors, Counter Sales, and Other Paid Distribution Outside USPS®	68	100
	(4) Paid Distribution by Other Classes of Mail Through the USPS (e.g., First-Class Mail®)	0	0
c. Total Paid Distribution (Sum of 15b (1), (2), (3), and (4)) ▶		242	333
d. Free or Nominal Rate Distribution (By Mail and Outside the Mail)	(1) Free or Nominal Rate Outside-County Copies included on PS Form 3541	35	68
	(2) Free or Nominal Rate In-County Copies Included on PS Form 3541	0	0
	(3) Free or Nominal Rate Copies Mailed at Other Classes Through the USPS (e.g., First-Class Mail)	0	0
	(4) Free or Nominal Rate Distribution Outside the Mail (Carriers or other means)	0	0
e. Total Free or Nominal Rate Distribution (Sum of 15d (1), (2), (3) and (4)) ▶		35	68
f. Total Distribution (Sum of 15c and 15e) ▶		277	401
g. Copies not Distributed (See Instructions to Publishers #4 (page #3)) ▶		13	25
h. Total (Sum of 15f and g) ▶		290	426
i. Percent Paid (15c divided by 15f times 100) ▶		87.36%	83.04%

* If you are claiming electronic copies, go to line 16 on page 3. If you are not claiming electronic copies, skip to line 17 on page 3.

16. Electronic Copy Circulation

	Average No. Copies Each Issue During Preceding 12 Months	No. Copies of Single Issue Published Nearest to Filing Date
a. Paid Electronic Copies ▶	0	0
b. Total Paid Print Copies (Line 15c) + Paid Electronic Copies (Line 16a) ▶	242	333
c. Total Print Distribution (Line 15f) + Paid Electronic Copies (Line 16a) ▶	277	401
d. Percent Paid (Both Print & Electronic Copies) (16b divided by 16c × 100) ▶	87.36%	83.04%

☒ I certify that 50% of all my distributed copies (electronic and print) are paid above a nominal price.

17. Publication of Statement of Ownership
☒ If the publication is a general publication, publication of this statement is required. Will be printed ☐ Publication not required
in the November 2018 issue of this publication.

18. Signature and Title of Editor, Publisher, Business Manager, or Owner

STEPHEN R. BUSHING - INVENTORY DISTRIBUTION CONTROL MANAGER   Date 9/18/2018

I certify that all information furnished on this form is true and complete. I understand that anyone who furnishes false or misleading information on this form or who omits material or information requested on the form may be subject to criminal sanctions (including fines and imprisonment) and/or civil sanctions (including civil penalties).

PS Form **3526**, July 2014 (Page 2 of 4)   PRIVACY NOTICE: See our privacy policy on www.usps.com

Moving?

Make sure your subscription moves with you!

To notify us of your new address, find your **Clinics Account Number** (located on your mailing label above your name), and contact customer service at:

Email: journalscustomerservice-usa@elsevier.com

800-654-2452 (subscribers in the U.S. & Canada)
314-447-8871 (subscribers outside of the U.S. & Canada)

Fax number: 314-447-8029

Elsevier Health Sciences Division
Subscription Customer Service
3251 Riverport Lane
Maryland Heights, MO 63043

*To ensure uninterrupted delivery of your subscription, please notify us at least 4 weeks in advance of move.

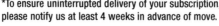

Printed and bound by CPI Group (UK) Ltd, Croydon, CR0 4YY

03/10/2024

01040302-0020